PUBLICATIONS OF THE NEWTON INSTITUTE

Models for Infectious Human Diseases:
Their Structure and Relation to Data

T0275775

Publications of the Newton Institute

Edited by J. Wright

Deputy Director, Isaac Newton Institute for Mathematical Sciences

The Isaac Newton Institute of Mathematical Sciences of the University of Cambridge exists to stimulate research in all branches of the mathematical sciences, including pure mathematics, statistics, applied mathematics, theoretical physics, theoretical computer science, mathematical biology and economics. The four six-month long research programmes it runs each year bring together leading mathematical scientists from all over the world to exchange ideas through seminars, teaching and informal interaction.

Associated with the programmes are two types of publication. The first contains lecture courses, aimed at making the latest developments accessible to a wider audience and providing an entry to the area. The second contains proceedings of workshops and conferences focusing on the most topical aspects of the subjects.

MODELS FOR INFECTIOUS
HUMAN DISEASES

Their Structure and Relation to Data

edited by

Valerie Isham

University College London

Graham Medley

University of Warwick

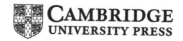
CAMBRIDGE
UNIVERSITY PRESS

CAMBRIDGE UNIVERSITY PRESS
Cambridge, New York, Melbourne, Madrid, Cape Town, Singapore, São Paulo

Cambridge University Press
The Edinburgh Building, Cambridge CB2 8RU, UK

Published in the United States of America by Cambridge University Press, New York

www.cambridge.org
Information on this title: www.cambridge.org/9780521453394

© Cambridge University Press 1996

First published 1996
This digitally printed version 2008

A catalogue record for this publication is available from the British Library

ISBN 978-0-521-45339-4 hardback
ISBN 978-0-521-05996-1 paperback

CONTENTS

Part 2   Dynamics of immunity (development of disease within individuals)

Invited papers

Invited Discussion

Contributed papers

Part 3   Population heterogeneity (mixing)

Invited papers

Contents   vii

Part 4   Consequences of treatment interventions

Invited papers

Invited Discussion

Contributed papers

Part 5   Prediction

Invited papers

Invited Discussion

Contributed papers

Introduction

Valerie Isham and Graham Medley

The epidemiology of infectious human diseases

Understanding and controlling the spread of infections is of vital importance
to society, and in the past century the epidemiology of human disease has
become a subject in its own right. Theory and applicable techniques have
been developed to study both the evolution of disease within individual people and the transmission of infections through populations. Mathematics has
an important role to play in these studies, which raise challenging problems
ranging from broad theoretical issues to specific practical ones, and in recent
years there have been significant advances in developing and analysing mathematical models of disease progression. For example, in human diseases in
particular, the problems of modelling population heterogeneity are especially
important.

Over the last decade there has been a great deal of work concerned with HIV
and AIDS. This has been concentrated mainly in two areas: the statistical
estimation of various parameters associated with HIV infection (for example,
the probability of vertical transmission; the description of the incubation
period from infection to clinical disease; the estimation from reported AIDS
cases of the number of people infected), and the description of transmission
of HIV within and between populations (for example, the characterisation of
networks of risk behaviour; the impact of different control strategies). To an
extent, the growth of studies in this area has become divorced from the study
of other infections, and therefore one of the primary purposes of this volume
is to bring together work on modelling a wide range of human diseases so as
to encourage cross-fertilisation between AIDS related research and research
of the epidemiology of other infections.

A second purpose is to encourage more constructive interaction between the
different areas within the epidemiology of human disease, especially between
those concerned with transmissible disease and non-transmissible disease.
The epidemiology of non-transmissible disease is a well-developed subject and
has helped define the risk of developing disease from exposure to environmental and other hazards. The spectrum of disease caused by HIV infection tends
to have a long incubation period, such that the population patterns of AIDS
are not directly related to those of HIV infection. Consequently, there should
be some sharing of techniques and ideas between these two areas. In the same
vein, there is now much interest in the description of the genetic evolution
of HIV within individuals that should be related to the study of within host
variation of other infections, such as malaria.

The development of mathematical theories of disease, especially transmissible disease, has largely occurred without the direct involvement of areas that rely on the application of the theory: community medicine and public health. A third purpose of the volume is to encourage theoretical and empirical researchers to confront each other, and to reveal areas where more positive collaboration is desirable, if not essential.

Finally, the epidemics of HIV and AIDS have highlighted the need for more rigorous use of quantitative techniques for the prediction of future trends and their health-care implications. This area has been short of theoretical study, and a fourth aim of the volume is to encourage researchers to consider the use to which predictive models may be put.

An ideal opportunity for leading research workers to collaborate in identifying and addressing current issues relating to the role of mathematical modelling in the epidemiology of human disease, has been provided by the Isaac Newton Institute for Mathematical Sciences (University of Cambridge), through its sponsorship of a six-month research programme entitled *Epidemic Models: Their Structure and Relation to Data*. This programme, which ran from January-June 1993, brought together scientists with a great variety of mathematical expertise (including applied probability, deterministic modelling and data analysis) and with close involvement in applied fields across the spectrum of social, medical and biological sciences. Its specific aim was to foster interdisciplinary cooperation in tackling problems relating to a wide range of human, animal and plant diseases. A priority was to encourage interaction between the development of theoretical results, the use of relevant expert knowledge from applied fields and the analysis of data.

During the *Epidemic Models* programme, three major workshops were held to promote this interdisciplinary interaction: the first dealt with general issues across the whole field, while the second and third were concerned with more specific topics, respectively the spread and persistence of animal and plant diseases, and of infectious human diseases. The papers in this volume were presented at the third of these, a week-long workshop focussing on human diseases, while two related volumes, Mollison (1995) and Dobson and Grenfell (1995), publish papers from the two earlier workshops. A general review of the area of mathematical models of epidemics with substantial discussion is also provided by the proceedings of a Discussion Meeting of the Royal Statistical Society (see Mollison, Isham and Grenfell, 1994).

The format of this volume

Following the aims described above, five themes were chosen. These were

- Transmissible diseases with long development times and vaccination strategies.

- Dynamics of immunity (the development of disease within individuals).

- Population heterogeneity (mixing).

- Consequences of treatment interventions.

- Prediction.

Within each theme there are between two and four main papers, invited specifically to contrast different aspects of the topic. Broadly, these aspects have been chosen to contrast work that is (a) theoretical/mathematical, (b) data-based, with regard to a specific disease, and (c) related to policy or control implications. These papers are followed by invited discussion and then by short papers on the same general theme, contributed at the workshop, together with further discussion.

The policy of inviting people to discuss the same topic from different view points is perhaps the most innovative aspect of this volume. At the workshop, this policy was a great success although there were often contrasts in communication and understanding between people from different disciplines supposedly studying the same natural phenomenon. In particular, the gulf that exists between the statistical science (stochastic) and mathematical modelling (deterministic) approaches to the transmission of infectious diseases was exposed. It is rare for these two areas to be equally represented at meetings such as this, and perhaps it will turn out that the most important results of this workshop will have been the informal discussions that took place between sessions, and the contacts, links and new collaborations that have been generated between these two areas. This aspect of the workshop cannot be documented here but we hope that it will surface in the future development of our subject.

In this volume, within each theme can be found the corresponding invited and contributed papers, a written version of the invited discussion together with an edited summary of some of the more important points made in the contributed discussion from the floor of the meeting, and the authors' responses to all the discussion. Where written versions were supplied for the contributed discussion, this is indicated by the symbol (**) by the discussant's name. Where no such symbol appears, the contribution has been written by the editors according to their understanding of what was said. We apologise to the discussants for any resulting misrepresentation of their questions or views.

Inevitably, individual contributed papers did not always fall neatly within one of our chosen themes but sometimes addressed issues related to two or more of them. The allocation of papers to themes has therefore resulted in a certain degree of overlap between the topics. Also, since many of the contributed papers describe work in progress, the level of detail and completeness of these varies considerably. However, the inclusion of all these papers adds to the picture of the wide range of diseases and approaches that come under the epidemic modelling umbrella. Where possible, especially in the case of very recent work, references have been added to indicate where further details may be found.

Following this Introduction, a list is given of all the registered participants at the Infectious Human Diseases Workshop, together with their permanent affiliations at the time of the meeting (some being temporarily affiliated to the Isaac Newton Institute). These affiliations will not be repeated on the individual papers, where only those of non-participating collaborators will be given.

We are grateful to all those whose active participation and enthusiasm contributed to the success of the Workshop, and especially to all the invited speakers, for all their efforts in giving stimulating, thought-provoking and timely verbal accounts of recent work and in providing excellent and carefully-prepared written accounts. All the participants will want to join us in thanking the Institute's Director, Sir Michael Atiyah, and then Deputy Director, Professor Peter Goddard, for the facilities and hospitality provided to us by the Isaac Newton Institute and, through them, all the staff of the Institute for their unfailingly cheerful and willing help in the face of the many demands made on them connected with the Workshop.

Finally, and most importantly, we wish to record our gratitude to the Wellcome Trust for the financial support that they provided for this Workshop. This help was invaluable in enabling us to contribute towards travelling and subsistence expenses, thereby allowing as wide as possible a participation in the meeting.

Valerie Isham and Graham Medley

References

Dobson, A. and Grenfell, B.T. (eds.) (1995) *Ecology of Infectious Diseases in Natural Populations*, Cambridge University Press, Cambridge

Mollison, D. (ed.) (1995) *Epidemic Models: their Structure and Relation to Data*, Cambridge University Press, Cambridge.

Mollison, D., Isham, V. and Grenfell, B.T. (1994) 'Epidemics: models and data (with Discussion)', *J. Roy. Statist. Soc. A* **157**, 115–149.

PARTICIPANTS

Professor Odd Aalen, Department of Medical Statistics, University of Oslo, PO Box 1122, Blindern, 0317 Oslo 3, Norway

Dr. Tony Ades, Department of Epidemiology, Institute of Child Health, 30 Guildford Street, London WC1N 1EH, UK

Professor Zvia Agur, Department of Applied Mathematics and Computer Science, Weizmann Institute, IL-76100 Rehovot, Israel

Dr. Michael Altmann, Box 511, UMHC, University of Minnesota, 420 Delaware Street, SE, Minneapolis MN 55455, USA

Professor Roy M. Anderson, Biology Department, Imperial College, London SW7 2BB, UK

Dr. R. Arca, Osservatario Epidemiologico, Via S. Costanza 53, 00198 Rome, Italy

Dr. Hannah Babad, Biology Department, Imperial College, London SW7 2BB, UK

Professor Peter Bacchetti, Department of Epidemiology and Biostatistics, University of California, San Francisco General Hospital, Bld 90, Ward 95, Room 512, 995 Potrero, San Francisco CA 94110, USA

Professor Norman T.J. Bailey, Chalet Chrine, Fang, 3782 Lauenen, Switzerland

Professor Frank Ball, Department of Mathematics, University Park, Nottingham NG7 2RD, USA

Ms. Maria Gloria Basanez, Biology Department, Imperial College, London SW7 2BB, UK

Professor Niels Becker, Department of Statistics, La Trobe University, Bundoora, Australia

Dr. R. Bellocco, Laboratorio di Epidemiologio e Biostatistica, Instituti Superiore di Sanita, Viale Regina Elena 299, 00161 Rome, Italy

Dr. Atit Ben-Salah, Biology Department, Imperial College, London SW7 2BB, UK

Dr. Valerie Beral, ICRF, Cancer Epidemiology Unit, Gibson Building, Radcliffe Infirmary, Oxford OX2 6HE, UK

Professor Lynne Billard, Department of Statistics, University of Georgia, Athens GA 30602, USA

Dr. P. Billingsley, Department of Biology, Imperial College, Prince Consort Road, London SW7 2BB, UK

Professor Sally Blower, Survey Research Center University of California at Berkeley, Berkeley, CA 94720, USA

Dr. Stephen Blythe, Department of Statistics, Strathclyde University, Livingstone Tower, 26 Richmond Street, Glasgow G1 1XH, Scotland

Dr. Ben Bolker Department of Zoology, University of Cambridge, Downing St., Cambridge CB2 3EJ, UK

Professor Ron Brookmeyer, Biostatistics Department, Johns Hopkins University, 615 North Wolfe Street, Baltimore MD 21205, USA

Dr. D.A.P. Bundy, Department of Zoology, Oxford University, South Parks Road, Oxford OX1 3PS, UK

Dr. Anthony Butterworth, Department of Pathology, University of Cambridge, Tennis Court Road, Cambridge CB2 1QP, UK

Dr. L. Carvalho, Dept. Estatistica, Investigacao Operacional Univ. de Lisboa, Fac. de Ciencias, Edificio C2, Campo Grande, 1700 LISBOA, Portugal

Professor Carlos Castillo-Chavez, Biometrics Unit, Cornell University, Ithaca NY 14853-7801, USA

Dr. Man-Suen Chan, Biology Department, Imperial College, London SW7 2BB, UK

Dr. Carole Clem, B3E Faculte de Medecine Saint-Antoine, 27 rue Chaligny, 75571 Paris Cedex 12, France

Dr. Andrew Cliff, Christ's College, Cambridge CB2 3BU, UK

Sir David R. Cox, Nuffield College, Oxford OX1 1NF

Ms. Julia Critchley, Biology Department, Imperial College, London SW7 2BB, UK

Dr. Brian Dangerfield, Centre for OR and Applied Statistics, University of Salford, Salford M5 4WT, UK

Dr. Sarah Darby, ICRF, Cancer Epidemiology Unit, Gibson Building, Radcliffe Infirmary, Oxford OX2 6HE, UK

Dr. Janet Darbyshire, HIV Clinical Trials Centre, Royal Brompton Hospital, London SW3 6NP, UK

Dr. Karen Day, Biology Department, Imperial College, London SW7 2BB, UK

Professor Nick Day, MRC Biostatistics Unit, Institute of Public Health, University Forvie Site, Robinson Way, Cambridge CB2 2SR, UK

Dr. Daniela de Angelis, MRC Biostatistics Unit, Institute of Public Health, University Forvie Site, Robinson Way, Cambridge CB2 2SR, UK

Dr. Raymundo de Azevedo Neto, Department of Pathology, Faculty of Medicine, University of Sao Paulo, Sao Paulo, Brazil

Dr. Rob de Boer, Theoretical Biology, University of Utrecht, Padualaan, 8, 3584 CH Utrecht, Netherlands

Professor Victor de Gruttola, Department of Biostatistics, Harvard University, School of Public Health, 677 Huntington Avenue, Boston MA 02115, USA

Dr. Mart de Jong, Centrall Diergeneeskundig Institute, Edelhertweg, 15, POBox 65, NL-8200 AB Lelystad, Netherlands

Professor Klaus Dietz, Institut fur Medizinische Biometrie, Universität Tübingen, Westbahnhofstrasse 55, D-7400 Tübingen 1, Germany

Dr. Andy Dobson, Biology Department, Princeton University, Princeton NJ, USA

Dr. Angela Downs, Unite de Recherches Biomath. et Biostat. (INSERM U263), Universite Paris 7, Tour 53, 2, place Jussieu, F-75251 Paris, CEDEX 05, France

Dr. Chris Dye, London School of Hygiene and Tropical Medicine, Keppel Street, London WC1E 7HT, UK

Mr. John Edmunds, Biology Department, Imperial College, London SW7 2BB, UK

Dr. Martin Eichner, Institut fur Medizinische Biometrie, Universität Tübingen, Westbahnhofstrasse 55, D-7400 Tübingen 1, Germany

Professor David Fan, Department of Genetics and Cell Biology, University of Minnesota, 1445 Gortner Avenue, St Paul MN 55108, USA

Professor Vern Farewell, Department of Statistics and Actuarial Science, University of Waterloo, Waterloo, Ontario, Canada

Dr. Katherine Fielding, MRC BIAS, Crew Building, Kings Buildings, West Mains Road, Edinburgh EH9 3JN, Scotland

Dr. Paul Fine, Department of Epidemiology and Population Health, London School of Hygiene and Tropical Medicine, Keppel Street, London WC1E 7HT, UK

Dr. Tony Fulford, Department of Pathology, University of Cambridge, Tennis Court Road, Cambridge CB2 1QP, UK

Dr. Geoff Garnett, Biology Department, Imperial College, London SW7 2BB, UK

Dr. Wally Gilks, MRC Biostatistics Unit, Institute of Public Health, University Forvie Site, Robinson Way, Cambridge CB2 2SR, UK

Dr. Noel Gill, PHLS AIDS Centre, CDSC, 61 Colindale Avenue, London NW9 5EQ, UK

Dr. Sheila Gore, MRC Biostatistics Unit, Institute of Public Health, University Forvie Site Robinson Way, Cambridge CB2 2SR, UK

Dr. J. Goudsmidt, Department of Medical Microbiology (Virology Section), University of Amsterdam, Meibergdreet, 15, 1105 AZ Amsterdam, Netherlands

Mr. Daryl Gove, Faculty of Mathematical Studies, The University, Highfield, Southampton SO9 5NH, UK

Dr. Simon Gregson, Biology Department, Imperial College, London SW7 2BB, UK

Dr. David Greenhalgh, Department of Statistics and Modelling Science, Livingstone Tower, 26 Richmond Street, Glasgow G1 1XH, Scotland

Dr. Bryan Grenfell, Department of Zoology, University of Cambridge, Downing St., Cambridge CB2 3EJ, UK

Dr. Sunetra Gupta, Biology Department, Imperial College, London SW7 2BB, UK

Professor Dik Habbema, Department of Public Health and Social Medicine, Erasmus University, 3000 DR Rotterdam, Netherlands

Professor Michael Haber, Emory University, School of Public Health, 1599 Clifton Road NE, Atlanta GA 30329, USA

Professor Karl Hadeler, Biologisches Institut, Auf der Morgenstelle 10, D-7400 Tübingen 1, Germany

Professor E. Halloran, Emory University, School of Public Health, 1599 Clifton Road NE, Atlanta GA 30329, USA

Dr. Günther Hasibeder, Abteilung fur Mathematische Biologie, Technische Universität Wien, Wiedner Hauptstr. 8/118, A-1040 Wien, Austria

Dr. D. Haydon, 16 Winchmore Drive, Trumpington, Cambridge CB2 2LW, UK

Dr. Hans Heesterbeek, CWI, PO Box 4079, 1009 AB Amsterdam, Netherlands

Dr. Siem Heisterkamp, RIVM, Antonie van Leeuwenhoeklaan, 9, PO Box 1, 3720 BA Bilthoven, Netherlands

Dr. J. Hendriks, Department of Medical Statistics, University of Nijmegen, 6500 HB, Nijmegen, Netherlands

Professor Herb Hethcote, Department of Mathematics, University of Iowa, Iowa City IA 52242, USA

Ms. Charlotte Hetzel, Department of Biology, Imperial College, Prince Consort Road, London SW7 2BB, UK

Dr. Peter Hudson, The Game Conservancy, Crubenmore Lodge, Newtonmore, Scotland

Dr. Valerie Isham, Department of Statistical Science, University College London, London WC1E 6BT, UK

Professor John A. Jacquez, Department of Physiology, University of Michigan, 7808 Med. Sci. II, Ann Arbor MI 48109-0622, USA

Dr. Harold Jaffe, Division of HIV/AIDS, National Center for Infectious Diseases, Centers for Disease Control, Atlanta GA 30333, USA

Professor Nicholas P. Jewell, Department of Biostatistics, University of California, School of Public Health, Berkeley CA 94720, USA

Dr. Anne M. Johnson, Department of Genito-Urinary Medicine, UC and Middlesex School of Medicine, James Pringle House, London W1N 8AA, UK

Dr. Lawrence Joseph, Department of Epidemiology and Biostatistics, McGill University, Montreal, Quebec, Canada

Professor Jack Kalbfleisch, Department of Statistics, University of Waterloo, Ontario, N2L 3G1, Canada

Professor Ed Kaplan, Yale School of Organisation and Management, Box 1A, Newhaven CT 06520, USA

Professor Jim Koopman, Department of Epidemiology, University of Michigan, 7808 Med. Sci. II, Ann Arbor MI 48109-0622, USA

Dr. Mirjam Kretzchmar, RIVM, Antonie van Leeuwenhoeklaan, 9, PostBus 1, 3720 BA Bilthoven, Netherlands,

Professor Dick Kryscio, Department of Statistics, University of Kentucky, Lexington KY 40506-0027, USA

Professor Jerry F. Lawless, Department of Statistics, University of Waterloo, Ontarion, N2L 3G1, Canada

Dr. Francoise le Pont, B3E Faculte de Medecine Saint-Antoine, 27 rue Chaligny, 75571 Paris Cedex 12, France

Dr. Mike Lloyd, 25 Union Square West, C1-4EA, New York NY 10003, USA

Professor Ira Longini, Emory University, School of Public Health, 1599 Clifton Road NE, Atlanta GA 30329, USA

Dr. Angela Mariotto, Laboratorio di Epidemiologia e Biostatistica, Istituto Superiore di Sanita', Viale Regina Elena, 299, 00161 Roma, Italy

Professor Anders Martin-Lof, Institute of Actuarial Mathematics and Actuarial Statistics, Stockholm University, Box 6701, S-11385 Stockholm, Sweden

Professor Robert May, Department of Zoology, University of Oxford, South Parks Road, Oxford OX1 3PS, UK

Dr. Angela McLean, Department of Zoology, University of Oxford, South Parks Road, Oxford OX1 3PS, UK

Mr. Alex McNeil, MRC Biostatistics Unit, Institute of Public Health, University Forvie Site Robinson Way, Cambridge CB2 2SR, UK

Dr. Graham Medley, Ecosystems Analysis and Management Group, Department of Biological Sciences, University of Warwick, Coventry CV4 7AL, UK

Dr. Colin Michie, Department of Paediatrics and Neonatal Medicine, Royal Postgraduate Medical School, Hammersmith Hospital, Du Cane Road, London W12 0NN, UK

Professor Denis Mollison, Department of Actuarial Mathematics and Statistics, Heriot-Watt University, Edinburgh EH14 4AS, Scotland

Professor Martina Morris, Department of Sociology, Columbia University, New York NY 10027, USA

Professor Andrew Moss, c/o Sergievsky Center, 630 West 168th Street, New York NY 10032, USA

Dr. Johannes Müller, Biologisches Institut, Auf der Morgenstelle 10, D-7400 Tübingen 1, Germany

Professor Ingemar Nåsell, Department of Mathematics, Royal Institute of Technology, S-100 44 Stockholm, Sweden

Dr. J.P. Nielsen, Laboratory of Actuarial Science, University of Copenhagen, 2100 Copenhagen 0, Denmark

Dr. James Nokes, Biology Department, Imperial College, London SW7 2BB, UK

Dr. Martin Nowak, Department of Zoology, University of Oxford, South Parks Road, Oxford OX1 3PS, UK

Professor Julian Peto, Institute of Cancer Research, Epidemiology, Block D, 15 Cotswold Road, Sutton, Surrey SM2 5NG, UK

Professor Richard Peto, ICRF, Cancer Studies Unit, Radcliffe Infirmary, Oxford OX2 6HE, UK

Dr. Tim Peto, Nuffield Department of Medicine, John Radcliffe Hospital, Headington, Oxford OX3 9DU, UK

Professor Tomas Philipson, Department of Economics, University of Chicago, 1126 East 59th street, Chicago, IL 60637, USA

Ms. K. Porter, PHLS AIDS Centre, CDSC, 61 Colindale Avenue, London NW9 5EQ, UK

Dr. Gillian Raab, MRC BIAS, Crew Building, Kings Buildings, West Mains Road, Edinburgh EH9 3JN, Scotland

Dr. A. Read, Department of Biology, Kings Buildings, West Mains Road, Edinburgh EH9 3JN, Scotland

Dr. Hans Remme, WHO, (TDR/TDE), CH-1211 Geneva 27, Switzerland

Dr. Wasima Rida, NIAID, Department of Biostatistics, Division of AIDS, Bethesda, Executive Boulevard 6001, Maryland, USA

Mrs Carole Roberts, Centre for OR and Applied Statistics, University of Salford, Salford M5 4WT, UK

Dr. Mick Roberts, MAF, Wallaceville Animal Research Centre, PO Box 40063, Upper Hutt, Wellington, New Zealand

Dr. E. Rott, Department of Genito-Urinary Medicine, UC and Middlesex School of Medicine, James Pringle House, London W1N 8AA, UK

Professor Carla Rossi, Dipartimento di Matematica, Universita degli Studi da Roma, Via Fontanile di Carcaricola, 00133 Roma, Italy

Dr. Glen Satten, Emory University, School of Public Health, 1599 Clifton Road NE, Atlanta GA 30329, USA

Professor Lisa Sattenspiel, Department of Anthropology, 200 Swallow Hall, University of Missouri, Columbia MO65211, USA

Professor Gian-Paolo Scalia-Tomba, Universita 'la Sapienza', Via A. Scarpa 16, I001 61 Rome, Italy

Professor Dieter Schenzle, Inst. fur Medizinische Biometrie, Universität Tübingen, Westbahnhofstrasse 55. 7400 Tübingen 1, Germany

Professor Norman Severo, Department of Statistics, SUNY at Buffalo, 249 Farber Hall, Buffalo, NY 14214, USA

Dr. Arjan Shahani, Faculty of Mathematical Studies, The University, Highfield, Southampton SO9 5NH, UK

Professor Carl Simon, Department of Mathematics, University of Michigan, 7808 Med. Sci. II, Ann Arbor, MI 48109-0622, USA

Professor R.E. Sinden, Biology Department, Imperial College, London SW7 2BB, UK

Dr. Gary Smith, University of Pennsylvania, New Bolton Center, Kennet Square, Pennsylvania, USA

Dr. Patty Solomon, Statistics Department, University of Adelaide, GPO Box 498, Adelaide, SA 5001, Australia

Professor Ann Stanley, Department of Mathematics, Iowa State University, 400 Carver, Ames IA 50011, USA

Mr. N. Stilianakis, Institut fur Medizinische Biometrie, Universität Tübingen, Westbahnhofstrasse 55, D-7400 Tübingen 1, Germany

Dr. Jonathan Swinton, Biology Department, Imperial College, London SW7 2BB, UK

Professor Jeremy M.G. Taylor, Division of Biostatistics, School of Public Health, UCLA, Los Angeles CA 90024-1772, USA

Dr. Hilary Tillett, PHLS AIDS Centre, CDSC, 61 Colindale Avenue, London NW9 5EQ, UK

Dr. David Tudor, Synthelabo Recherche, 31, avenue Paul Vaillant-Couturier, F-92225 Bagneux CEDEX, France

Dr. Mike Turner, Laboratory for Biochemical Parasitology, Department of Zoology, University of Glasgow, University Gardens, Glasgow G12 8Q1, Scotland

Ms. Chinma Uche, Biology Department, Imperial College, London SW7 2BB, UK

Dr. Odette van der Heijden, RIVM, Antonie van Leeuwenhoeklaan, 9, PostBus 1, 3720 BA Bilthoven, Netherlands

Dr. Hans van Druten, Department of Medical Statistics, University of Nijmegen, Toernooiveld 1, 6526 ED Nijmegen, Netherlands

Dr. Gerrit van Oortmarssen, Department of Public Health and Social Medicine, Erasmus University, 3000 DR Rotterdam, Netherlands

Dr. Lyn Watson, Department of Statistics, La Trobe University, Bundoore, Australia

Mr. John Williams, Biology Department, Imperial College, London SW7 2BB, UK

Dr. Sue R. Wilson, Centre for Mathematics and its Applications, Australian National University, PO Box 4, Canberra, ACT 2601, Australia

Dr. Mark Woolhouse, Department of Zoology, University of Oxford, South Parks Road, Oxford OX1 3PS, UK

Dr. Alastair Young, Statistical Laboratory, University of Cambridge, 16 Mill Lane, Cambridge CB2 2SB, UK

NON-PARTICIPANT CONTRIBUTORS

Dr. Mario Abundo, Dipartimento di Matematica, Universita degli Studi da Roma, Via Fontanile di Carcaricola, 00133, Rome, Italy

Dr. R. Bailey, London School of Hygiene and Tropical Medicine, Keppel Street, London WC1E 7HT, UK

Dr. P. Billingsley, Biology Department, Imperial College, London SW7 2BB, UK

Dr. A.G. Bird, Churchill Hospital, Oxford OX3 7LJ, UK

Dr. Maarten C. Boerlijst, University of Utrecht, 3584 CH, Utrecht, Netherlands

Dr. S.C. Brailsford, Faculty of Mathematical Studies, The University, Highfield, Southampton SO9 5NH, UK

Dr. R.P. Brettle, City Hospital Edinburgh, Regional Infectious Disease Unit, Edinburgh EH10 5SB, Scotland

Dr. D.A.P. Bundy, Biology Department, Imperial College, London SW7 2BB, UK

Dr. A.E. Butterworth, Department of Pathology, University of Cambridge, Cambridge CB2 1QP, UK

Dr. Robert H. Byers, Division of HIV/AIDS, Center for Disease Control and Prevention, Atlanta GA 30329, USA

Dr. W. Scott Clark, Division of Biostatistics, School of Public Health, Emory University, Atlanta GA 30329, USA

Dr. W.G. Cumberland, Department of Biostatistics, UCLA, Los Angeles CA 90024, USA

Dr. I. de Vincenzi, European Centre for Epidemiological Monitoring of Aids, Saint-Lawrence, France

Dr. D.W. Dunne, Department of Pathology, University of Cambridge, Cambridge CB2 1QP, UK

Dr. Elizabeth Halloran, Division of Biostatistics, Emory University, School of Public Health, Atlanta, GA 30329, USA

Dr. J.M. Hyman, Theoretical Division, B284, Centre for Nonlinear Studies, Los Alamos National Laboratory, Los Alamos NM 87545, USA

Dr. John M. Karon, Division of HIV/AIDS, Center for Disease Control and Prevention, Atlanta GA 30329, USA

Dr. D.C.W. Mabey, London School of Hygiene and Tropical Medicine, Keppel Street, London WC1E 7HT, UK

Dr. S.E. Meacock, Faculty of Mathematical Studies, The University, Highfield, Southampton SO9 5NH, UK

Dr. J.A.J. Metz, Institute of Theoretical Biology, PO Box 9516, 2300 RA, Leiden, Netherlands

Dr. R.T. Mitsuyasu, Department of Medicine, UCLA, Los Angeles CA 90024, USA

Dr. J.H. Ouma, Division of Vector-Borne Diseases, Ministry of Health, PO Box 20750, Nairobi, Kenya

Dr. A.P. Plaisier, Centre for Decision Sciences in Tropical Disease Control, Department of Public Health, Erasmus University, Rotterdam, Netherlands

Dr. R.B. Roy, Genito–Urinary Department, Royal Bournemouth Hospital, Bournemouth, Dorset, UK

Dr. R.E. Sinden, Biology Department, Imperial College, London SW7 2BB, UK

Dr. Daphne Smith, Department of Statistics, University of Georgia, Athens GA 30602, USA

Dr. C.J. Struchiner, Division of Biostatistics, Emory University, School of Public Health, Atlanta, GA 30329, USA

Dr. R.F. Sturrock, Department of Medical Parasitology, London School of Hygiene and Tropical Medicine, London WC1E 7HT, UK

Dr. J.P. Sy, Department of Biostatistics, UCLA, Los Angeles CA 90024, USA

Dr. H.H.J. van der Hoorn, Faculty of Mathematical Studies, The University, Highfield, Southampton SO9 5NH, UK

Dr. G. van Griensven, Department of Public Health, Amsterdam Municipal Health Service, 1000 HE Amsterdam, Netherlands

Dr. M.E. Ward, Faculty of Medicine, The University, Highfield, Southampton SO9 5NH, UK

Dr. Stefan Zehnder, Institut fur Medizinische Biometrie, Universität Tübingen, Westbahnhofstrasse 55, D-7400 Tübingen 1, Germany

Part 1
Transmissible diseases with long development times and vaccination strategies

Overview of Data Analysis: Diseases with Long Development Times

Sheila M. Gore

1 Introduction

Among diseases with long development times – from inception to diagnosis, from diagnosis to death, or both – feature breast and cervical cancer, end-stage organ failure and cardiovascular disease; all four have aspects in common with HIV disease, but its transmissibility by many routes sets it apart from the rest.

Breast and cervical cancers are detectable when asymptomatic (or precancerous) by screening; treatment of screen-detected lesions saves lives. Blood pressure lowering drugs reduce the incidence of stroke and coronary heart disease. An HIV antibody positive test leads to consideration of personal measures to prevent onward transmission of HIV disease and, from clinical management, to a better quality and length of HIV infected life, but as yet no cure. Cervical cancer, like HIV disease, is viral in origin and sexual transmission is implicated in its spread. Transplantation shares with HIV disease an immunological basis, recency, and unusual intensity of patient monitoring through laboratory markers.

Section 2 reviews the statistical problems posed by these other four applications, all of high public health or political profile, before consideration in Section 3 of chronic disease processes generally, and the transmissibility of HIV disease. Section 4 focusses on three data analytic themes in HIV disease – progression markers, incubation distribution and infectivity – and briefly reviews how they have been tackled. Future statistical directions in HIV disease are outlined in Section 5 with emphasis on transmission study design and overview, and on the non-proportionality over time of covariate influences. This includes unmeasured (frailty) as well as measured (and appropriately parametrized) covariates.

2 Review of applications: statistical problems posed

2.1 Breast cancer

Based on cases whose maximum follow-up from onset was six years, Greenwood (1926) wrote of breast cancer: 'At no observed epoch from onset is the

rate of mortality of the same order of magnitude as normal mortality' and
noted also that the time-specific risk of death, or hazard, increased during
the first three years after onset and was then constant or slowly declined.
Boag (1949) observed that late relapse was not infrequent after five years in
many forms of cancer and so 5-year survival rate, however defined, was an un-
satisfactory estimate of the proportion permanently cured. Boag's view was
that a proportion C of patients was cured by treatment and so liable only to
causes of death other than the original cancer, but for the remaining patients
time to death from breast cancer, distributed lognormally, was not modified
by unsuccessful treatment. In 1975, Brinkley and Haybittle reported on the
Addenbrooke's breast cancer series in which overall mortality was similar to
that in the normal population after 21 years, but deaths from breast cancer
were 16 times more likely in the study group (eight deaths reported). Because
careful follow-up of breast cancer patients may bring benefit by the early detection and treatment of intercurrent illness, they warned: 'to define cure in
terms of the general population mortality may have its limitations' (see also
Langlands *et al.* 1979). And so, more than 50 years after Greenwood's astute
observations on the 'National Duration of Cancer', no satisfactory description
of the natural history of treated breast cancer had emerged. Curability was in
doubt. Breast cancer is a chronic disease and age-related intercurrent deaths
are not infrequent.

Standard regression models – Weibull, proportional hazards (Cox 1972),
log-logistic – failed to represent the survival of patients with breast cancer
in the Western General series (Gore *et al.* 1984) despite *agreement* on the
relative influence of clinical covariates. The latter finding has been generalized by Solomon (1986), and by d'Agostino *et al.* (1990) to time-dependent
covariates. The proportional hazards model accommodated neither the observed convergence of hazard functions nor diversity of times to peak hazard
in breast cancer (see Figure 1). To investigate whether the influence of baseline covariates diminished in time, proportional hazards models were applied
in three distinct epochs of follow-up, a different constant of proportionality
being estimated for each. This led to a modified Cox model in which the influence of covariates was allowed to change smoothly with time according to a
prescribed function. Differential frailty, through unmeasured covariates such
as 'viable metastases' or otherwise, is a possible explanation for the observed
hazard patterns, see Aalen (1988).

In the Western General series, covariate information was elicited only at
the time of diagnosis so that patients' menopausal status, for example, was
not updated during follow-up. Besides date and cause of death, only the
date of first recurrence or metastasis (together with site(s)) was recorded
– but not analysed because of retrospective data retrieval from case-notes.
Recently, Zedeler *et al.* (1992) have considered the differential influence of

prognostic factors on the simultaneous occurrence of metastases at various anatomical sites in human breast cancer.

In the early 1980s breast cancer management was different between countries, between specialties, and by prognosis – with only one third of doctors claiming that treatment plans were distinguishable in terms of patient survival (Gore *et al.* 1988). Statistical overview of randomized trials in breast cancer had only just begun; it has now dispelled the need for radical surgery, shed light on increased long-term mortality associated with radiotherapy, and revealed a persistent survival advantage for women treated systemically by hormonal, cytotoxic or immune therapy (Early Breast Cancer Trialists' Collaborative Group 1992). Meanwhile, reduction in mortality from breast cancer after mass screening with mammography had also been established in randomized trials. Breast screening, at 3 year intervals, is now offered throughout the UK to women aged 50–65 years; research continues to optimize both screening interval and the management of screen-detected cancers, and to investigate screening at younger ages (Breast Cancer Screening 1986). Tabar *et al.* (1992) argue that approaches to therapy based on results obtained in clinically diagnosed, so-called 'early', breast cancers may be inappropriate for most screen-detected cancers – because the disease becomes systemic with viable metastases between the time at which it can be diagnosed by mammography and the time at which clinical diagnosis usually occurs.

The links between diet and breast cancer, randomized trial of systemic hormonal prophylaxis for women at high risk of breast cancer, and determining the genetics of familial breast cancer (Aalen 1992, Clayton 1991), are outstanding problems.

2.2   Cervical cancer

Cervical cancer is thought to originate with viral infection. It is rare in celibate women. Young age at first vaginal intercourse is a risk factor for disease progression, for reasons that may be associated with pubertal cervical physiology. Cervical screening aims to identify women with treatable cervical lesions which, if ignored, may develop into invasive cancer. Critical considerations in designing screening programmes include: smear accuracy in detecting underlying precursors, rates of progression, and the possibility of spontaneous regression. The management of women with mild or moderate dyskaryotic cervical smears remains controversial.

Kirby *et al.* (1992) concluded that mild or moderate dyskaryotic smears should not be an indication for immediate referral for colposcopy, since under Grampian's conservative management policy most women returned to normal without needing treatment, but the increased risk associated with abnormal smears justified rigorous surveillance. They had identified 500 women with mild or moderate cervical dyskaryosis in 1978 or 1979 and 500, matched by age, who had had a normal smear at the same time. The standard statistical technique of censoring at the time of last smear could have led to serious bias in comparison of biopsy rates because last known smear result is to a certain extent informative about a woman's prognosis. After a negative smear, women were therefore assumed negative for three further years, the approximate mean inter-smear interval for control women, and censored thereafter. Analysis of the full screening history for these women included the use of graphical models and Gibbs sampling. Gilks *et al.* (1993) characterized woman i, who has had n_i smears, at time intervals t_{ij} between the $(j-1)$th and jth smear, as having smear results y_{ij} when the true underlying disease state was x_{ij}. The x_{ij} were unobserved realizations of a discrete state, continuous time, time-homogeneous Markov process, except for the last state $x_{i\,n_i+1}$ which was *observed* as a result of biopsy.

2.3   Transplantation for end-stage organ failure

The antecedents of organ failure vary: inborn errors of metabolism such as α_1-antitrypsin deficiency, progressive disease of adult onset such as diabetes, or acute events such as corneal trauma. Acceptance criteria for patients awaiting transplantation, and for donors, have changed dramatically over time and by centre; so too have results. Cadaveric kidney donors up to 70 years and heart donors up to 55 years are now accepted in the UK. Since 1985 patients with hepatic carcinoma have only been accepted for liver transplantation in Cambridge after laparotomy to exclude pre-existing metastases. However, before 1980, 45 out of 92 liver transplants were to patients with hepatic carcinoma and this diagnostic group had the highest risk of dying from three months after transplantation (Gore *et al.* 1987). In the second half of the 1980s, immunosuppression with Cyclosporin brought marked improvements in one year survival for all types of transplanted organ, as did beneficial matching in renal transplantation, and was therefore established as the immunological basis of kidney exchange in the UK.

Epoch-specific proportional hazards regression identified both the transient immunodominance of HLA matching (see Gilks *et al.* 1990 with corroboration by Thorogood *et al.* 1990) and that the risk of early renal graft failure (in the first two weeks post-transplant) was not reduced by Cyclosporin but was alleviated by beneficial matching. Neither tissue matching nor Cyclosporin has substantially reduced the 5% per annum hazard of late renal graft failure (that is: after the first year). Accelerated failure of regrafts (Gore and Bradley 1988), ascertainment bias and measurement error in DR typing were other features of note in transplantation studies. Ascertainment bias occurred at the inception of DR-typing, which was first applied in investigation of patients who had a failed renal graft. HLA-DR types, which were unknown at the time

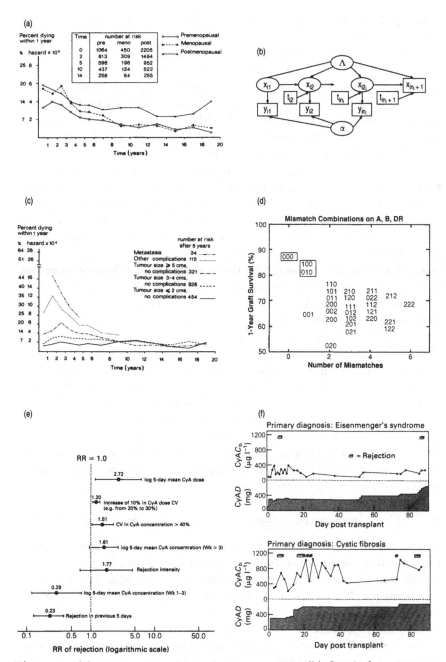

Figure 1: (a) Western General breast cancer series; (b) Cervical cancer: Gibbs sampling; (c) Western General breast cancer series; (d) HLA matching in kidney transplantation; (e) Risk of lung graft rejection; (f) Cyclosporin dose and blood levels.

of first graft, were subsequently infilled on the national database so that the strongest predictor of graft failure became knowledge of the recipient DR type! Such data-management errors are not uncommon in registry or clinical databases; moreover, it is often the case that new tests or drugs are used first in high risk patients. Unless due care is exercised, similar problems recur. Investigating the influence of HLA-phenotype on progression of HIV disease has been complicated by preferment for HLA typing of patients whose life expectancy is short. Moreover, there is serological failure of DR typing in 20% of patients whose HIV disease has progressed.

Reciprocal creatinine has been used successfully, but retrospectively, in Kalman-filter monitoring of post-transplant renal function (Smith and West 1983): slope change signalled imminent kidney graft rejection. But in liver transplantation, so-called 'biochemical rejection' is no longer a basis for bolus steroids being used, unless rejection is confirmed by liver biopsy. Short-term risks of nephrotoxicity and acute graft rejection in Papworth heart-lung transplantees are being assessed by the monitoring of Cyclosporin dose and blood levels, together with reciprocal creatinine (retrospectively in the first instance, but with a view to development of an online clinical decision aid). High coefficient of variation of individual Cyclosporin dose (and blood level) over the previous 10 days significantly increased the risk of lung graft rejection (Best *et al.* 1992).

In heart transplantation, patients who survive the short-term competing hazards of acute graft rejection, infection and nephrotoxicity – and 80% do – are then at risk of developing coronary occlusive disease, and so are monitored at predetermined intervals by angiographic assessment (see Gilks *et al.* 1993). The narrowing of major coronary arteries is graded on a three-point scale: normal, mild stenosis (50% or less narrowing) or severe stenosis; and analysis has featured a discrete state, continuous time, time-homogeneous Markov process with irreversible disease states.

2.4   Cardiovascular disease prevention and treatment

Assessment of the real strength of the relation between 'usual' blood pressure and the primary incidence of coronary vascular disease has required correction for the biassing effects of purely random variations in baseline blood pressure measurements. MacMahon *et al.* (1990) gave a lucid account of how to correct indirectly for regression dilution bias in prospective observational studies, but stressed the importance for future studies of remeasuring risk factors at a later follow-up in at least a representative proportion of survivors so that internal correction for regression dilution could be made.

After correction for regression dilution, and by considering several studies in combination, MacMahon *et al.* (1990) showed that usual blood pressure was positively related to the risk of stroke and of coronary heart disease, not only among individuals who might be considered 'hypertensive' but also among those who would usually be considered 'normotensive'; and that these relations were at least 60% stronger than previously thought. MacMahon *et al.* thus set in an epidemiological context their subsequent overview of randomized drug trials involving short-term reductions in blood pressure (see Collins *et al.* 1990). Whereas the incidence of strokes was significantly reduced in randomized trials of blood pressure lowering drugs to the extent suggested by epidemiological studies, a lesser short-term effect was reported in respect of coronary heart disease: 14% reduction (but with wide confidence interval from 4% to 22%) instead of the 20 to 25% reduction suggested by observational epidemiological data. Whether intervention or follow-up was too short to observe the full epidemiologically-expected benefit, or the drugs insufficiently effective remains to be resolved. Correction for regression dilution biasses (by using repeat measurement of risk factors to determine usual levels) is, of course, relevant to other risk factors that may be subject to substantial measurement error, such as dietary characteristics (salt reduction for example: see Frost *et al.* 1991 and Law *et al.* 1991a,b).

Cardiovascular disease prevention and treatment has demonstrated cohesive interplay of epidemiology, statistical overview and trial design leading to good accounts of the scientific rationale for chosing between clinical trials (see Sandercock *et al.* 1986), advocacy of factorial designs, and *a priori* determination of plausible treatment effect sizes, thus ensuring that appropriate numbers of patients are randomized , on occasion over 40,000 as by ISIS-3 Collaborative Group (1992). Increasingly, strategies for preventing ischaemic heart disease are directed towards whole populations, with emphasis on changes in national diets, reduction in cigarette smoking and control or prevention of hypertension (but see also Shaper *et al.* (1986) and the OX-CHECK Study Group (1991)).

2.5 Summary

Statistical science has contributed importantly to understanding the natural history of breast and cervical cancer, to the design and implementation of interventions such as mass screening and organ exchange policy, and to quantification of existing evidence from therapeutic trials, as well as to directing attention to treatment options which merit sound evaluation. Statisticians have also shown the importance of dealing with ascertainment and measurement error in assessing risk relationships; and that risk relationships commonly change over time, because of heterogeneity of frailty (Aalen 1988) or for other reasons including unmodelled treatment by covariate interaction. Statistical monitoring of marker processes for individualized acute patient managements remains largely a research activity; prospective evaluations and implementation are rare.

Other diseases with long development times are likely to pose interesting statistical problems in the 1990s. Besides HIV disease, there are the demographically compelling problems of aging, particularly dementia; the conundrum of early 'programming' by nature or nurture; and the esoteric prion diseases (proteinaceous infectious particle: see Brown *et al.* 1993). In humans, prion diseases include Creutzfeldt–Jakob disease (Weber *et al.* 1993) and, in animals, scrapie (affecting sheep and goats and prevalent in most sheep rearing countries except Australasia or Japan) and bovine spongiform encephalopathy (currently a major epidemic confined almost entirely to the cattle of the British Isles: Hughes (1993)).

3   Chronic disease processes generally, and HIV disease

3.1   Chronic disease processes

The applications of the previous section were chosen to illustrate in context some major data analytic themes which have exercised statisticians. These are now drawn out schematically in Figure 2 with chronic disease processes generally in mind. Briefly, from *inception* of the disease process there is an interval until the disease, or its progression, is detectable by *screening* (such as by cervical smear, blood pressure, HIV test or CD4 count). Inevitably screening is an imperfect (and often indirect) measure of the *true underlying disease state*, but the intensity of subsequent screening, behaviour modification (such as condom use, diet or exercise) and drug prophylaxis (to reduce blood pressure) may depend upon what was observed. *Clinical signs* are another insight to the underlying disease state, and the signs which manifest (Kaposi's sarcoma, for example) may both determine the speed of (clinical) *diagnosis* and anticipate future transitions between underlying disease states. There may be a choice of patient managements, medical or surgical, some of which are *major interventions* in the sense that the progression marker which has been monitored hitherto is removed (tumour size by mastectomy) or its relevance alters (reciprocal creatinine in dialysed or transplanted renal recipient). Moreover, after such major interventions the focus of patient monitoring may shift to include the *monitoring of drug toxicity* as well as efficacy (as in the case of Cyclosporin) or of *new disease processes*, such as coronary occlusive disease in long-term survivors of heart transplantation. It may thus be anticipated that *covariates exert different influences* in distinct epochs of follow-up in which different outcomes, or markers thereof, are relevant. Finally *external data*, such as from clinical trials or epidemiological studies, may be adduced to infer the likely size of treatment effects, or the times of infection (in the case of HIV disease). Covariates and marker processes may be *measured with error* and important but unknown influences may be *unmeasured*.

3.2   Progression of HIV disease

Figure 2 is now interpreted in the context of HIV disease: inception is the time of infection, which is seldom known exactly but often an interval can be defined in which the individual must have become infected – the start of this interval being determined epidemiologically (by when HIV infections began in the region) or individually (according to behavioural or serological history). Antibodies to HIV disease form within weeks or few months of infection – so-called seroconversion – and can be tested for in blood, urine or saliva. A flu-like seroconversion illness may occur, but is either rare or recognised rarely for what it is. Individuals differ in their susceptibility to HIV infection. Those with the haplotype A1 B8 DR3, for example, have been reported as more susceptible to infection and, once infected, indeed progress more rapidly to AIDS (Steel *et al.* 1988). There may be differences in the virulence of the virus strain by which individuals were infected, and this may have implications for their disease progression, or infectivity (see below). External epidemiological studies (such as contact tracing), or self referral to 'check out' HIV status, or clinical symptoms may lead to an individual's being HIV tested, the result of which (positive or negative) may modify risk behaviours. Once HIV disease has been diagnosed, the patient's CD4 count – and other markers such as IgA, β_2-microglobulin and haemoglobin – are monitored at irregular intervals. Irregularity is occasioned, for example, by 20% failure to attend appointments (Brettle *et al.* 1992), intensification of monitoring for clinical trials (Ellenberg *et al.* 1992), or alteration in three-monthly schedule because of good (or poor) prognosis (Munoz *et al.* 1992). Prophylaxis against pneumocystis carinii pneumonia is instituted according to CD4 count, the underlying true disease state being unobserved. Clinical symptoms and opportunistic infections, tumours and HIV encephalopathy are managed as they manifest – for example foscarnet is given to avert cytomegalovirus retinitis, a cause of blindness (Studies of Ocular Complications of AIDS 1992). No major intervention in the sense described above for breast cancer or end-stage-organ failure is yet applicable in HIV disease (Stablein 1990). Treatment with zidovudine, initially offered only to patients with ARC or AIDS, is now advertised for patients whose CD4 count is 'less than 500 and rapidly falling'. Optimal strategy for zidovudine use is unclear from clinical trials, and so is also being investigated in clinical cohorts (McNeil 1993). Intercurrent death rate is around 2.5% per annum among HIV infected drug users, but some suicides and deaths by overdose may be HIV-related.

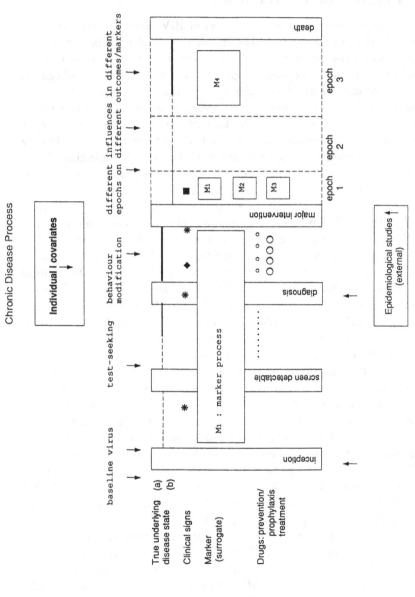

Figure 2. Chronic Disease Process. The symbols *, ◆, ■ represent different clinical signs; the symbols o, ◯ indicate different intensities of prevention/prophylaxis treatment.

3.3   Transmissibility of HIV disease

Description of the consequences of HIV disease must take account of its transmissibility. Inherited susceptibility, for example to breast cancer, and the destruction of a donor organ by the same disease process which compromised the recipient's are examples of a sort of transmissibility. There may be barriers to transmissibility, such as cross-species (baboon to human liver xenotransplantation because the baboon liver is thought to be resistant to human hepatitis B virus infection: see Starzl 1993), or the opposite may hold, namely accelerated incubation (as in some prion diseases: Hughes 1993).

After HIV *infection* of the index case, an interval (possibly of zero length) elapses before the index becomes infectious; thereafter infectiousness may wax and wane – either independently of, or in association with, the true underlying disease state of the index (Jewell and Shiboski 1990, Shiboski and Jewell 1992). In the latter circumstance, markers of disease progression for the index illuminate true infectiousness; in the former case they will not, but other measures of infectiousness, such as in vitro characterisation of the *virus*, may be relevant. For HIV disease it has been suggested that infectiousness is highest around seroconversion and again in late disease, but empirical support for the former is difficult to obtain, see Shiboski and Jewell (1992); and as with hepatitis B virus (Masuko *et al.* 1985), some HIV infected individuals may be less highly viraemic than others (Learmont *et al.* 1992).

Until the index is aware of having been HIV infected – that is, after both seroconversion and HIV antibody positive test – temporal changes in needle sharing or sexual behaviour may be uninfluenced by local and national public health initiatives. *After diagnosis of the index case*, specific changes in behaviour may follow, and the index's response to public health initiatives in the future may be conditioned by awareness of HIV positivity. Thus the *opportunity for transmission* within an existing partnership, or new ones, is time-inhomogeneous and needs to be elicited; further behavioural changes may follow *disclosure* within an existing or new partnership of the index case's HIV diagnosis. The opportunity for transmission may be further *affected by the index's underlying disease state*.

A final consideration is *susceptibility* of the contact(s) to the virus of the index case. This susceptibility may vary over time, for example because the virus changes itself or for other reasons related to the contact's defence against infection (see Learmont *et al.* 1992), or be fixed, such as the contact's HLA phenotype (Steel *et al.* 1988).

4   Data analytic themes in HIV disease

Major statistical issues in HIV disease concern progression markers, incubation distribution and infectivity: see Jewell (1990) and Gail (1991) for extensive bibliography. The extent to which progression markers give information about time since infection and time to AIDS diagnosis is important in public health terms: for deciding whether anonymized serosurveillance of HIV disease can be extended to infer sero-incidence (Satten and Longini 1993) and whether AIDS drugs can be licensed by being shown to affect surrogate endpoints (Ellenberg *et al.* 1992, Freedman *et al.* 1992).

Incubation distribution (see Bacchetti and Jewell 1992) is one of three key components in backcalculation (reported AIDS cases and assumptions about past HIV incidence being the other two). Backcalculation (see Bacchetti *et al.* 1993, de Angelis *et al.* 1993, Rosenberg *et al.* 1992) has provided satisfactory short-term planning estimates of AIDS diagnoses, but with bounds of uncertainty which have remained wide. The extent to which incubation distribution is affected by treatment, or is different between risk groups, is part of that uncertainty. Forecasting the health care needs of HIV infected individuals (Brookmeyer and Liao 1990, Longini *et al.* 1992) increasingly requires estimation also of the stage-specific numbers of HIV infections, and associated incubation times.

Dynamic modelling of HIV sub-epidemics in homosexuals (Heisterkamp *et al.* 1992), injecting drug users, and other heterosexuals (Blower *et al.* 1991, Arca *et al.* 1992) requires assumptions about infectivity. Assumptions about infectivity also determine public health education policy on how to minimize the risks of HIV transmission (Gail *et al.* 1989), personal decisions on implementation of safe(r) sex or HIV test uptake, and public health action in the follow-up of persons who have been potentially exposed to HIV infection – for example, by being operated on by an HIV infected surgeon (see Bird *et al.* 1991, Royal College of Pathologists 1992).

4.1   Markers of HIV progression

Jewell and Kalbfleisch (1992) suggested that a start could be made, in considering statistical models for the joint distribution of a marker process $\{x(t) : 0 < t < T\}$ and time to AIDS, T, by focussing on the three component problems of: the link between realization of the marker process and AIDS hazard; the relationship between other factors and AIDS hazard; and the influence of background factors on the stochastic properties of the marker process. They suggested a Poisson process representation for the marker process together with an additive hazard model.

More usually, as we shall see, the marker process has been analysed as longitudinal data (see Zeger and Liang (1992) and Vonesh (1992) for general accounts of the analysis of longitudinal data) without regard to the time of AIDS diagnosis, but preferably with seroconversion as the time origin. Interest has focussed on a suitable functional form for the marker process, after transformation if necessary. Or, the marker process has been utilized as a time-dependent covariate in a relative risks regression with rather little attention to covariate coding. Also, constancy of relative risk has been little questioned. Some attention has been paid to measurement error (Raboud *et al.* 1993) but little account has been taken in AIDS or infectivity regression models of unmeasured covariates, that is of frailty.

CD4 count, like blood pressure (see Berkey *et al.* 1992, Gaffney *et al.* 1993), is subject to diurnal and other sources of measurement error, but unlike blood pressure its measurement is invasive. Moreover, restricting the times of CD4 clinic visits increases non-attendance, especially by HIV infected injecting drug users whose lifestyle is chaotic. Nakamura (1992) provides a simple correction (based on the variance of measurement error) for asymptotically biased regression coefficients from a maximized proportional hazards partial likelihood for the case that measurement errors are additive and normally distributed. The case of correlated time-dependent HIV covariates subject to different measurement error is considered by Raboud *et al.* (1993). Phillips *et al.* (1992) warned about bias in relative odds estimation owing to imprecise measurement of correlated exposures – HDL cholesterol and triglycerides in the genesis of coronary heart disease, in their example. The extent to which this caution applies when several marker processes – CD4 count, β_2-microglobulin, IgA – are utilized as time-dependent covariates in proportional hazards models is unclear, but a concern.

Hastie and Tibshirani (1990, 1993) have explored the nature of covariate effects in proportional hazards models, first featuring $\exp\{\sum_{j=1}^p f_j(x_{ij})\}$ instead of $\exp\{\sum_{j=1}^p \beta_j x_{ij}\}$ for patient i where $f_j(\ )$ are unspecified smooth functions that are estimated using scatterplot smoothers and can be used to suggest covariate transformations. More recently, they focussed on varying coefficient models, where the regression coefficient could be a function, for example, of time: $\exp\{\sum_{j=1}^p \beta_j(t)x_{ij}\}$. Non-proportionality of hazards can also be suggested by Aalen plots or other diagnostics (Henderson and Milner 1991, Gray 1990); accommodated by adaptive weighted logrank tests (Self 1992); and for time-dependent covariates explored by fitting relative risks regression in distinct epochs of follow-up. Stratification for epoch k allows a check on whether $\beta_k = \beta$ for all k. Hughes *et al.* (1992) chose to update covariate values at the start of each epoch, preferring to use software for non-time-dependent covariates to facilitate short-term prediction and hazard plots.

The above methods of checking for covariate transformation or non-proportionality have been little used in modelling HIV progression. Even the question of whether it is CD4 level or CD4 change that matters (see Cain *et al.* 1992) is not well addressed. Assessing the differential influence of prognostic factors – either on the simultaneous occurrence of one or more manifestations of HIV disease or on the repeated occurrence of the same opportunistic infection or clinical sign (see Abu-Libdeh *et al.* 1990) – has not been tackled. The reason may be that the diversity of such signs has posed a daunting data-management problem prospectively, and only few, like Kaposi's sarcoma, could be reliably retrieved from case-notes.

Frailty models in survival analysis acknowledge that the hazard function $\lambda_i(t)$ for individual i with observed covariates $\mathbf{x}_i$ may depend also on some unknown, or unmeasured, other characteristics. This unknown factor is thought of as individual heterogeneity, so-called frailty, but could be shared (ζ_s) – being common to households (some aspect of diet or environment: see Klein 1992), to families (genetic) or to HIV transmission networks (some aspect of the virus: denoting individuals who are believed to have been infected by a common source). Thus

$$\lambda_i(t) = \lambda(t|\mathbf{x}_i, \zeta_s) = \lambda_0(t)\zeta_s \exp\{\sum_{j=1}^{p} \beta_j x_{ij}\} = \lambda_0(t)\zeta_s \exp\{\boldsymbol{\beta}\mathbf{x}_i\}.$$

Aalen (1988) considered gamma, Poisson and inverse Gaussian mixing distributions for ζ_s but commented that statistical inference would have less ambiguity if repeated events could be observed per individual, the better to characterize ζ_s (see McGilchrist and Aisbeth (1991) for a cardiovascular application). Abu-Libdeh *et al.* (1990) have considered the case of multi-type recurrent events, such as infections following bone marrow transplantation which may be bacterial, fungal or viral in origin, with differential frailties according to the type of recurrent event.

Clayton (1991) provided a Monte Carlo method for Bayesian inference in frailty models. This easily extends to the case that an unmeasured characteristic exerts a different influence in distinct epochs of follow-up – just as measured covariates often do – or is modified by known covariates. A generalized frailty model for consideration in HIV disease could thus be written as

$$\lambda_i(t) = \lambda(t|\mathbf{x}_{1i}(t), \mathbf{x}_{2i}(t), \zeta_s) = \lambda_0(t) \exp\{\beta_1 \mathbf{x}_{1i}(t) + \zeta_s(\beta_2 \mathbf{x}_{2i}(t))\}$$

where $\mathbf{x}_{2i}(t)$ could indicate distinct follow-up epochs or initiation of treatment, for example.

Carlin *et al.* (1992) presented hierarchical Bayesian analyses of change-point problems: changing regressions, changing Poisson processes and changing Markov chains. From Lange *et al.* (1992) there is a detailed account of their hierarchical Bayes models for the progression of HIV infection using longitudinal CD4 counts. Analysis was on the square root scale, CD4 counts (for 327 subjects) were all prior to the start of zidovudine, and external data on seroconversion times were used in offset estimation of Υ_i, the time from seroconversion to cohorting of individual i. Individual level random effects (intercept, slope, time since seroconversion of slope change) allowed for random deviation of an individual's trajectory from the expected trajectory for the population to which the individual belonged. Model choice was based on goodness of prediction when the most recent observation was left out. Using an inverse prediction approach, posterior distributions of time for CD4 count to reach a specified level were computed.

McNeil (1993) extended this approach to model the impact of zidovudine therapy on individual loss of root CD4 count, using 1992 data from the Edinburgh City Hospital cohort to assess the predictive fit of models based on CD4 counts to the end of 1991. The models envisaged change in level (proportional to intervention CD4 level) and change in slope after zidovudine. 164 HIV infected injecting drug users with well estimated seroconversion times and at least 10 CD4 counts were studied.

Neither Lange, Carlin and Gelfand nor McNeil imposed an explicit correlation structure (see Munoz *et al.* 1992) in their hierarchy to allow for short-term fluctuations in individual CD4 count, Lange *et al.* having noted that exchangeable random effects result anyway in correlations between measurements that typically decrease with increasing time between measurements.

McNeil (1993) added survival to the regression tier of his hierarchical Bayesian model by assuming an extreme value distribution for the time to AIDS. For individual i with baseline cofactor x_{2i} and true root CD4 marker path $\alpha_i + \phi_i x_i(t)$, the hazard of AIDS onset was related to CD4 marker path by

$$\lambda_i(t) = \lambda(t; [\alpha_i, \phi_i], x_{2i}) = (\nu + \beta_1 \phi_i) e^{(\nu + \beta_1 \phi_i)t} e^{\beta_1 \alpha_i + \beta_2 x_{2i}}.$$

The shape of McNeil's extreme value survival distribution thus varies between individuals depending upon ϕ_i, the rate of loss of root CD4 count. The same parameter β_1 that explains how slope modifies shape also explains how intercept modifies scale; other cofactors like x_{2i} may also modify scale. Applied to observations on the 164 individuals from the Edinburgh City Hospital Cohort with 10 or more serial CD4 counts, the McNeil model estimated median incubation time to AIDS onset of more than 20 years for 20 of these patients. Essentially model dependent, these predictions must await longer follow-up of the Edinburgh City Hospital Cohort for validation. The model is notable for accommodating heterogeneity of distributional shape; and it fitted more readily using Monte Carlo methods than a Weibull survival model with ϕ_i as scale modifier and no dependence on α_i, the individual immuno-competence at seroconversion.

4.2   Incubation distribution

Brookmeyer and Gail (1987) seminally defined the biases in prevalent cohorts, amongst them onset confounding, of which the cofactor 'sexual activity' was an example, because individuals with many sexual partners were likely to have become HIV infected earlier than those who had few partners. Retrospective ascertainment, which applies to transfusion associated AIDS cases (see Wang and See 1992), under-samples long incubation times, necessitating conditional estimation; whereas prevalent cohorts, especially those instituted several years after the start of the HIV epidemic, undersample short incubation times. Bacchetti (1990) ingeniously used deconvolution from AIDS diagnoses together with good information on the distribution of HIV infection times to estimate the incubation period distribution; see also Bacchetti and Jewell (1992) and Chiarotti *et al.* (1992). De Gruttola and Lagakos (1989) gave non-parametric and weakly structured parametric methods for analysing survival data in which both time origin and failure event can be right or interval censored, with application to HIV infected haemophiliacs. Law and Brookmeyer (1992) investigated the effect of mid-point estimation on the analysis of doubly censored data and concluded that the procedure was reasonable for seroconversion intervals up to two years in width when the incubation time was typically 10 years, as in HIV disease. Munoz *et al.* (1992) made use of markers of maturity of infection, specifically percent CD4 lymphocytes, in estimation of the time since exposure for a prevalent cohort.

Solomon and Wilson (1990) suggested accommodating change due to treatment in backcalculation by changing the density function for the incubation period from f_1 before calendar time T to f_2 after T, whereas Rosenberg *et al.* (1992) parametrized treatment impact on the incubation distribution by specifying the relative hazard for AIDS in treated and untreated individuals as a function of their duration of HIV infection; and also modelled the prevalence of treatment, see also de Angelis *et al.* (1993) and Lim (1992). Uncertainty about how zidovudine affects the incubation distribution has not been resolved by randomized controlled trials because short-term benefits have led to early stopping of these trials, and the offering of zidovudine to patients originally randomized to placebo (Ellenberg *et al.* 1992). The 'natural' history of HIV disease has not been observed beyond 10 years; prophylaxis against pneumocystis carinii pneumonia, antiretroviral therapy, and experience in patient care have extended the incubation distribution of HIV disease. Incubation times are shorter for older individuals but there is great uncertainty about whether the route of transmission and size of inoculum affect the incubation period.

4.3   Infectivity

The infectivity of HIV for a given route of transmission has been defined as the per-contact probability of infection, but Wiley *et al.* (1989) have suggested that the risk of acquiring HIV infection sexually depends primarily on the number of sexual partnerships formed and not on the frequency of intercourse within the partnership. Routes of transmission include by percutaneous injury or mucous membranes (to health care workers), transfusion of HIV infected blood (after 1985 only if HIV antibody negative), unprotected vaginal or anal intercourse, orogenital transmission, by maternal breast milk, or from mother to child in utero or at birth, and by needle sharing (among HIV infected injecting drug users). Shiboski and Jewell (1992) remark that little is known about HIV transmission probabilities for various modes of contact, or about the role of cofactors in promoting or suppressing transmission. Based on partner study data, they modelled the time dependence of HIV infectivity as determined by the time, u, since infection of the index case, i. Thus:

$$\lambda_i(u) = \lambda_i \lambda(u)$$

where λ_i summarized the biological heterogeneity in infectiousness of the index case i, susceptibility of the partner, and nature of contacts. They fitted a binary regression (involving cofactors and rate of contacts as well as infectivity) with log-log link and smoothness constraints via a penalized likelihood. However, in this context the random effect λ_i is unlikely to be constant over time, which provides further motivation for generalized frailty, as introduced in Section 3 and alluded to by Jewell and Kalbfleisch (1992).

Typically in partner studies, seroconversion dates are interval censored for the index case and partner (if applicable); also, more attention in data collection has been given to retrospective behavioural than to prospective biological data. The Edinburgh Heterosexual Partner Study is an exception. Not only is there good immunological follow-up of HIV infected participants, intentional HLA typing of all couples, but also retrospective HIV testing (for known HIV infected individuals) of sera which have been stored since 1983. This has resulted in narrow seroconversion intervals for 302 out of 577 patients (to end December 1991) recruited to the Edinburgh City Hospital Cohort, who include index cases and infected partners in the heterosexual partner study. Further work is in hand to ascertain IgA and β_2-microglobulin levels in the stored HIV positive sera which predate the patient's HIV diagnosis. This will provide immunological staging prior to patients' entering clinical follow-up. Characterization of the virus at diverse times after HIV infection remains a data deficiency in this and other studies, which single partner designs are unable to resolve analytically. Progress could be made in studies of virus-sharing-networks if individual susceptibility were also measurable.

5 Future statistical directions in HIV disease

Comparative review of data analysis in diseases with long development times shows that only modest attention has been paid in HIV disease to careful parametrization of covariate influences and to checks for non-proportionality of those influences over time. The availability and serial measurement of several immunological progression markers – an unusual phenomenon – has perhaps induced a certain complacency. The invasiveness of blood sampling limits, but does not obviate, practicable designs for assessing measurement error.

In HIV disease, Bayesian hierarchical models have been deployed to good effect to estimate individual trajectories from short time series of CD4 counts. This has importance not least for understanding the longer term effects of antiretroviral therapy. Unusually, zidovudine has been adopted on the basis of short-term benefit established in randomized controlled trials, which have stopped early on that account. Regression methods for survival, notably successful in identifying prognostic factors, are conspicuously little used for individual counselling in any of the diseases considered. Bayesian methods for modelling HIV progression using longitudinal CD4 counts are pretenders for that fiefdom.

External data have been drawn into backcalculation to limit the range of uncertainty of AIDS forecasts by restricting to convolutions which breach none of a series of plausibility constraints. Raab *et al.* (personal communication) made constraints explicit as prior distributions for the incubation distribution's mean and shape, numbers HIV infected in Scotland by 1989, and for the impact of treatment. The posterior distributions which resulted after taking into account diagnosed cases of AIDS or severe HIV related immunodeficiency in Scotland to the end of 1991 suggest greater attention to the shape of the incubation distribution, as do the hazard models of McNeil (1993); and to differential impact of treatment by risk group. de Angelis *et al.* (1993) outlined a graphical modelling approach to the propagation of uncertainty in backcalculation.

Particularly in respect of HIV infectivity, statistical science has made rather little impact, despite some very fine individual contributions to the analysis of limited data. The reason appears two-fold: failure to draw together the sundry data sources on HIV infectivity by different transmission routes, even to ensure that these data are collected systematically; and failure to design studies which tackle HIV transmission in sexual or injecting networks linked to an index case, rather than in single partnerships. In studies of infectivity, it is very likely that unmeasured attributes (viral, infectiousness of index, susceptibility of contact) differ importantly between and within networks. Consideration of HIV infectivity, and also of HIV progression, motivates a generalized notion of frailty for which Monte Carlo methods would be appropriate. Their use is recommended when sharing networks can be identified amongst HIV infected patients, for example in progression studies, and in the more general problem of HIV infectivity according to different modes of transmission.

The Acquired Immunodeficiency Syndrome (AIDS) manifests clinically in so many ways that it has been expedient to concentrate statistical effort on immunological markers of HIV disease rather than its clinical signs. Nonetheless, studies of how the disease manifests clinically, and of how the patient's immune system recovers from successive illnesses may be important, remembering that in transplantation the individual's response to rejection episodes is indeed informative about future risks.

References

Breast Cancer Screening (1986) *Report to the Health Ministers of England, Wales, Scotland and Northern Ireland by a working group chaired by Professor Sir Patrick Forrest*, HMSO, London.

Aalen, O.O. (1988) 'Heterogeneity in survival analysis', *Stats. Med.* **7**, 1121–1137.

Aalen, O.O. (1992) 'Modelling the influence of risk factors on familial aggregation of disease', *Biometrics* **47**, 933–946.

Abu-Libdeh, H., Turnbull, B.W. and Clark, L.C. (1990) 'Analysis of multi-type recurrent events in longitudinal studies; application to a skin cancer prevention trial', *Biometrics* **46**, 1017–1034.

Andersen, P.K. (1991) 'Survival analysis 1982–1991: the second decade of the proportional hazards regression model', *Stats. Med.* **10**, 1931–41.

Andersen, P.K. (1992) 'Repeated assessment of risk factors in survival analysis', *SMMR* **1**, 297–315.

Arca, M., Perucci, C.A. and Spadea, T. (1992) 'The epidemic dynamics of HIV-1 in Italy: modelling the interaction between intravenous drug users and heterosexual population', *Stats. Med.* **11**, 1657–1684.

Bacchetti, P. (1990) 'Estimating the incubation period of AIDS by comparing population infection and diagnosis patterns', *JASA* **85**, 1002–1017.

Bacchetti, P. and Jewell, N.P. (1992) 'Non-parametric estimation of the incubation period of AIDS based on a prevalent cohort with unknown infection times', *Biometrics* **47**, 947–960.

Bacchetti, P., Segal, M.R. and Jewell, N.P. (1993) 'Backcalculation of HIV infection rates', *Statistical Science* **8**, 82–101.

Berkey, C.S., Laird, N.M., Valadian, I. and Gardner, J. (1992) 'Modelling adolescent blood pressure patterns and their prediction of adult pressures', *Biometrics* **47**, 1005–1018.

Best, N.G., Trull, A.K., Tan, K.K.C., Hue, K.L., Spiegelhalter, D.J., Gore, S.M. and Wallwork, J. (1992) 'Blood cyclosporin concentrations and the short-term risk of lung rejection following heart-lung transplantation', *Br. J. Clin. Pharmac.* **34**, 513–520.

Bird, A.G., Gore, S.M., Leigh-Brown, A. and Carter, D. (1991) 'Escape from collective denial: HIV transmission during surgery', *BMJ* **303**, 351–352.

Blower, S.M., Hartel, D., Dowlatabadi, H., Anderson, R.M. and May, R.M. (1991)
'Drugs, sex and HIV: a mathematical model for New York City', *Phil. Trans.
Royal Soc. London B* **331**, 171–187.

Boag, J.W. (1949) 'Maximum likelihood estimates of the proportion of patients
cured by cancer therapy (with discussion)', *JRSS (B)* **11**, 15–53.

Brettle, R.P., Gore, S.M. and McNeil, A.J. (1992) 'Outpatient medical care of
injection drug use related HIV', *Inter. J. of STD and AIDS* **3**, 96–100.

Brinkley, D. and Haybittle, J.L. (1975) 'The curability of breast cancer', *Lancet* **ii**,
95–96.

Brookmeyer, R. and Gail, M. (1987) 'Biases in prevalent cohorts', *Biometrics* **43**,
739–749.

Brookmeyer, R. and Liao, J. (1990) 'Statistical modelling of the AIDS epidemic
for forecasting health care needs', *Biometrics* **46**, 1151–1163.

Brown, P., Kaur, P., Sulima, M.P., Goldfarb, L.G., Gibbs, C.J. Jnr. and Gajdusek,
D.C. (1993) 'Real and imagined clinico-pathological limits of *prion dementia*',
Lancet **341**, 127–129.

Cain, K.C., Kronmal, R.A. and Kosinski, A.S. (1992) 'Analysing the relationship
between change in a risk factor and risk disease', *Stats. Med.* **11**, 783–797.

Carlin, B.P., Gelfand, A.E. and Smith, A.F.M. (1992) 'Hierarchical Bayesian analysis of changepoint problems', *Applied Stats.* **41**, 389–408.

Chiarotti, F., Polombi, M., Schinaia, N., Ghirardini, A. and Prospero, L. (1992)
'Effects of different parametric estimates of seroconversion time on analysis of
progression to AIDS among Italian HIV+ve haemophiliacs', *Stats. Med.* **11**,
591–601.

Clayton, D.G. (1991) 'A Monte Carlo method for Bayesian inference in frailty
models', *Biometrics* **47**, 467–485.

Collins, R., Peto, R., MacMahon, S., *et al.* (1990) 'Blood pressure, stroke and coronary heart disease. Part 2, short-term reductions in blood pressure: overview of
randomized drug trials in their epidemiological context', *Lancet* **335**, 827–38.

Cox, D.R. (1972) 'Regression models and life tables (with discussion)',
JRSS (B) **34**, 187–200.

d'Agostino, R.B., Lee, M.-L., Belanger, A.J., Cupples, L.A., Anderson, K. and
Kannel, W.B. (1990) 'Relation of pooled logistic regression to time dependent
Cox regression analysis: the Framingham heart study', *Stats. Med.* **9**, 1501–
1516.

de Angelis, D., Day,N.E., Gore, S.M., Gilks, W.R. and McGee, M.A. (1993) 'AIDS:
the statistical basis for public health', *SMMR* **2**, 75–91.

de Gruttola, V. and Lagakos, S.W. (1989) 'Analysis of doubly censored survival
data, with application to AIDS', *Biometrics* **45**, 1–11.

Early Breast Cancer Trialists' Collaborative Group (1992) 'Systemic treatment of
early breast cancer by hormonal, cytotoxic, or immune therapy', *Lancet* **339**,
1–15, 71–85.

Ellenberg, S.S., Finkelstein, D.M. and Schoenfeld, D.A. (1992) 'Statistical issues arising in AIDS clinical trials (with discussion)', *JASA* **87**, 562–583.

Freedman, L.S., Graubard, B.I. and Schatzkin, A. (1992) 'Statistical validation of intermediate endpoints for chronic diseases', *Stats. Med.* **11**, 167–178.

Frost, C.D., Law, M.R. and Wald, N.J. (1991) 'By how much does dietary salt reduction lower blood pressure? II – Analysis of observational data within populations', *BMJ* **302**, 815–818.

Gail, M.H. (1991) 'A bibliography and comments on the use of statistical models in epidemiology in the 1980s', *Stats. Med.* **10**, 819–1885.

Gail, M.H., Preston, D. and Piantadosi, S. (1989) 'Disease prevention models of volunatry confidential screening for human immunodeficiency virus (HIV)', *Stats. Med.* **8**, 59–82.

Gilks, W.R., Gore, S.M. and Bradley, B.A. (1990) 'Renal transplant rejection – transient immunodominance of HLA mismatches', *Transplantation* **50**, 141–146.

Gilks, W.R., Clayton, D.G., Spiegelhalter, D.J., Best, N.G., McNeil, A.J., Sharples, L.D. and Kirby, A.J. (1993) 'Modelling complexity: applications of Gibbs sampling in medicine', *JRSS (B)* **55**, 39–52.

Gore, S.M. and Bradley, B.A. (1988) *Renal Transplantation: Sense and Sensitization*, Kluwer, Dordrecht, 162–790.

Gore, S.M., Barroso, E. and White, D.J.G. (1987) 'Risk factors in orthotopic first liver transplantation'. In *Liver Transplantation*, Sir Roy Y. Calne (ed.) Grune and Stratton, London, 513–530.

Gore, S.M., Langlands, A.O., Spiegelhalter, D.J. and Stewart, H.J. (1988) 'Treatment decisions in breast cancer'. In *Recent Results in Cancer Research Vol. III*, Springer-Verlag, Heidelberg, 149–170.

Gore, S.M., Pocock, S.J. and Kerr, G.R. (1984) 'Regression models and nonproportional hazards in the analysis of breast cancer survival', *Applied Statistics* **33**, 176–195.

Gray, R.J. (1990) 'Some diagnostic methods for Cox regression models through hazard smoothing', *Biometrics* **46**, 93–102.

Greenwood, M. (1926) 'A Report on the Natural Duration of Cancer'. In *Report on Public Health and Medical Subjects* **33** HMSO, London.

Hastie, T. and Tibshirani, R. (1990) 'Exploring the nature of covariate effects in the proportional hazards model', *Biometrics* **46**, 1005–1016.

Hastie, T. and Tibshirani, R. (1993) 'Varying-coefficient models (with discussion)', *JRSS (B)*, **55**, 757–796.

Heisterkamp, S.H., de Haan, B.J., Jager, J.C., van Druten, J.A.M. and Hendriks, J.C.M. (1992) 'Short and medium term projections of the AIDS/HIV epidemic by a dynamic model with an application to the risk group of homo/bisexual men in Amsterdam', *Stats. Med.* **11**, 1425–1441.

Henderson, R. and Milner, A. (1991) 'Aalen plots under proportional hazards', *Applied Stats.* **40**, 401–410.

Hughes, J.T. (1993) 'Prion diseases. Depend on transmissable and sometimes heritable agents', *BMJ* **306**, 288.

Hughes, M.D., Raskino, C.L., Pocock, S.J., Biagini, M.R. and Burroughs, A.K. (1992) 'Prediction of short-term survival with an application in primary biliary cirrhosis', *Stats. Med.* **11**, 1731–45.

ISIS-3 Collaborative Group (1992) 'ISIS-3: a randomized comparison of streptokinase vs. tissue plasminogen activator vs. anistreplase and of aspirin plus heparin vs. aspirin alone among 41299 cases of suspected acute myocardial infarction', *Lancet* **339**, 753–769.

Jewell, N.P. (1990) 'Some statistical issues in studies of the epidemiology of AIDS', *Stats. Med.* **9**, 1387–1416.

Jewell, N.P. and Kalbfleisch, J.D. (1992) 'Marker models in survival analysis and applications to issues associated with AIDS'. In *AIDS Epidemiology: Methodological Issues* N.P. Jewell, K. Dietz and V. Farewel (eds.), Birkhauser, Boston, 211–230.

Jewell, N.P. and Shiboski, S.C. (1990) 'Statistical analysis of HIV infectivity based on partner studies', *Biometrics* **46**, 1133–1150.

Kirby, A.J., Spiegelhalter, D.J., Day, N.E., Fenton, L., Swanson, K., Mann, E.M.F. and Macgregor, J.E. (1992) 'Conservative treatment of mild/moderate cervical dyskaryosis: long-term outcome', *Lancet* **339**, 828–831.

Klein, J.P. (1992) 'Semiparametric estimation of random effects using the Cox model based on the EM algorithm', *Biometrics* **48**, 795–806.

Lange, N., Carlin, B.P. and Gelfand, A.E. (1992) 'Hierarchical Bayes models for the progression of HIV infection using longitudinal CD4 T-cell counts. *JASA* **87**, 615–632.

Langlands, A.O., Pocock, S.J., Kerr, G.R. and Gore, S.M. (1979) 'Long-term survival of patients with breast cancer: a study of the curability of the disease', *BMJ* **ii**, 1247–1251.

Law, C.G. and Brookmeyer, R. (1992) 'Effects of mid-point imputation on the analysis of doubly censored data', *Stats. Med.* **11**, 1569–1578.

Law, M.R., Frost, C.D. and Wald, N.J. (1991a) 'By how much does dietary salt reduction lower blood pressure? III – Analysis of data from trials of salt reduction', *BMJ* **302**, 819–824.

Law, M.R., Frost, C.D. and Wald, N.J. (1991b) 'By how much does dietary salt reduction lower blood pressure? I – Analysis of observational data among populations', *BMJ* **302**, 811–815.

Learmont, J., Tindall, B., Evans, L., Cunningham, A., *et al.* (1992) 'Long-term symptomless HIV-1 infection in recipients of blood products from a single donor', *Lancet* **340**, 869–867.

Lim, L. L.-Y. (1992) 'Estimating compliance to study medication from serum drug levels: application to an AIDS clinical trial of zidovudine', *Biometrics* **48**, 619–630.

Longini, I.M. Jnr., Byers, R.H,, Hessol, N,A. and Tan, W.Y. (1992) 'Estimating the stage-specific numbers of HIV infection using a Markov model and back-calculation', *Stats. Med.* **11**, 831–844.

MacMahon, S., Peto, R., Culter, J., Collins, R. *et al.* (1990) 'Blood pressure, stroke and coronary heart disease. Part I, prolonged differences in blood pressure: prospective observational studies corrected for the regression dilution bias', *Lancet* **335**, 765–774.

Mackisack, M., Dobson, A.J. and Heathcote, C.R. (1992) 'Predicting the prevalence of a disease in a cohort at risk', *Stats. Med.* **11**, 295–305.

Masuko, K., Mitsui, T., Iwano, K., Yamazaki, C., *et al.* (1985) 'Factors influencing post exposure immunoproplylaxis of hepatitis B virus infection with hepatitis B immune globulin', *Gastroenterology* **88**, 151–155.

McGilchrist, C.A. and Aisbeth, C.W. (1991) 'Regression with frailty in survival analysis', *Biometrics* **47**, 461–466.

McNeil, A.J. (1993) *Statistical Methods in AIDS Progression Studies with an Analysis of the Edinburgh City Hospital Cohort*, PhD thesis, University of Cambridge.

Munoz, A., Carey, V., *et al.* (1992) 'A parametric family of correlation structures for the analysis of longitudinal data', *Biometrics* **48**, 733–742.

Munoz, A., Carey, V., Taylor, J.M.G., *et al.* (1992) 'Estimation of time since exposure for a prevalent cohort', *Stats. Med.* **11**, 939–952.

Nakamura, T. (1992) 'Proportional hazards models with covariates subject to measurement error', *Biometrics* **48**, 829–838.

OXCHECK Study Group, Imperial Cancer Research Fund (1991) 'Prevalence of risk factors for heart disease in OXCHECK trial: implications for screening in primary care', *BMJ* **302**, 1057–1060.

Phillips, A.N. and Davey Smith, G. (1992) 'Bias in relative odds estimation owing to imprecise measurement of correlated exposures', *Stats. Med.* **11**, 953–961.

Raboud, J., Reid, N., Coates, R.A. and Farewell, V.T. (1993) 'Estimating risks of progressing to AIDS when covariates are measured with error', *Statistics in Society (JRSS (A)* **156**, 393–406.

Report of a Working Group of the Royal College of Pathologists (Chairman: J.E. Banatvala) (1992) *HIV Infection: Hazards of Transmission to Patients and Health Care Workers during Invasive Procedures*, Royal College of Pathologists, London.

Rosenberg, P.S., Gail, M.H. and Carroll, R.J. (1992) 'Estimating HIV prevalence and projecting AIDS incidence in the United States: a model that accounts for therapy and changes in the surveillance definition of AIDS', *Stats. Med.* **11**, 1633–1655.

Sandercock, P., Bamford, J., Warlow,C., Peto, R. and Starkey, I. (1986) 'Is a controlled trial of long-term oral anticoagulants in patients with stroke and non-rheumatic atrial fibrillation worthwhile?', *Lancet* **i**, 788–792.

Satten, G.A. and Longini, I.M. Jnr. (1993) 'Estimation of incidence of HIV infection using cross-sectional marker surveys', *Biometrics*, submitted.

Self, S.G. (1991) 'An adaptive weighted log-rank test with application to cancer prevention and screening trials', *Biometrics* **47**, 976–986.

Shaper, A.G., Pocock, S.J., Phillips, A.N. and Walker, M. (1986) 'Identifying men at high risk of heart attacks: strategy for use in general practice', *BMJ* **293**, 474–479.

Shiboski, S.C. and Jewell, N.P. (1992) 'Statistical analysis of the time dependence of HIV infectivity based on partner study data', *JASA* **87**, 360–372.

Smith, A.F.M. and West, M. (1983) 'Monitoring renal transplants: an application of the multi-process Kalman filter', *Biometrics* **39**, 867–878.

Solomon, P.J. (1984) 'Effect of misspecification of regression models in the analysis of survival data', *Biometrika* **71**, 291–298.

Solomon, P.J. and Wilson, S.R. (1990) 'Accommodating change due to treatment in the method of backprojection for estimating HIV infection incidence', *Biometrics* **46**, 1165–1170.

Stablein, D.M. (1990) 'Challenges of HIV vaccine development', *Stats. Med.* **9**, 1425–1431.

Starzl, T.E., Fung, J., Tzakis, A., Todo, S., *et al.* (1993) 'Baboon-to-human liver transplantation', *Lancet* **341**, 65–71.

Steel, C.M., Ludlam, C.A., Beatson, D., Peutherer, J.F., *et al.* (1988) 'HLA haplotype A1B8DR3 as a risk factor for HIV-related disease', *Lancet* **i**, 1185–1188.

Studies of Ocular Complications of AIDS Research Group and AIDS Clinical Trials Group. (1992) 'Mortality in patients with the acquired immunodeficinency syndrome treated with either foscarnet or ganciclovir for cytomegalovirus retinitis', *NEJM* **326**, 213–220.

Tabar, L., Fagerberg, G., Day, N.E., Duffy, S.W. and Kitchin, R. (1992) 'Breast cancer treatment and natural history: new insights from results of screening', *Lancet* **339**, 412–414.

Thorogood, J., Persijn, G.G., Schreuder, G.M.Th., *et al.* (1990) 'The effect of HLA matching on kidney graft survival in separate post transplantation intervals', *Transplantation* **50**, 146–150.

Vonesh, E.F. (1992) 'Non-linear models for the analysis of longitudinal data', *Stats. Med.* **11**, 1929–1954.

Wang, M.-C. and See, L.-C. (992) 'N-estimation from retrospectively ascertained events with application to AIDS', *Biometrics* **48**, 129–142.

Weber, T., Tumani, H., Holdorff, B., Collinge, J., Palmer, M., Kretzschmar, H.A. and Felgenhauer, K. (1993) 'Transmission of Creutzfeldt-Jakob disease by handling of dura mater', *Lancet* **341**, 123–124.

Wiley, J.A., Herschkorn, S.J. and Padian, N.S. (1989) 'Heterogeneity in the probability of HIV transmission per sexual contact: the case of male-to-female transmission in penile-vaginal intercourse', *Stats. Med.* **8**, 93–102.

Zedeler, K., Keiding, N. and Kamby, C. (1992) 'Differential influence of prognostic factors on the occurrence of metastases at various anatomical sites in human breast cancer', *Stats. Med.* **11**, 281–294.

Zeger, S.L. and Liang, K-Y. (1992) 'An overview of methods for the analysis of longitudinal data', *Stats. Med.* **11**, 1825–1839.

Discussion

LONGINI Diseases with long development times can usually be divided quite naturally into clinical stages. In the case of people with HIV infection, the hazard rate of AIDS development increases exponentially to a plateau, and this pattern arises from staged models. It would seem natural to model such diseases as staged processes.

SHAHANI** It seems to me that clinically meaningful early events, during the course of a disease, which have serious effects on the quality of life of an individual have received insufficient statistical attention. The statistical work seems to focus mainly on important late events. Two examples of such late events are death due to breast cancer and time to AIDS in studies of HIV infection.

REPLY Herpes zoster may qualify as such an event in the early course of HIV disease, at least among injecting drug users.

HPV and Cervical Cancer

Julian Peto

1   Introduction

Cervical cancer is the second commonest female cancer worldwide. Over the last few years, the evidence that sexually transmitted human papillomavirus (HPV) infection is involved in the development of most cases of cervical cancer has become virtually conclusive (Howley 1991, Schiffman 1992). HPV is therefore among the most important targets for practical cancer prevention. Screening for HPV is cheap and reliable, and animal studies suggest that vaccination may prove effective both in curing established infection and in preventing re-infection (Campo *et al.* 1993).

Against this background, formal modelling of the transmission and persistence of HPV infection would be a useful next step towards understanding the epidemic. The data required for preliminary simple models are beginning to emerge from case-control and prospective studies, but it is already clear that the natural history of infection is complex and heterogeneous. Statistical models of the natural history of various chronic diseases are reviewed by Gore (this volume). As for HIV, HPV susceptibility and infectiousness may be significantly influenced by other sexually transmitted infections as well as by genetic and immunological host factors.

The aim of this paper is to summarise the evidence that HPV is the cause of most cervical cancers, and to indicate what data should now be collected to elucidate its transmission dynamics. There have been rapid advances over the last few years in HPV diagnostic methods and our understanding of the relationship between HPV, dysplasia and malignancy. Much of the material summarised below is described in the recent IARC Scientific Report entitled The Epidemiology of HPV and Cervical Cancer (IARC 1992).

2   The epidemiology of cervical cancer

Cervical cancer risk is strongly related to number of regular sexual partners, and in monogamous women to the husband's number of partners. The risk may also be increased by early age at first intercourse, parity, smoking, oral contraceptive use, other genital infections, and low dietary intake of beta-carotene and vitamins A, C and E (Brinton 1992). Non-invasive cervical lesions (cervical intra-epithelial neoplasia, or CIN) are associated with more or

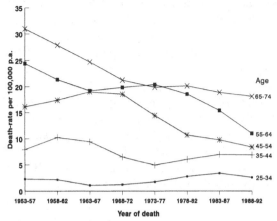

Figure 1. Cervical cancer mortality trends (England and Wales)

less the same risk factors, with the possible exception of age at first intercourse (Schneider and Koutsky 1992, Ley *et al.* 1991).

Successive generations of British women have suffered very different lifetime risks of cervical cancer. The risk was high in women born before 1880, those born around 1920 and those born since 1945, with substantially lower rates in intervening birth cohorts. The death rate below age 35 in Britain thus increased rapidly from 1965 to about 1985, since when it has fallen slightly, probably due mainly to improvements in the national cervical screening programme (Figure 1). At current rates, the lifetime risk of developing invasive cervical cancer in the U.K. is about 1.4% and the risk of dying from it is about 0.7%, but the recent increase at young ages suggests that British women born since 1945 will suffer considerably higher lifetime risks.

3   Precancerous cervical lesions

The Papanicolaou ('Pap') cervical smear test provides one of the most useful and effective cancer screening tests. Since 1954, when Papanicolaou first described the spectrum of cervical dysplasia, from cells which are atypical without malignant changes to those suggestive of malignancy, there have been various attempts to develop a standard reproducible cytological classification. Cytology is by definition based only on the morphology of individual cells seen on a cervical smear, whereas histology, which requires a biopsy, is based primarily on the thickness of the dysplastic lesion within the epithelial layer. Unfortunately this distinction has not been consistently observed, and grade of CIN (cervical intra-epithelial neoplasia), which is a histological diagnosis, is often incorrectly used to describe the cellular morphology seen on a cervical

smear. The Bethesda system, introduced in 1989, is the most recent attempt
to establish a simple cytological classification which correlates reasonably well
with histological findings. Under this system moderate and severe dysplasia
and carcinoma-in-situ are combined as a single group called HSIL (high-grade
squamous intra-epithelial lesions). HSIL corresponds more or less to the histological classifications CIN 2 and 3, where undifferentiated basal cells extend
beyond the bottom third of the epithelial layer. The Bethesda low-grade lesion group LSIL includes both CIN 1 and 'cellular changes suggestive of HPV
infection', as inter-observer studies suggest that this distinction is inconsistent and perhaps meaningless. The third and least severe Bethesda group,
atypical squamous cells of undetermined significance (ASCUS), includes other
mild cellular abnormalities not due to identified infections.

4   HPV and cervical neoplasia

Over 60 human papillomaviruses have already been detected. Different types
infect different epithelial tissues, ranging from those that cause various types
of wart on the hands and feet to those that are almost exclusively genital. The
commonest non-carcinogenic genital types are HPV 6 and HPV 11. These
can cause genital warts as well as mild cervical dysplasia, but they are not associated with cancer. HPV 16 and HPV 18 are the commonest genital types
associated with cancer, but many rarer genital types are also carcinogenic
(HPV 31, 33, 35, 39, 45, 51, 52, 56 and 58). It has been known for many
years that women whose cervical smears show koilocytosis (cellular changes
suggestive of HPV infection) are at high risk of developing more severe cervical dysplasia (Zur Hausen *et al.* 1981). Until 1990, however, a substantial
proportion of dysplasias and cancers could not be shown to contain HPV.
Moreover, in some studies the majority of normal smears from women in the
general population were reported to contain HPV. Researchers were therefore
not certain whether HPV played any causal role in cervical carcinogenesis.
These ambiguous findings have been shown to be due to four distinct errors
of classification or measurement, all of which can now be routinely avoided.

1. *HPV detection.* The HPV detection method now used, the polymerase
chain reaction (PCR), is so sensitive that it can detect less than one virus per
cell. Earlier methods were much less sensitive, and often gave a substantial
false negative rate.

2. *HPV typing.* Two common HPV types, HPV 6 and HPV 11, are
frequently associated with dysplasia but almost never with cancer. Many
early studies presented results for all HPV types combined.

3. *Sample contamination.* Because PCR is so sensitive, extreme care is
required to avoid cross-contamination of samples. Many laboratories mistak-
enly reported very high HPV rates in normal samples (Manos *et al.* 1990).

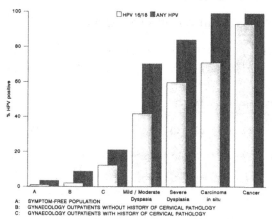

Figure 2. Cervical HPV prevalence in various patient groups (van den Brule *et al.* 1991)

4. *Misclassification of cervical dysplasia.* In some studies, cases of severe dysplasia which have been confirmed as CIN 3 by a panel of pathologists show a considerably higher prevalence of HPV than cervical smears classified as 'severe' by one cytologist. Since 1990 these methodological difficulties have been recognised and overcome (Manos *et al.* 1990), and many laboratories have now reported the striking correlation between grade of cervical neoplasia and HPV infection illustrated in Figure 2. Over the same period, it has been shown that the HPV E6 and E7 proteins bind to the products of two major human tumour suppressor genes (p53 and Rb1 respectively), which accounts for the transforming and carcinogenic effects of HPVs (Howley 1991).

The correlation between HPV type and severity of neoplasia is remarkably specific. In a large series from the US (Table 1) the ratio of HPV prevalence in invasive cancer compared with that in CIN 3 was zero for HPV types 6, 11, 43 and 44 (the non-carcinogenic types), 1.1 or less for most other types, and about 5 for types 18 and 45. The same three subgroups have been identified by phylogenetic analysis of DNA sequence homology. Types 6, 11, 42, 43 and 44 are members of a distinct group, and the other (carcinogenic) types form a separate group within which 18 and 45 (and 39) form a clear subgroup (Table 2).

A remarkable and unexplained feature of genital HPV is the stable co-existence of so many closely similar but distinct types. HPV 16 is the commonest type in most areas, but the relative frequency of the other types varies considerably. HPV appears to have been present in most populations for thousands of years, and HPV 16 exhibits minor mutational variants characteristic of its region of origin (Ho *et al.* 1991). Structurally similar papillomaviruses are also endemic in many other species.

HPV TYPES DETECTED

	NONE	6/11	42/43/44	16	31	33	35	51	52	56	18	45	X†	TOTAL
Normal cervix	1465 (94%)	8	6	16	7	3	2	6	8	1	5	2	33	1562
Low-grade SIL	115 (31%)	63	13	61	19	13	10	9	7	8	15	4	35	372
High-grade SIL	33 (13%)	8	3	123	27	12	11	5	6	3	13	1	15	260
Cancer	16 (11%)	0	0	72	8	2	2	1	1	2	36	3	8	151
Cancer: HSIL* prevalence ratio		0.0	0.0	1.0	0.5	0.3	0.3	0.3	0.3	1.1	4.8	5.2	0.9	

*HSIL: High-grade squamous intra-epithelial lesion

†X: Unidentified HPV types

Table 1. Prevalence of HPV types in cervical samples (Lorincz *et al.* 1992).

I	HPV 1	Cutaneous warts
II	HPV 5, 8, 14, 20, 21, 25, 47	Cutaneous epidermodysplasia verruciformis
III	HPV 2, 57	Cutaneous/mucosal
IVa	HPV 6, 11, 13, 42, 43, 44	Genital non-carcinogenic
IVb(i)	HPV 16, 31, 33, 35, 51, 52, 56, 58	Genital carcinogenic subgroup (i)
IVb(ii)	HPV 18, 39, 45	Genital carcinogenic subgroup (ii)

Table 2. Phylogenetic HPV classification based on the E6 gene DNA sequence (Van Ranst *et al.* 1992).

5 Natural history of CIN and HPV infection

The high prevalence of HPV in all grades of cervical dysplasia suggests that most of these lesions are merely clinical manifestations of HPV proliferation. Most mild dysplasia (or CIN 1) regresses and disappears within a few months, but women whose mild dysplasia persists for several months frequently progress to severe dysplasia which is histologically classified as CIN 3. Moreover, the HPV viral load in CIN 3 is often very much higher than in CIN 1 (Cuzick *et al.* 1992). It is not known whether HPV proliferation

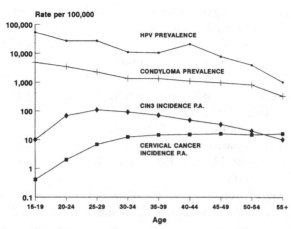

Rate per 100,000

Figure 3. Age-specific cervical HPV and neoplasia rates (Schiffman 1992)

in CIN 3 has a specific cellular basis, such as a mutation permissive of HPV replication. Indeed, it is still not known whether CIN 3 is monoclonal. For the practical purpose of epidemic modelling, however, HPV infections can be classified as either newly acquired or recurrent, and as transient or persistent, irrespective of the underlying immunological or other mechanisms which inhibit or facilitate viral proliferation.

There are thus four main stages in the progression from HPV infection to malignancy: subclinical HPV infection (detected by PCR); condyloma (any detectable manifestation of cervical HPV infection, including warts, flat white areas, and most mild dysplasias detected by a Pap smear); CIN 3 (severe dysplasia, often associated with a very high HPV load); and cervical cancer. These show striking differences in age distribution in Western populations (Figure 3). The prevalence of HPV infection is about 10%–20% between ages 15 and about 40, but much lower above age 45. Condylomata show a similar pattern, although at each age the cross-sectional prevalence of CIN 1 (mild dysplasia) is 5–10 times lower than that of detectable HPV infection. CIN 3 is rare below age 20, commonest at about age 30, then declines sharply. In contrast, the incidence of cervical cancer rises steeply up to about age 50 and subsequently remains roughly constant.

Among young women, number of recent sexual partners is strongly predictive of HPV infection (Ley *et al.* 1991). It has been generally assumed that the frequent appearance and disappearance of both detectable HPV and mild cervical dysplasia in young women (Schneider *et al.* 1992) reflect a persistent infection which undergoes cycles of latency and proliferation. However, preliminary results of a prospective study in the U.S. suggest that most women

who are initially HPV negative but who are HPV positive when a second
smear is taken 18 months later have been recently infected by a new partner
(M. Schiffman, personal communication) The natural history of infection in
young women may therefore involve repeated reinfections which disappear
completely within a few months, rather than latency and recurrence.

The lower prevalence of HPV in women aged over 40 is probably due at
least in part to their lower number of new partners. In addition, however,
repeated previous exposure may induce effective immunity. Several studies
have found that the presence of HPV in older women is unrelated to numbers
of sexual partners (Schneider and Koutsky 1992) although this could be due
to errors of HPV detection.

A major obstacle to a better understanding of HPV transmission dynamics
is the difficulty in obtaining reliable information on HPV prevalence in men.
Population-based prevalence data for men are not available, partly because
men do not have routine periodic screening analogous to the cervical smear
test, but also because a penile or urethral swab provides far fewer cells than
a cervical smear.

6   Significance of HPV infection in older women

The prevalence of HPV infection varies widely between different populations,
but in Western countries the prevalence of carcinogenic types in the general
population from a single cervical smear is of the order of 5% at age 45. Such
infection may have little prognostic significance, as a far higher proportion
may be transiently infected at some time between the ages of 40 and 50.
On the other hand, it is possible that some are persistently infected and will
remain so, and that most cervical cancers will occur in this group. As the
lifetime risk of developing invasive cancer is about 1% for a woman aged 45,
the risk to older women with persistent infection could thus be extremely high.
This can be resolved only by repeated cervical smears and long follow-up in
a large prospective study.

7   Vaccination and immunology

Vaccination of cattle can both prevent and eliminate infection with bovine
papillomavirus (BPV) (Campo *et al.* 1993). This raises the possibility that
HPV vaccination could be used to prevent or treat HPV infection and perhaps even cervical neoplasia (Crawford 1993). Several human vaccination
trials are now beginning, using either specific HPV proteins or a live vector incorporating one or more HPV genes which have been inactivated by
mutation.

HPV serology is still in its infancy, and only a minority of women who have been infected are seropositive with currently available tests (Galloway 1992). Even insensitive methods may be useful epidemiologically, however (Jha *et al.* 1993), and much better tests are likely to be developed in the near future. The determinants of persistent HPV infection in older women are not understood but are likely to be immunological, and there is evidence of HLA association in cervical neoplasia (Wank and Thompson 1991).

8 Conclusion

Genital HPV is an extremely well-adapted virus, being very common, highly infectious and virtually asymptomatic. As for any endemic infection, parameters of interest include the role (if any) of supercarriers, age-specific changes in natural history, infectiousness, co-factors for transmission, and heterogeneity of prevalence between population subgroups. HPV immunology promises exciting developments in our understanding of the natural history of HPV infection, and vaccination may be effective in preventing infection, and perhaps even for the treatment of both HPV infection and cervical neoplasia. A great deal remains to be done in measuring these parameters, in modelling their effects, and, most important of all, in conducting large trials of both preventive and therapeutic vaccination.

References

Brinton, L.A. (1992) 'Epidemiology of cervical cancer – overview'. In *IARC (1992)*, 3–23.

Campo, M.S., Grindlay, G.J., O'Neil, B.W., Chandrachdud, L.M., McGarvie, G.M. and Jarrett, W.F.H. (1993) 'Prophylactic and therapeutic vaccination against a mucosal papillomavirus', *J. Gen. Virol.* **74**, 945–953.

Crawford, L. (1993) 'Prospects for cervical cancer vaccines', *Cancer Surveys* **16**, 215–229.

Cuzick, J., Terry, G., Ho, L., Hollingworth, T., and Anderson, M. (1992) 'Human papillomavirus type 16 DNA in cervical smears as predictor of high-grade cervical cancer', *Lancet* **339**, 959–960.

Galloway, D. (1992) 'Serological assays for the detection of HPV antibodies'. In *IARC (1992)*, 147–161.

Ho, L., Chan., S-Y., Chow, V., Chong, T., Tay, S-K., Villa, L.L. and Bernard, H-U. (1991) 'Sequence variants of human papillomavirus type 16 in clinical samples permit verification and extension of epidemiological studies and construction of a phylogenetic tree', *Journ. Clin. Microbiology* **29**(9), 1765–72.

Howley, P.M. (1991) 'Role of the human papillomaviruses in human cancer', *Cancer Research* (suppl.) **51**, 5019s–5022s.

IARC (1992) *The Epidemiology of HPV and Cervical Cancer*, N. Munoz, F.X. Bosch, K.V. Shah and A. Meheus (eds.), International Agency for Research on Cancer, Scientific Publication no. 119, IARC, Lyon.

Jha. P.K.S., Beral, V., Peto, J., Hack, S., Hermon, C., Deacon, J., Mant, D., Chilvers, C., Vessey, M.P., Pike, M.C., Muller, M. and Gissmann L. (1993) 'Antibodies to human papillomavirus and to other genital infectious agents and invasive cervical cancer risk', *Lancet* **341**, 116–118.

Ley, C., Bauer, H.M., Reingold, A., Schiffman, M.H., Chambers, J.C., Tashiro, C.J. and Manos, M.M. (1991) 'Determinants of genital HPV infection in young women', *J. Nat. Cancer Inst.* **83**, 997–1003.

Lorincz, A.T., Reid, R., Jenson, A.B., Greenberg, M.D., Lancaster, W. and Kurman R.J. (1992) 'Human papillomavirus infection of the cervix: relative risk associations of 15 common anogenital types', *Obstet. and Gynaecol.* **79**(3), 328–337.

Manos, M., Lee, K., Greer, C., Waldman, J., Kiviat, N., Holmes, K. and Wheeler, C. (1990) 'Looking for HPV type 16 by PCR', *Lancet* **i**, 734.

Schiffman, M.H. (1992) 'Recent progress in defining the epidemiology of human papillomavirus infection and cervical neoplasia', *J. Nat. Cancer Inst.* **84**, 6, 394–398.

Schneider, A., Kirchhoff, T., Meinhardt, G. and Gissmann, L. (1992) 'Repeated evaluation of human papillomavirus 16 status in cervical swabs of young women with a history of normal Papanicolaou smears', *Obstet. and Gynaecol.* **79**, 683–688.

Schneider, A., and Koutsky, L. (1992) 'Natural history and epidemiological features of genital HPV infection'. In *IARC (1992)*, 25–52.

Van den Brule, A.J.C., Walboomers, J.M.M., du Maine, M., Kenemans, P. and Meuer, C.J.L.M. (1991) 'Difference in prevalence of human papillomavirus genotypes in cytomorphologically normal cervical smears is associated with a history of cervical intraepithelial neoplasia', *Int. J. Cancer* **48**, 404–408.

Van Ranst, M., Kaplan, J.B. and Burk, R.D. (1992) 'Phylogenetic analysis of human papillomaviruses : correlation with clinical manifestations', *J. Gen. Virol.* **73**, 2653–2660.

Wank, R. and Thompson, C. (1991) 'High risk of squamous cell carcinoma of the cervix for women with HLA-DQw3', *Nature* **352**, 723–725.

Zur Hausen, H., de Villiers, E.M., Gissmann, L. (1981) 'Papillomavirus infections and human genital cancer', *Gynecol. Oncol.* **12**(2), S124–128.

Discussion

HADELER** Peto has shown that empirical evidence indicates that the on-off pattern in virus presence in regularly observed patients is not related to variable latency but due to a process of recovery and reinfection. Is the possibility of successive reinfections related to the virus existing in several different types?

REPLY The HPV types involved in successive infections have not been studied systematically. As repeated episodes of infection are common and HPV 16 accounts for the majority of infections, repeated episodes must often involve HPV 16. Whether this indicates transient immunity or whether such episodes reflect recurrence rather than reinfection has not been established.

GORE Human papilloma virus has been implicated in other cancers such as anal cancers. How important do you think that this is, and would you expect the spectrum of cofactors influencing the development of cancers to differ between cancers?

REPLY HPV appears to be involved in a number of other cancers, including anal, laryngeal and oral. Oral and laryngeal infection can occur during birth. Oral and anal sexual contact are also modes of transmission, and anal cancer is commoner among homosexual men. Smoking is a major risk factor for oral and laryngeal cancers, but this is presumably a direct carcinogenic effect. It is not known how smoking causes cervical cancer. There is evidence of both immunological deficit and the presence of carcinogens in the cervical epithelium of smokers.

DIETZ I find the high prevalence of viral infection of up to 50% difficult to reconcile with transmission via the sexual route only. Could vertical transmission from mother to infant be playing a role in the epidemiology of HPV?

REPLY There is no doubt that most genital HPV infection in young women is sexually transmitted. Ley *et al.* (1991) reported a steady increase in prevalence with increasing numbers of sexual partners up to 69% in women with 10 or more partners. They observed 20% prevalence (3/15) in women reporting no partners. It is not clear whether this reflects inaccuracy of reporting or assay, or other routes of transmission.

ADES Data derived from polymerase chain reaction (PCR) methodologies requires considerable care in interpretation. In particular, does a positive result from this technique really represent infection, and is there is any correspondence between PCR results and clinical symptoms? What is the relevance of the term 'prevalence' of infection when the detection of virus seems to alternate between positive and negative on such a short time scale.

REPLY PCR methodology is now virtually free from the problems of contamination and insensitivity which plagued earlier studies. Visible lesions are not always present, but PCR results are highly correlated both with increasing severity of cervical dysplasia and with Southern blot results. The transience of most infections is a major problem in HPV epidemiology, however, and can be overcome only by improvements in HPV serology.

An Age-structured Model for Measles Vaccination

Martin Eichner, Stefan Zehnder and Klaus Dietz

1 Introduction

If a fraction of a population is vaccinated, the spread of the infective agent is slowed down and consequently the incidence of infection for non-vaccinated persons is reduced. If the vaccine itself carries some risk then the risk of illness for a non-vaccinated person can drop below that for a vaccinated one. This occurs when the spread of infection has been greatly reduced by vaccination. It then becomes questionable whether people will agree to be vaccinated and whether, therefore, an infectious disease can be eliminated by vaccination on a voluntary basis. With smallpox vaccination it was shown that in the final years of the campaign more cases of illness were caused in the US by vaccination than by infections (CDC 1971) and nowadays there is a lively discussion about the oral poliomyelitis vaccines which have been incriminated in causing more paralytic cases in the US than the rare wild viruses do (Beale 1990, Begg *et al.* 1987, Cossart 1977, McBean and Modlin 1987). Fine and Clarkson (1986) were the first to compare the risk of illness of vaccinated persons with that of non-vaccinated ones from a theoretical point of view. To estimate the incidence of infection that results from a given vaccination coverage, they made arbitrary assumptions which imply that an infection can only be eliminated if 100 percent of the population are effectively immunized. Moreover, they did not take into consideration an age-specific conditional probability of illness or death upon infection. Many of the so-called 'childhood diseases' tend to be more serious in adults than in infants. By vaccinating a fraction of the population, the immunized individuals are protected against infection, but the mean age of infection for non-immunized ones is increased. This may cause more cases of serious disease. In this study we compute the risk of death due to measles under more realistic assumptions. Using standard epidemiological modelling, we examine the effect of vaccination coverage on the lifetime risk of measles for non-vaccinated individuals. The efficacy of the vaccine is taken into account. The fixed risk of disease and death as it was used by Fine and Clarkson is generalized to an age-dependent risk.

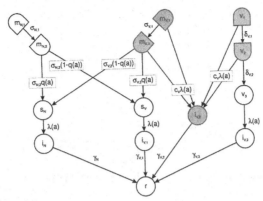

Figure 1. Graphical illustration of the model structure. For abbreviations see Appendix.

2 Model assumptions

The paper concentrates on equilibrium conditions for the population and for the force of infection under a given vaccination coverage. This approach avoids the difficulties that are associated with transient phenomena that depend on the initial conditions and the time horizon chosen. See Figure 1 for an illustration of the states and transitions before and after vaccination.

2.1 Demographic structure

Deaths are compensated for by an equal number of newborns per unit of time (leading to constant population size). The total size of the population is set to one. Since one of the main features of the model is the age-dependent probability of complications after infection, a realistic age-structure is incorporated. The age- and sex-specific mortality is fitted to data from Germany (Statistisches Bundesamt 1992; survival function see Figure 2). The impact of measles mortality on the age distribution is very small and has, therefore, been neglected (if this model were applied to developing countries, this would have to be modified; McLean and Anderson (1988)).

2.2 Age-specific contact rates

In order to describe age-specific contact rates we adapt a model, proposed by Pretorius (1930) and described by Mode and Busby (1982), which uses a bivariate lognormal distribution (Figures 3a–b). This continuous bivariate contact rate is used as it can be modified by changing only two parameters.

2.3 Protection by maternal antibodies

Figure 4 depicts the annual number of births of a cohort of 10,000 women. Newborns of immune mothers are protected by maternal antibodies. This pro-

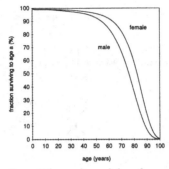

Figure 2. Survival function of the male and female population.

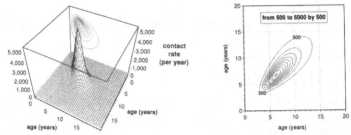

Figures 3. Age-specific contact rate: (a) surface plot; (b) contour plot.

tection is completely lost in a two-step process (corresponding to a gamma distributed period of protection). Newborns of naturally immune mothers are fully protected against infection. Those of mothers with only vaccination-derived antibodies can become infected and have a reduced period of maternal protection. The probability that a contact leads to infection is reduced. Infection does not result in disease (silent infection) and has reduced infectivity and duration. Figure 5 depicts the decline of maternal antibodies and the rise of naturally acquired immunity for a non-vaccinated population.

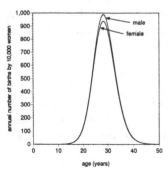

Figure 4. Age-specific birth rate (per year) for a cohort of 10,000 women.

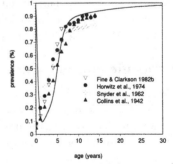

Figure 5. Comparison of the age-specific prevalence of measles antibodies in the absence of vaccination (model result) with the observed history of measles infection (dots).

2.4 Vaccination

It is assumed that vaccinations take place independently (i.e. neither the fraction vaccinated nor the individual success of further vaccinations depends on the outcome of previous vaccinations). For the results shown below, a vaccination age of 1.5 years is chosen. By this age nearly all infants have lost their maternal protection.

Once an individual has been successfully vaccinated, he or she becomes partially and temporarily protected against infection and fully and permanently protected against disease. Vaccination is of no consequence to naturally immunes, infectives and maternally protected individuals. The vaccinated fraction of individuals who still have maternal protection at the age of vaccination is, therefore, added to the group of non-successfully vaccinated individuals. The only effect of booster vaccination to successfully vaccinated individuals is to restore their protection against infection if it has been lost.

Those who are successfully vaccinated can still become infected, but the probability that a contact leads to infection is reduced. Infection then does not lead to disease (silent infection) and has reduced infectivity and duration.

Vaccination derived immunity is lost in a two-step process (again corresponding to a gamma distributed period of protection) which finally leads to a stage where protection against infection (but not against disease) is completely lost.

2.5 Infection and disease

Infection occurs if full or partial susceptibles come into sufficiently close contact with infectives. The contact rate depends on the age of both the susceptible and the infective. All fully susceptible individuals who become infected develop measles symptoms and bear the risk of complications. Partial susceptibles develop silent infection (see above). Figure 6 shows the age-dependent probability of dying as a consequence of measles infection (case fatality rate). Infectivity is lost at a constant rate and results in fully protective and permanent immunity. Using the parameter values given in the Appendix, the force of infection has a maximum at early school age (Figure 7) and the total fraction of immunes is 92% in a non-vaccinated population.

3 Results

In order to assess the effect of vaccination at age 1.5 years we calculate the number of individuals who acquire clinical measles or die as a result of measles (Figures 8a–b and Figures 9a–b). The number of measles infections and deaths is broken down into three categories:

1. Cases occuring before the age of vaccination. These cases are not preventable using the given strategy.

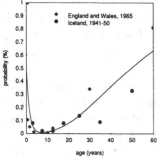
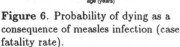
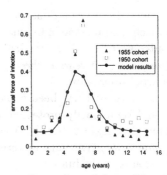

Figure 6. Probability of dying as a consequence of measles infection (case fatality rate).

Figure 7. Comparison of the model results of the annual force of infection of infection with data calculated by Fine and Clarkson (1982).

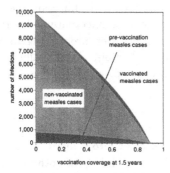
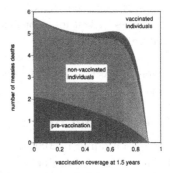

Figure 8. Lifetime number of (a) measles infections and (b) measles deaths of a cohort of 10,000 individuals. Vaccination causes full and permanent immunity.

2. Cases among vaccinated individuals (due to vaccine failure).

3. Cases among non-vaccinated individuals.

In Figures 8a–b it is assumed that successful vaccination leads to full and permanent immunity. As the force of infection decreases with increasing vaccination coverage, the mean age of infection increases. Infants (especially those without maternal antibody protection) benefit from this age shift. They have less risk of dying from measles if they are infected later (Figure 6). The number of deaths due to measles before the age of vaccination, therefore, strongly decreases with increasing vaccination coverage (Figure 8b). On the other hand, children and adults who are not successfully vaccinated are likely to become infected later and therefore have a higher risk of dying from measles (Figure 8b). The increased risk to the non-vaccinated (or not successfully vaccinated) individuals results in there being no dramatic decrease in the

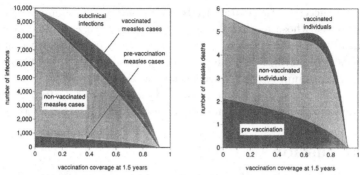

Figures 9. Lifetime number of (a) measles infections and (b) measles deaths of a cohort of 10,000 individuals. Vaccination causes partial and temporary immunity, but protects against the disease.

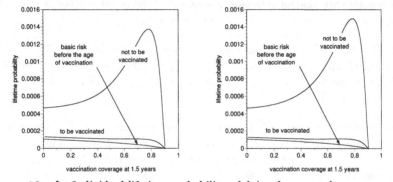

Figure 10a, b. Individual lifetime probability of dying from measles.

number of deaths due to measles. This is true for a wide range of vaccination coverage (Figure 8b). Only if the vaccination coverage exceeds 75%, does the number of measles deaths after the age of vaccination decrease.

Figures 10a–b depict the life time probabilities of dying from measles for a vaccinated and a non-vaccinated individual. Both individuals have the same basic probability of dying from measles before the vaccination age. The risk for vaccinated children is then reduced to 5%, while the non-vaccinated ones remain at full risk. The vaccination of the population decreases the force of infection, which in turn leads to a higher age of infection. This increases the probability of dying from measles after the vaccination age. Only if the vaccination coverage exceeds 75%, does the life-time probability for non-vaccinated individuals reduce again (Figures 10a–b).

According to the observations made about a recent measles epidemic (van Binnendijk *et al.* 1992), it might be over-optimistic to assume that vaccinated individuals are completely protected against infection. We thus include the chance that successful vaccination leads to only partial and temporary protection (newborns whose mothers have vaccination derived antibodies are also only partially protected in this case). Even if the susceptibility of vaccinated individuals is reduced to 10%, there is a large incidence of subclinical infections for the medium range of vaccination coverage (Figure 9a). Subclinical infectives have only a short infective period and reduced infectivity, so they have little impact on the incidence of measles cases and deaths (Figure 9b).

4   Discussion

The present model takes into account age- and sex-dependence of vaccination, birth, death, contact and case-fatality rates. The duration of protection by maternal antibodies depends on the immunity status of the mother (naturally immune or immune due to vaccination). Vaccination protects only partially and temporarily against infection whereas it protects completely and permanently against disease. Several conclusions emerge:

1. The number of infections decreases approximately linearly with increasing vaccination coverage. The incidence of measles deaths, however, is little affected up to a coverage of about 75%, above which a steep decline is achieved.

2. Whilst only about 10% of the infections occur before the age of vaccination, these give rise to nearly 40% of the deaths. These deaths are non-preventable using vaccination at the recommended age of 18 months.

3. The individual lifetime probability of death due to measles for newborns who are destined to be vaccinated decreases monotonically with increasing vaccination coverage. The corresponding probability for non-vaccinated individuals nearly doubles before it is steeply reduced to zero at very high vaccination coverage.

The last conclusion contradicts the usually stressed beneficial effect of vaccination to those who are not vaccinated. For the total population the mortality is decreasing. This decreasing function represents a weighted average between the risks of vaccinated and non-vaccinated individuals. In many countries vaccination coverage is around the value at which those who are not vaccinated have the highest risk, i.e. where coverage is clearly insufficient to eliminate measles.

In many countries there are sizeable groups who oppose vaccination for various reasons. They usually stress the potential risks associated with vaccination and play down the risks from infection. For the individual it is only rational to refuse vaccination if the risk of non-vaccinated individuals acquiring the disease is less than the vaccine associated risk. This is only true near the vaccination coverage required for elimination.

Anderson and May (1990) discussed these issues as follows: 'We believe the answer to these dilemmas, where individual and group interests ineluctably conflict, are programmes of compulsory immunisation, backed by an analytical understanding of the effects of herd immunity and by publicly funded compensation for side-effects'. Mathematical models are undoubtedly necessary for the evaluation of vaccination programmes. It appears, however, that both the state of the art modelling of infectious diseases and the availability of the necessary data are overestimated. Even the complicated model presented in this paper represents a considerable oversimplification of reality and it reveals uncertainty about important basic aspects of measles epidemiology. In many countries even the minimal parameters such as the incidence of infection and disease are not available.

The attitude towards compulsory vaccination in Western democracies varies considerably: it is performed in the U.S. and in France, but in the U.K. and in Germany it does not appear to be acceptable (in former East Germany it was performed, but has now been terminated). Such overriding political constraints have to be respected in making recommendations for vaccination strategies.

Acknowledgements

Martin Eichner received financial support from Evangelisches Studienwerk eV, Haus Villigst, Schwerte. Klaus Dietz and Martin Eichner acknowledge the support by the Prudential Fellowship during their stay at the Isaac Newton Institute. Klaus Dietz thanks the University of Tübingen for granting leave of absence. Partha Dasgupta, Department of Applied Economics, Cambridge University, provided stimulating suggestions.

Appendix

Variables and parameters

Epidemiological status

$m_{N,1}^{(\text{sex})}$, $m_{N,2}^{(\text{sex})}$	newborns protected by naturally acquired maternal antibodies in each of two stages during which protection is lost
$m_{V,1}^{(\text{sex})}$, $m_{V,2}^{(\text{sex})}$	newborns protected by vaccine derived maternal antibodies in each of two stages during which protection is lost

$s_N^{(\text{sex})}$ susceptibles who never have been vaccinated

$s_V^{(\text{sex})}$ susceptibles (individuals who were vaccinated unsuccessfully)

$i_N^{(\text{sex})}$ infectives (non-vaccinated individuals)

$i_{V,1}^{(\text{sex})}$ infectives (unsuccessfully vaccinated individuals)

$i_{V,2}^{(\text{sex})}$ infectives (partially protected by vaccine derived antibodies)

$i_{V,3}^{(\text{sex})}$ infectives (individuals who have lost their vaccination derived protection)

$v_1^{(\text{sex})}, v_2^{(\text{sex})}$ vaccinated individuals (partially and temporarily immune) in each of two stages during which protection is lost

$v_3^{(\text{sex})}$ vaccinated individuals who have lost their immunity (only protected against disease)

$r^{(\text{sex})}$ individuals with full and permanent protection against infection

Loss rates of maternal protection

$\sigma_{N,1}, \sigma_{N,2}$ rates of loss of protection by (naturally acquired) maternal antibodies during each stage of loss

$\sigma_{V,1}, \sigma_{V,2}$ rates of loss of protection by (vaccine derived) maternal antibodies during each stage of loss

Parameters for infection and disease

$\kappa(\tilde{a}, a)$ effective contact rate of individuals of age $\tilde{a}$ with individuals of age a

$\lambda(a)$ age-specific force of infection acting on individuals of age a

γ_N rate of loss of infectivity of non-vaccinated individuals

$\gamma_{V,2}$ rate of loss of infectivity of individuals protected by vaccine derived antibodies

$\gamma_{V,3}$ rate of loss of infectivity of vaccinated individuals who have lost their immunity

$f^{(\text{sex})}(a)$ age-specific risk of death at infection

Parameters related to vaccination

$a_{V,1}, \ldots, a_{V,n}$	ages at vaccination
$p_1^{(\text{sex})}, \ldots, p_n^{(\text{sex})}$	fractions vaccinated at age $a_{V,1}, \ldots, a_{V,n}$
E	probability that a susceptible individual is successfully vaccinated
c_V	susceptibility of individuals with vaccine-derived antibodies
k_V	infectivity of individuals with vaccine-derived antibodies
$\delta_{V,1}, \; \delta_{V,2}$	rates of loss of vaccination immunity
$q^{(\text{sex})}(a)$	function for directing individuals after loss of their maternal protection to different susceptible stages (see 'boundary conditions')

Demographic parameters

$N(a)$	total size of the population at age a
$N^{(\text{sex})}(a)$	total size of the population at age a by sex
$\mu^{(\text{sex})}(a)$	age-specific mortality rate
$\beta^m(a)$	rate at which women of age a give birth to boys
$\beta^f(a)$	rate at which women of age a give birth to girls
$\beta_0^{(\text{sex})}$	birth rates of boys and girls
$L^{(\text{sex})}$	life expectancy

Model equations

Individuals protected by maternal antibodies

$$\frac{\partial m_{N,1}^{(\text{sex})}}{\partial a} + \frac{\partial m_{N,1}^{(\text{sex})}}{\partial t} = -(\sigma_{N,1} + \mu^{(\text{sex})}(a))m_{N,1}^{(\text{sex})}, \tag{1}$$

$$\frac{\partial m_{N,2}^{(\text{sex})}}{\partial a} + \frac{\partial m_{N,2}^{(\text{sex})}}{\partial t} = \sigma_{N,1}m_{N,1}^{(\text{sex})} - (\sigma_{N,2} + \mu^{(\text{sex})}(a))m_{N,2}^{(\text{sex})}, \tag{2}$$

$$\frac{\partial m_{V,1}^{(\text{sex})}}{\partial a} + \frac{\partial m_{V,1}^{(\text{sex})}}{\partial t} = -(\sigma_{V,1} + c_V\,\lambda(a) + \mu^{(\text{sex})}(a))m_{V,1}^{(\text{sex})}, \tag{3}$$

$$\frac{\partial m_{V,2}^{(\text{sex})}}{\partial a} + \frac{\partial m_{V,2}^{(\text{sex})}}{\partial t} = \sigma_{V,1}m_{V,1}^{(\text{sex})}$$
$$-(\sigma_{V,2} + c_V\,\lambda(a) + \mu^{(\text{sex})}(a))m_{V,2}^{(\text{sex})}. \tag{4}$$

Susceptibles

$$\frac{\partial s_N^{(\text{sex})}}{\partial a} + \frac{\partial s_N^{(\text{sex})}}{\partial t} = q^{(\text{sex})}(a)(\sigma_{N,2} m_{N,2}^{(\text{sex})} + \sigma_{V,2} m_{V,2}^{(\text{sex})}) \tag{5}$$
$$-(\lambda(a) + \mu^{(\text{sex})}(a)) s_N^{(\text{sex})},$$

$$\frac{\partial s_V^{(\text{sex})}}{\partial a} + \frac{\partial s_V^{(\text{sex})}}{\partial t} = (1 - q^{(\text{sex})}(a))(\sigma_{N,2} m_{N,2}^{(\text{sex})} + \sigma_{V,2} m_{V,2}^{(\text{sex})}) \tag{6}$$
$$-(\lambda(a) + \mu^{(\text{sex})}(a)) s_V^{(\text{sex})}.$$

Successfully vaccinated individuals

$$\frac{\partial v_1^{(\text{sex})}}{\partial a} + \frac{\partial v_1^{(\text{sex})}}{\partial t} = -(c_V \lambda(a) + \delta_{V,1} + \mu^{(\text{sex})}(a)) v_1^{(\text{sex})}, \tag{7}$$

$$\frac{\partial v_2^{(\text{sex})}}{\partial a} + \frac{\partial v_2^{(\text{sex})}}{\partial t} = \delta_{V,1} v_1^{(\text{sex})} - (c_V \lambda(a) + \delta_{V,2} + \mu^{(\text{sex})}(a)) v_2^{(\text{sex})}, \tag{8}$$

$$\frac{\partial v_3^{(\text{sex})}}{\partial a} + \frac{\partial v_3^{(\text{sex})}}{\partial t} = \delta_{V,2} v_2^{(\text{sex})} - (\lambda(a) + \mu^{(\text{sex})}(a)) v_3^{(\text{sex})}. \tag{9}$$

Infectives

$$\frac{\partial i_N^{(\text{sex})}}{\partial a} + \frac{\partial i_N^{(\text{sex})}}{\partial t} = \lambda(a) s_N^{(\text{sex})} - (\gamma_N + \mu^{(\text{sex})}(a)) i_N^{(\text{sex})}, \tag{10}$$

$$\frac{\partial i_{V,1}^{(\text{sex})}}{\partial a} + \frac{\partial i_{V,1}^{(\text{sex})}}{\partial t} = \lambda(a) s_V^{(\text{sex})} - (\gamma_{V,1} + \mu^{(\text{sex})}(a)) i_{V,1}^{(\text{sex})}, \tag{11}$$

$$\frac{\partial i_{V,2}^{(\text{sex})}}{\partial a} + \frac{\partial i_{V,2}^{(\text{sex})}}{\partial t} = c_V \lambda(a)(m_{V,1}^{(\text{sex})} + m_{V,2}^{(\text{sex})} + v_1^{(\text{sex})} + v_2^{(\text{sex})})$$
$$-(\gamma_{V,2} + \mu^{(\text{sex})}(a)) i_{V,2}^{(\text{sex})}, \tag{12}$$

$$\frac{\partial i_{V,3}^{(\text{sex})}}{\partial a} + \frac{\partial i_{V,3}^{(\text{sex})}}{\partial t} = \lambda(a) v_3^{(\text{sex})} - (\gamma_{V,3} + \mu^{(\text{sex})}(a)) i_{V,3}^{(\text{sex})}. \tag{13}$$

Immunes

$$\frac{\partial r^{(\text{sex})}}{\partial a} + \frac{\partial r^{(\text{sex})}}{\partial t} = \gamma_N (i_N^{(\text{sex})} + i_{V,1}^{(\text{sex})})$$
$$+ \gamma_{V,2} i_{V,2}^{(\text{sex})} + \gamma_{V,3} i_{V,3}^{(\text{sex})} - \mu^{(\text{sex})}(a) r^{(\text{sex})}. \tag{14}$$

Boundary conditions

(A) The system is solved for $0 \le a \le a_{V,1}$ with boundary conditions for $a = 0$

$$m_{N,1}^{(\text{sex})}(0) = \int_{14}^{45} (i_N^{\text{f}}(a) + i_{V,1}^{\text{f}}(a) + i_{V,2}^{\text{f}}(a) + i_{V,3}^{\text{f}}(a) + r^{\text{f}}(a)) \beta^{(\text{sex})}(a) da,$$

$$m_{V,1}^{(\text{sex})}(0) = \int_{14}^{45} (v_1^{\text{f}}(a) + v_2^{\text{f}}(a)) \beta^{(\text{sex})}(a) da,$$

$$s_N^{(\text{sex})}(0) = \int_{14}^{45} (s_N^{\text{f}}(a) + s_V^{\text{f}}(a) + v_3^{\text{f}}(a)) \beta^{(\text{sex})}(a) da,$$

$$m_{N,2}^{(\text{sex})}(0) = 0, \quad m_{V,2}^{(\text{sex})}(0) = 0, \quad s_V^{(\text{sex})}(0) = 0,$$
$$i_N^{(\text{sex})}(0) = 0, \quad i_{V,2}^{(\text{sex})}(0) = 0 \quad i_{V,2}^{(\text{sex})}(0) = 0, \quad i_{V,3}^{(\text{sex})}(0) = 0,$$
$$v_1^{(\text{sex})}(0) = 0, \quad v_2^{(\text{sex})}(0) = 0, \quad v_3^{(\text{sex})}(0) = 0, \quad r^{(\text{sex})}(0) = 0.$$

(B) The system is solved for $a_{V,i} \le a \le a_{V,i+1}$ or $a_{V,i} \le a < \infty$ ($i \ge 2$) with boundary conditions for $a = a_{V,i}$

$$
\begin{aligned}
s_N^{(\text{sex})}(a_{V,i}) &:= (1 - p_i^{(\text{sex})}) s_N^{(\text{sex})}(a_{V,i}) \\
s_V^{(\text{sex})}(a_{V,i}) &:= (1 - p_i^{(\text{sex})}) s_V^{(\text{sex})}(a_{V,i}) \\
&\quad + (1 - E) p_i^{(\text{sex})}(s_N^{(\text{sex})}(a_{V,i}) + s_V^{(\text{sex})}(a_{V,i})), \\
v_1^{(\text{sex})}(a_{V,i}) &:= v_1^{(\text{sex})}(a_{V,i}) + p_i^{(\text{sex})} E(s_N^{(\text{sex})}(a_{V,i}) + s_V^{(\text{sex})}(a_{V,i}) \\
&\quad + v_2^{(\text{sex})}(a_{V,i}) + v_3^{(\text{sex})}(a_{V,i})), \\
v_2^{(\text{sex})}(a_{V,i}) &:= (1 - p_i^{(\text{sex})} E) v_2^{(\text{sex})}(a_{V,i}), \\
v_3^{(\text{sex})}(a_{V,i}) &:= (1 - p_i^{(\text{sex})} E) v_3^{(\text{sex})}(a_{V,i}),
\end{aligned}
\tag{15}
$$

$$
\begin{aligned}
m_{N,1}^{(\text{sex})}(a_{V,i}) &:= m_{N,1}^{(\text{sex})}(a_{V,i}), & i_N^{(\text{sex})}(a_{V,i}) &:= i_N^{(\text{sex})}(a_{V,i}) \\
m_{N,2}^{(\text{sex})}(a_{V,i}) &:= m_{N,2}^{(\text{sex})}(a_{V,i}), & i_{V,1}^{(\text{sex})}(a_{V,i}) &:= i_{V,1}^{(\text{sex})}(a_{V,i}) \\
m_{V,1}^{(\text{sex})}(a_{V,i}) &:= m_{V,1}^{(\text{sex})}(a_{V,i}), & i_{V,2}^{(\text{sex})}(a_{V,i}) &:= i_{V,2}^{(\text{sex})}(a_{V,i}) \\
m_{V,2}^{(\text{sex})}(a_{V,i}) &:= m_{V,2}^{(\text{sex})}(a_{V,i}), & i_{V,3}^{(\text{sex})}(a_{V,i}) &:= i_{V,3}^{(\text{sex})}(a_{V,i}) \\
r^{(\text{sex})}(a_{V,i}) &:= r^{(\text{sex})}(a_{V,i}). &
\end{aligned}
$$

The right hand sides of the equations denote the solutions of the system which was solved in $a_{V,i-1} \le a \le a_{V,i}$.

(C) Loss of maternal protection after the age of first vaccination
Individuals who still have maternal protection cannot be vaccinated successfully. The fraction of them that is vaccinated, is therefore added to the group of unsuccessfully vaccinated individuals when maternal protection is lost. The function $q^{(\text{sex})}(a)$ denotes the fraction which is added to the non-vaccinated individuals. In a population, where n different age groups are vaccinated, it is

$$
q^{(\text{sex})}(a) = \begin{cases}
1 & \text{for } a < a_{V,1}, \\
(1 - p_1^{(\text{sex})}) & \text{for } a_{V,1} \le a < a_{V,2}, \\
\quad \cdots\cdots\cdots \\
\prod_{i=1}^{k}(1 - p_i^{(\text{sex})}) & \text{for } a_{V,k} \le a < a_{V,k+1},
\end{cases}
$$

with $k \le n$ ($a_{V,n+1}$ is set to ∞).

(D) Force of infection

The force of infection is given by

$$\lambda(a) = \int_0^\infty \kappa(\tilde{a},a)(i_N^m(\tilde{a}) + i_{V,1}^m(\tilde{a}) + k_V\, i_{V,2}^m(\tilde{a}) + i_{V,3}^m(\tilde{a}))d\tilde{a}$$
$$+ \int_0^\infty \kappa(\tilde{a},a)(i_N^f(\tilde{a}) + i_{V,1}^f(\tilde{a}) + k_V\, i_{V,2}^f(\tilde{a}) + i_{V,3}^f(\tilde{a}))d\tilde{a}.$$

Infectives with protection from maternal antibodies or vaccination $(i_{V,2}^{(\text{sex})})$ do not become fully infective and therefore have to be multiplied by the factor $k_V < 1$, whereas those who have completely lost their immunity become infective with the same probability as susceptibles and develop a full infectivity $(i_{V,3}^{\cdot(\text{sex})})$.

Parameter values chosen

Age-independent parameters

infectivity of vaccine-immunity protected individuals after infection	$k_V = 0.5$
rate of loss of infectivity of non-protected individuals	$\gamma_N = \gamma_{V,1} = \gamma_{V,3} = 52/\text{year}$
rate of loss of infectivity of vaccine-immunity protected individuals	$\gamma_{V,2} = 5\gamma_N$
first vaccination age	$a_{V,1} = 1.5$ years
vaccine efficacy	$E = 0.95$
rate of loss of (naturally acquired) maternal antibody protection	$\sigma_{N,1} = \sigma_{N,2} = 4$ per year
rate of loss of (vaccination derived) maternal antibody protection	$\sigma_{V,1} = \sigma_{V,2} = 8$ per year
rate of loss of vaccine-immunity	$\delta_{V,1} = \delta_{V,2} = 1/200$ per year

Age-dependent functions

(a) Age- and sex-specific mortality rates are fitted to official data from Germany by using cubic splines (data from Statistisches Bundesamt 1992); see Figure 2.

With this the life expectancies

$$L^{(\text{sex})} = \int_0^\infty e^{-\int_0^a \mu^{(\text{sex})}(\alpha)d\alpha}da \quad \text{are} \quad \begin{array}{l} L^m = 72.25 \text{ years,} \\ L^f = 78.68 \text{ years.} \end{array}$$

As the total size of the population is set to 1, we must have $\beta_0^m L^m + \beta_0^f L^f = 1$.

With the sex ratio of newborns $\beta_0^m/\beta_0^f = 1.053$ one gets the sex-specific birth rates

$$\beta_0^m = 0.006805 \text{ per year},$$
$$\beta_0^f = 0.006462 \text{ per year},$$

and the total male and female fractions of the population are

$$\int_0^\infty N^m(a)da = \beta_0^m L^m = 0.492,$$
$$\int_0^\infty N^f(a)da = \beta_0^f L^f = 0.508.$$

(b) The age- and sex-specific birth rate of women aged a is fitted to data published by Statistisches Bundesamt (1992; Figure 4).

(i) Fitted function: $\beta^{(\text{sex})}(a) = c^{(\text{sex})}e^{c_1 a + c_2 a^2 + c_3 a^3 + c_4 a^4 + c_5 a^5 + c_6 a^6}$ with

$$\begin{cases} c^m = 1.45515 \times 10^{-6} & c^f = 1.3891 \times 10^{-6} \\ c_1 = 0 & c_2 = 3.9 \times 10^{-2} \\ c_3 = 0 & c_4 = -6.826 \times 10^{-5} \\ c_5 = 1.615 \times 10^{-6} & c_6 = -1.098 \times 10^{-8} \end{cases}$$

(ii) The sex ratio of newborns is equal to $c^m/c^f = 1.053$.

(c) Age-specific contact rate as depicted in Figures 3a–b.

$$\kappa(\tilde{a}, a) = \begin{cases} K(\tilde{a}, a) & \text{for } \tilde{a} \le a, \\ K(\tilde{a}, a)\frac{N(\tilde{a})}{N(a)} & \text{for } \tilde{a} \ge a \end{cases}$$

with $N(a) = N^m(a) + N^f(a)$ and

$$K(\tilde{a}, a) = \frac{\exp\left((\ln \tilde{a} - M)^2 - 2\rho(\ln \tilde{a} - M)(\ln a - M) + (\ln a - M)^2\right) / \left(-2\sigma^2(1 - \rho^2)\right)}{k_1 \tilde{a} a} + k_2,$$

$$M = 2, \quad \sigma = 0.3, \quad \rho = 0.8,$$
$$k_1 = 2\pi\sigma^2\sqrt{1 - \rho^2}/75000, \quad k_2 = 325.$$

(d) Age-specific risk of dying from measles fitted to data published by (Black 1989; see Figure 6).

$$f^m(a) = f^f(a) = \int_0^a \frac{c_1^{c_2} \alpha^{c_2 - 1} e^{-c_1 a}}{c_0 \Gamma(c_2)} d\alpha + c_3 e^{-c_4 a} \text{ with } \begin{cases} c_0 = 0.01 \\ c_1 = 0.0611 \\ c_2 = 3.3611 \\ c_3 = 0.005 \\ c_4 = 0.7 \end{cases}$$

with the Gamma function Γ.

Calculation of Various Output Variables

(a) Age-specific prevalence of serum antibodies in a non-vaccinated population (Figure 5)

$$\Big((m_{N,1}^m(a) + m_{N,1}^f(a) + m_{N,2}^m(a) + m_{N,2}^f(a)) $$
$$+ (i_N^m(a) + i_N^f(a)) + (r^m(a) + r^f(a)) \Big) \Big/ N(a).$$

(b) Cumulative incidence of clinical and subclinical infections (see Figures 8a and 9a)

of pre-vaccination measles cases $\quad = \int_0^{a_{V,1}} \frac{\lambda(a)}{\beta_0^m + \beta_0^f} (s_N^m(a) + s_N^f(a)) da,$

of non-vaccinated measles cases $\quad = \int_{a_{V,1}}^{\infty} \frac{\lambda(a)}{\beta_0^m + \beta_0^f} (s_N^m(a) + s_N^f(a)) da,$

of vaccinated measles cases $\quad = \int_{a_{V,1}}^{\infty} \frac{\lambda(a)}{\beta_0^m + \beta_0^f} (s_V^m(a) + s_V^f(a)) da,$

of subclinical infections $\quad = \int_0^{\infty} \frac{\lambda(a)}{\beta_0^m + \beta_0^f} (t_V^m(a) + t_V^f(a)) da$

with

$$t_V^{(sex)}(a) = c_V (m_{V,1}^{(sex)}(a) + m_{V,2}^{(sex)}(a) + v_1^{(sex)}(a) + v_2^{(sex)}(a)) + v_3^{(sex)}(a)$$

(c) Cumulative incidence of deaths due to measles infections before the first vaccination is I_{pre}, of non-vaccinated individuals I_N and of vaccinated individuals I_V, where

$$I_{pre} = \int_0^{a_{V,1}} \frac{\lambda(a)}{\beta_0^m + \beta_0^f} (s_N^m(a) f^m(a) + s_N^f(a) f^f(a)) da,$$

$$I_N = \int_{a_{V,1}}^{\infty} \frac{\lambda(a)}{\beta_0^m + \beta_0^f} (s_N^m(a) f^m(a) + s_N^f(a) f^f(a)) da,$$

$$I_V = \int_{a_{V,1}}^{\infty} \frac{\lambda(a)}{\beta_0^m + \beta_0^f} (s_V^m(a) f^m(a) + s_V^f(a) f^f(a)) da.$$

(d) Individual lifetime probability of dying from measles (see Figures 10a–b)

In the case of one vaccination only, the individual lifetime probability of dying from measles of individuals not to be vaccinated is

$$I_{pre}^{(sex)} + \frac{I_N^{(sex)}}{1 - p_1^{(sex)}},$$

and of individuals to be vaccinated is

$$I_{\text{pre}}^{(\text{sex})} + \frac{I_V^{(\text{sex})}}{p_1^{(\text{sex})}},$$

with

$$I_{\text{pre}}^{(\text{sex})} = \int_0^{a_{V,1}} \lambda(a) \frac{s_N^{(\text{sex})}(a)}{\beta_0^{(\text{sex})}} f^{(\text{sex})}(a) da,$$

$$I_N^{(\text{sex})} = \int_{a_{V,1}}^\infty \lambda(a) \frac{s_N^{(\text{sex})}(a)}{\beta_0^{(\text{sex})}} f^{(\text{sex})}(a) da,$$

$$I_V^{(\text{sex})} = \int_{a_{V,1}}^\infty \lambda(a) \frac{s_V^{(\text{sex})}(a)}{\beta_0^{(\text{sex})}} f^{(\text{sex})}(a) da.$$

If an individual is destined never to be vaccinated in a population where vaccinations are performed at n different ages, the individual lifetime risk can be calculated as follows: Let $I_{N,k}^{(\text{sex})}$ denote the cumulative incidence of deaths due to measles of non-vaccinated individuals in the age group $[a_{V,k}, a_{V,k+1})$ (with $a_{V,n+1} = \infty$):

$$I_{N,k}^{(\text{sex})} = \int_{a_{V,k}}^{a_{V,k+1}} \lambda(a) \frac{s_N^{(\text{sex})}(a)}{\beta_0^{(\text{sex})}} f^{(\text{sex})}(a) da.$$

Then the average individual lifetime risk that has to be expected by an individual destined not to be vaccinated, is calculated as

$$I_{\text{pre}}^{(\text{sex})} + \sum_{k=1}^n \left(\frac{I_{N,k}^{(\text{sex})}}{\prod_{i=1}^k (1 - p_i^{(\text{sex})})} \right).$$

Short description of the computer program

Unless mentioned otherwise, all calculations are performed with a computer program written in the Pascal programming language. The model is examined in endemic equilibrium ($\partial/\partial t = 0$) and therefore the differential equations are only solved with respect to age.

(1) In the first step the system of differential equations is solved without vaccination ($p_1^{(\text{sex})} = p_2^{(\text{sex})} = 0$). Values for the boundary conditions ($m_{N,1}^{(\text{sex})}(0) + s_N^{(\text{sex})}(0) = \beta_0^{(\text{sex})}$) and for the force of infection function $\lambda(a)$ in the first step are chosen arbitrarily and kept fixed while the system of differential equations is solved numerically. An algorithm with adaptive step size, using the formula of England of 4th and 5th order, is used. The source code of the differential equation solving routine, of the integration routine and of the cubic splines interpolation was published by Engeln-Müllges and Reutter (1991).

(2) New boundary values and a new force of infection are calculated from this 'first guess' solution. These again are kept fixed to solve the differential

equations and to calculate new values. This procedure is repeated until the system is in equilibrium.

(3) Then a (small) vaccination coverage is added to the system. The boundary values and the force of infection which result from the first calculation loop are used at the beginning and the above calculations are then repeated until the system is again in equilibrium. The vaccination coverage is then increased etc.

(4) When the system is in equilibrium for a given vaccination coverage, relative risks and cumulative incidences are calculated as described above and results are written to a file for graphical presentation.

Program parameters

- The maximum age of individuals is set to 100 years.

- At the beginning of the calculations, all newborns are regarded as being protected by maternal antibodies $(m_{N,1}^{(\text{sex})}(0) = \beta_0^{(\text{sex})})$.

- The (arbitrarily chosen) initial force of infection is constant for all ages $(\lambda(a) \equiv 0.1)$.

- The differential equation system is evaluated in steps of one week before the age of vaccination, in steps of two weeks between the age of 1.5 years and 20 years and half a year for all older ages. All 'intermediate' values are interpolated by cubic splines.

- Vaccination coverage is varied between 0 and 100% by steps of 1%.

- After setting a new vaccination coverage, an initial Norm M_0 is calculated:

$$M_0 := \max_{i=1}^{n} |(r_{\text{old}}^{\text{m}}(a_n) + r_{\text{old}}^{\text{f}}(a_n)) - (r_{\text{new}}^{\text{m}}(a_n) + r_{\text{new}}^{\text{f}}(a_n))|.$$

- The system is regarded as being in equilibrium, if

$$\max_{i=1}^{n} |(r_{\text{old}}^{\text{m}}(a_n) + r_{\text{old}}^{\text{f}}(a_n)) - (r_{\text{new}}^{\text{m}}(a_n) + r_{\text{new}}^{\text{f}}(a_n))| < \epsilon M_0$$

with $\epsilon = 0.075$.

References

Anderson, R.M. and May, R.M. (1990) 'Modern vaccines. Immunization and herd immunity', *Lancet* **335**, 641–45.

Beale, A.J. (1990) 'Polio vaccines: time for a change in immunisation policy?', *Lancet* **335**, 839–42.

Begg, N.T., Chamberlain, R. and Roebuck, M. (1987) 'Paralytic poliomyelitis in England and Wales, 1970–84', *Epidemiol. Inf.* **99**, 97–106.

van Binnendijk, R.S., Rümke, H.C., van Eijdhoven, M.J.A., Bosman, A., Hirsch, R., van Loon, A.M., Benne, C.A., van Dijk, W.C., Rima, B.K., vd Heijden, R.W.J., UytdeHaag, F.G.C.M., and Osterhaus, A.D.M.E. (1992) 'A measles outbreak in vaccinated schoolaged children in the Netherlands: Identification of clinically and subclinically infected children by evaluation of virus-specific antibody and T cell responses'. In *T cell function in measles*, R.S. van Binnendijk (ed.), Proefschrift, Rijksuniversiteit te Utrecht. 27–44.

Black, F. (1989) 'Measles'. In *Viral Infection of Humans. Epidemiology and Control*, third edition, A.S. Evans (ed.), Plenum, New York, 457.

CDC (1971) 'Vaccination against smallpox in the United States. A reevaluation of the risks and benefits', *Morb. Mortal. Weekly Report* **20**, 339–345.

Collins, S.D., Wheeler, R.E. and Shannon, R.D. (1942) *The occurrence of whooping cough, chicken pox, mumps, measles and German measles in 200,000 surveyed families in 28 large cities*, United States Public Health Service Division of Public Health Methods Special Study Series 1, Washington, DC.

Cossart, Y.E. (1977) 'Evolution of poliovirus since introduction of attenuated vaccine', *BMJ* I, 1621–3.

Engeln-Müllges, G. and Reutter, F. (1991) *Formelsammlung zur Numerischen Mathematik mit Turbo Pascal Programmen*, B.I. Wissenschaftsverlag, Mannheim, Wien, Zürich.

Fine, P.E.M. and Clarkson, J.A. (1982) 'Measles in England and Wales—II: The impact of the measles vaccination program on the distribution of immunity in the population', *Int. J. Epidemiol.* **11**, 15–25.

Fine, P.E.M. and Clarkson, J.A. (1986) 'Individual versus public priorities in the determination of optimal vaccination policies', *Am. J. Epidemiol.* **124**, 1012–20.

Horwitz, O., Grünfeld, K., Lysgaard-Hansen, B. and Kjeldsen, K. (1974) 'The epidemiology and natural history of measles in Denmark', *Am. J. Epidemiol.* **100**, 136–149.

McBean, A.M. and Modlin, J.F. (1987) 'Rationale for the sequential use of inactivated poliovirus vaccine and live attenuated poliovirus vaccine for routine poliomyelitis immunization in the United States', *Ped. Inf. Dis. J.* **6**, 881–7.

McLean, A.R., Anderson, R.M. (1988a) 'Measles in developing countries. Part I: Epidemiological parameters and patterns', *Epidemiol. Infect.* **100**, 111–33.

McLean, A.R. and Anderson, R.M. (1988b) 'Measles in developing countries. Part II: The predicted impact of mass vaccination', *Epidemiol. Infect.* **100**, 419–42.

Mode, C.J. (1985) *Stochastic Processes in Demography and their Computer Implementation*, Lecture Notes in Biomathematics 14, Springer Verlag, Berlin, Heidelberg, New York, Tokyo.

Mode, C.J. and Busby, R.C. (1982) 'An eight-parameter model of human mortality – the single decrement case', *Bull. Math. Biol.* **44**, 647–59.

Pretorius, S.J. (1930) 'Skew bivariate frequency surfaces examined in the light of numerical illustrations', *Biometrika* **22**, 109–223.

Snyder, M.J., McCrumbl, F.R., Bigbee, T., Schluederberg, A.E. and Togo, Y. (1962) 'Observations on the seroepidemiology of measles', *Am. J. Dis. Child.* **103**, 250–51.

Statistisches Bundesamt (1992) *Statistisches Jahrbuch für die Bundesrepublik Deutschland*, Metzler and Poeschel.

Discussion

SHAHANI The various functions of vaccine coverage obtained from the model provide quantitative guidance for evolving public health policies. The possibility of an increased risk to non-vaccinated individuals is included. Perhaps it would be helpful to include, explicitly, a state in the model that accounts for the damage which may be inflicted on a vaccinated individual. The model could then provide some measure of the number of damaged individuals that result from a vaccination policy. This information could help in an explicit consideration of suitable compensation to the individuals who are damaged for the protection of society as a whole.

Invited Discussion

V. T. Farewell

In the first session of this conference, we have heard three very different papers on three very interesting topics. I wish, however, to claim the prerogative granted to me by the organizers to comment in detail on the paper by Dr. Gore and to make only brief reference to the other papers. This approach is primarily motivated by the prior availability of Dr. Gore's manuscript and is no reflection on the other presentations.

Dr. Gore has provided an impressive survey of data analysis methods which have been employed for the study of a variety of diseases with long development times. In my comments, I hope to elaborate on some of the issues raised rather than to offer specific criticisms.

Time to event regression models have played a major role in the analysis of longitudinal data. Dr. Gore has placed some stress on the need for further consideration of the covariate codings in such models, in particular with respect to HIV disease. I have five comments on this issue.

(1) When using time dependent variables, it is almost essential that lagged covariates be used. It is unlikely that, for example, interest is directed towards the predictive role of CD4 counts at the time of AIDS diagnosis. In an analysis of the Toronto Sexual Contact Cohort (TSCC) data (Coates *et al.* 1992), we adopted the approach of lagging immunological markers by one year so that the developed models used covariates of the form $X(t-1)$ rather than $X(t)$. The need for this is sometimes not recognized because covariates are not updated continuously and therefore an effective lagging takes place because the last available measurement is used in the regression models.

(2) Non-linear covariate effects might be examined in a variety of ways. The concept of frailty represents one formal departure but it is worth stressing that simple codings can be quite informative. Dr. Gore alludes to period specific covariate effects. Another example, derived from analysis of TSCC data (Coates *et al.* 1992), is the use of simple covariate by time interactions and the comparison of fixed and time dependent covariates. In this prevalent cohort, with information on the estimated time of seroconversion, a regression analysis relating time to AIDS to immunological measures taken at the time of enrolment demonstrated a significant effect for PHA and marginal significance for IgA. However, a significant PHA × time interaction was identified which indicated that the predictive value of this marker declined over time. When these two variables were also examined as time dependent covariates lagged by one year, IgA was highly significant and PHA had a much more marginal role. These simple analyses indicated that the results observed were consistent with

57

biological insight since PHA can be regarded as a measure of the functional integrity of the lymphocytes and thus as a qualitative measure of immune deficiency useful for long term prediction. IgA, on the other hand, may have greater importance as a serial marker of current immune function.

(3) The disentanglement of the role of the current level and the rate of change of time dependent covariates is difficult and Dr. Gore indicates that it is an open question in the study of CD4 counts and HIV disease. I should simply like to suggest the rather simple first step of looking at the combination of covariate values lagged by different amounts. For example, in the TSCC cohort, covariates lagged by one and two years were examined, i.e. $X(t-1)$ and $X(t-2)$. Such variables will be less correlated in general than current level and slope. In this analysis only the value lagged by one year was a significant predictor. In contrast, Prentice *et al.* (1982) used this approach in a study of cardiovascular disease and demonstrated a variety of more complicated relationships.

(4) As suggested earlier, most time dependent covariates are derived from periodic monitoring and frequently the last observed value is taken as current. If however the monitoring interval and/or the rate of change of such covariates are different for individuals experiencing the event of interest at a time t and the remainder of individuals in the risk set, then biased regression coefficient estimates can arise. This is discussed in Raboud *et al.* (1992) and is illustrated in the abstracted results in the following table which shows how the coefficient estimates for three immunological markers changed when time dependent covariates were updated after every visit (visits were scheduled to be three months apart), every second visit and so on.

	Every visit	Every 2nd visit	Every 3rd visit	Enrolment value
CD4/CD8	-.431	-.347	-.259	-.214
IgA	.445	.432	.365	.262
PHA	-.174	-.166	-.122	-.122

(5) Finally, it is wise to note that most presented regression analyses do not reflect the uncertainty due to variable selection procedures.

The value, perhaps indeed the necessity, of augmenting regression analyses of prognostic factors for diseases with long development times with some form of multi-state models is being increasingly recognized. The choice of states is often suggested by regression modelling and can be quite influential. For example, HPV infection subdivided by type might be a critical component of a model for cervical cancer.

Consider the following simple multi-state model which might be used in kidney transplantation.

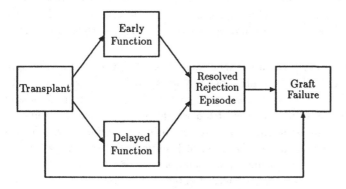

It has been suggested (Halloran *et al.* 1988a) that early function, which is defined as function of the transplanted kidney within one week of transplantation, may be a critical component of the graft failure process. For example, this work demonstrated that the inclusion of an indicator of early function in a regression model for graft failure explained much of the well established effect of transplant number on this response variable. Also, since more transitions to the early states of such a model are often observed, more information may be derived by examining prognostic factors for such transitions. For example, Dr. Gore has indicated that it was not possible to demonstrate that cyclosporin reduced the rate of early graft failure. However, Halloran *et al.* (1988b) showed that the probability of early function was significantly reduced by the early use of cyclosporin compared with initial use of a polyclonal preparation followed by cyclosporin. Thus the relationship between cyclosporin and early graft failure is not surprising and is perhaps better understood in light of this examination of early model states.

As well as providing a more comprehensive and, perhaps, a better causal understanding of a process, multi-state models are also much better suited than regression models for prediction, particularly with time dependent covariates. In fact, this is why, as Dr. Gore indicates, regression models have been little used for individual counselling which is essentially predictive. While certain limitations are at present necessary, notably Markov-like dependencies on time dependent factors, useful work should be possible. Arjas and Eerola (1993) examine the issue of prediction from time to event regression models and Klein *et al.* (1993) illustrate some useful methodology with data from a marrow transplant programme.

Dr. Gore has highlighted that understanding markers of disease progression is of considerable importance and raises the specific issue of using markers such as CD4 counts in clinical trials involving HIV infected individuals.

For this particular application, the generalizability of the conclusions may be of particular importance. Much longitudinal data is collected in a relatively uncontrolled manner particularly with respect to characteristics such as treatment assignment. While much can be learned from such data, the findings may not be applicable in other settings, notably in the evaluation of new therapies.

Prentice (1989) has given a stringent definition of a surrogate marker and it is clear that CD4, for example, does not satisfy this definition. Recently, Cook (1992) has investigated the combined use of a surrogate marker and a primary endpoint which incorporates a weighting which involves the estimated correlation between the surrogate and primary endpoint. While this might be expected to allow a relaxation of Prentice's criteria, the approach still appears to retain problems under some scenarios. I suggest that surrogate markers are being adopted with limited justification and I hope that the statistical modelling of marker behaviour in what is essentially historical data will not give uncritical encouragement to reliance of these models for treatment evaluation. The situation appears to have some parallel with the arguments that the availability of regression models which adjust for covariate effects renders randomization unnecessary in clinical trials.

Finally, I would like to comment on a possible application of the type of investigation presented by Dr. Dietz. Identification of the possible impact of various vaccination scenarios might provide guidance on the choice of explanatory variables when the effects of vaccination are being investigated in particular applications. For example, in the recent design of a case-control study following a measles outbreak in Kitchener-Waterloo, Canada, a major concern was the specification of testable hypotheses which might provide information on the apparent failure of some vaccination strategies.

Both the organizers and the speakers are to be commended for providing us with such an interesting opening session for this conference.

References

Arjas, E. and Eerola, M. (1993) 'On predictive causality in longitudinal studies', *J. Stat. Plan. Inf.* **34**, 361–384.

Coates, R.A., Farewell, V.T., Raboud, J., Read, S.E., Klein, M., MacFadden, K., Calzavara, L.M., Johnson, J.K., Fanning, M.M. and Shepherd, F.A. (1992) 'Using serial observations to identify predictors of progression to AIDS in the Toronto Sexual Contact Study', *J. Clin. Epidemiol.* **45**, 245–253.

Cook, R.J. (1992) *Group Sequential Methods for Bivariate Responses in Clinical Trials*, PhD thesis, University of Waterloo.

Halloran, P.F., Aprile, M., Farewell, V., Ludwin, D., Kinsey Smith, E., Tsai, S.Y., Bear, R.A., Cole, E.H., Fenton, S.S. and Cattran, D.C. (1988a) 'Multivariate analysis of 200 consecutive cadaveric renal transplants treated by a protocol incorporating antilymphocyte globulin, cyclosporine and azathioprine: the principal factor determining graft survival is early function', *Transplantation* **46**, 223–228.

Halloran, P., Aprile, M. and Farewell, V. (for the Ontario Renal Transplant Group) (1988b) 'Factors influencing ealy renal function in cadaver kidney transplants. A case control study', *Transplantation* **45**, 122–127.

Klein, J.P., Keiding, N. and Copelan, E.A. (1993) 'Plotting summary predictions in multistate survival models: Probabilities of relapse and death in remission for bone marrow transplantation patients', *Stat. Med.* **13**, 2315-2332.

Prentice, R.L. (1989) 'Surrogate endpoints in clinical trials: definition and operational criteria', *Stat. Med.* **8**, 431–440.

Prentice, R.L., Shimizu, Y., Lin, C.H., Petersen, A.V., Kato, H., Mason, M.W. and Szatrowski, T.P. (1982) 'Serial blood pressure measurements and cardiovascular disease in a Japanese cohort', *Am. J. Epi.* **116**, 1–28.

Raboud, J.M., Coates, R.A. and Farewell, V.T. (1992) 'Estimating risks of progression to AIDS using serially measured immunologic markers'. In *Multiple Comparisons and Selection in Biometry*, F.M. Hoppe (ed.), Marcel Dekker, New York, 415–425.

Invited Discussion

James S. Koopman

We have heard from a biostatistician, an epidemiologist, and a mathematical modeller. This is the combination that is necessary to advance our enterprise of analyzing the reality that transmits infections through populations. It was great to have them on the same podium. It is great to have them meeting in discussions over tea. It would be even greater to have them working together on joint projects.

Julian Peto has presented us with an example of a chronic infectious disease where the need to combine the principles of infectious and chronic disease analysis is clear. HPV is a chronic infection where the course and outcome of the infection are dependent upon numerous host and agent specific factors. Even before the agent of cervical cancer was determined, the sexual mode of transmission was made clear as the number of partners of the victim and of the victim's spouse were both related to the risk of disease. Now that the agent has been determined, we can proceed to work out the determinants of transmission of that agent in ways that should help better to orient prevention programmes. We can begin to assess what aspects of sexual contact patterns and of host immune responses affect the level of disease in a population. We can then begin to plan both behavioural and biological interventions to prevent disease.

To work out transmission dynamics, we also need to understand the natural history of infection and how infection gets translated into disease and into contagiousness. As Julian Peto suggests, the natural history of HPV is complex and heterogenous. Therefore we are going to need the best modelling tools we can muster to the task. But just as it is necessary to work out the natural history in order to determine transmission dynamics, so also we need a better understanding of transmission dynamics in order to work out the natural history. The observation that recent partners but not those more distant in time are associated with HPV infection illustrates some of the problems to be encountered. Are more distant infections associated with both immunity and risk and do these two elements cancel out. To resolve this question, we need to specify both the natural history of immunity and the determinants of infection risk. That risk, like the risk for all STDs, needs to be specified in terms of the risk presented to the study subject by the risk of infection in their partners, and not just in terms of what acts the study subject has performed or how many partners they may have had.

Much of Sheila Gore's presentation centred around new statistical approaches to clarify the natural history of disease progression. Many of the advances she discussed relate to the analysis of dynamic data. The dynamics of disease progression and how risk factors affect that progression is a relatively new, but now central, preoccupation of chronic disease epidemiology. Epidemiologists are increasingly collecting serial observations to examine disease dynamics and statisticians are developing ever more appropriate and useful ways to analyze these data. Significant advances have been made in accounting for both measured and unmeasured sources of variation in rates of progression.

The time and age patterns of disease onset in a population are determined both by the nature of the pathogenic process and by how much variation there is in the population with regard to the determinants of that process. To understand the determinants of the disease progression, we separate these effects in our analysis. To do this, we must use models of the disease process that incorporate population variability. Frailty models and new parameter estimation procedures for these have made significant advances toward that goal. Dr. Gore illustrated the phenomenon involved with the time dependent hazard rates used to model breast cancer, transplant survival, and HIV outcomes.

To date, models of disease progression have not taken transmission dynamics into account as a determinant of disease progression. The usual assumption has been that nothing in a population outside what directly affects an individual, influences the course of infection progression in that individual. That is to say, chronic disease epidemiology usually proceeds using the assumption that the outcome in one individual is independent of the outcomes in other individuals. Dependence resulting from the sampling process is the only source of dependence between individuals addressed in chronic disease models.

Even for infectious diseases, we can often make this assumption of independence. Any risk assessment for infectious diseases that includes the infection process will have to account for the dependence of outcomes between individuals that arises from the infection process. But when examining the natural history of infection *given infection status*, independence across individuals might be a reasonable assumption for some, but not all, infectious diseases. Let us consider when it might not be a reasonable assumption.

Immune responses to multiple cross reacting infections could be involved in disease progression. In the case of HP, for example, the sequential order and timing of infections could affect the nature of the immune response. This would mean that the outcome dependence between individuals generated by transmission dynamics would carry over into survival analyses given infection status. Also the initial dose which is transmitted is likely to determine the natural history of infection. The different progression rates of HIV infection in different risk groups is a case in point. In the model presented by Klaus Dietz, the natural history of measles progression was assumed to be dependent upon prior vaccination status. Natural measles infection was viewed as inducing solid immunity. For most agents there is no such thing as perfect immunity. The case of HPV, for infection, immunity must certainly be viewed in the context of the degree of cross reaction between different viruses.

Measles is viewed by epidemiologists as a classic infectious disease. But the all or none phenomenon of complete immunity under which measles and measles immunization is often characterized is in fact not characteristic of almost any other infectious disease, especially not chronic infectious diseases. Thus I hope Dietz's treatment of measles helps establish a new paradigm for infectious processes, one where immunity is relative and where the major effects of an immune response are on the natural history of infection.

One of the big holes in the integration of modern statistics into the analysis of infectious disease data was brought out by Sheila Gore. As she pointed out, we are really doing a poor job of estimating transmission probabilities. We are doing an especially poor job in figuring how different elements of the infection and the immune process affect transmission probabilities. To do a better job, I think we need to integrate modern statistical approaches and the use of transmissions models like those presented by Klaus Dietz. We need to establish a science of transmission system analysis that uses transmissions models to analyze data collected upon a transmission system so as to estimate the parameters of those models. We also then need to use transmission models to design better the collection of data so that the important elements of the transmission system can be determined.

Transmission models are too often viewed as policy devices rather than scientific theories. We can't advance our understanding of transmission systems without models of those transmission systems. Even given appropriate models, we still can't develop a science of transmission system analysis if our models depend upon ad hoc parameter values. Just as new statistical methods applicable to dynamic data are helping us take important steps in working out the natural history of disease processes, we need new statistical methods applicable to the dynamic process of infection transmission. There is a system which generates the infection phenomenon which we observe in epidemiological studies. What we need to do better to understand that system is to develop means of estimating system parameters from our observations and then to define what observations can help us select between alternative system formulations.

Natural history of infection and immunity, of course, plays a key role in a transmission system. How transmission probabilities are affected by that natural history is crucial. But equally crucial is the determination of contact patterns and how these translate into core groups. If modern statistical advances in chronic diseases are to be integrated into the analysis of infectious disease data, I think we must pay more attention to contact patterns. Sheila Gore pointed out that estimating transmission probabilities through the examination of individual exposures to infected individuals is not a very productive undertaking. I am not sure if her suggestion about examining transmission in networks corresponds to my suggestion here that we fit population patterns of infection to transmission models. She might more likely be referring to the examination of transmission in smaller units akin to the approaches that Longini and I developed for estimating transmission probabilities from data that are available in the end stage distribution of infection in families.

The approach that I suggest with regard to fitting transmission models to infection patterns in populations has some significant advantages that I will deal with when I get my turn to talk later in the week. One of those advantages is that the approach extracts information from the population phenomenon generated by transmission dynamics. Standard epidemiological techniques do not do this.

Dietz pointed out in his presentation that vaccination has effects in the population that go considerably beyond effects in individuals. If we model those population effects, presumably our models could capture the information regarding vaccination effects upon transmission probabilities that are intrinsic to the population patterns generated. Since contact patterns are one determinant of the population infection pattern, we will gain power to estimate transmission probabilities as we increase our abilities to describe contact patterns.

If we could improve our ability to estimate transmission probabilities by improving our ability to model and estimate the parameters of the natural history of infection and model and estimate the parameters of the contact process, then we would not have to use speculative values for parameters in models like those presented by Dietz. We could use data relevant parameters. For example, we could estimate relative transmission risk from unvaccinated and previously vaccinated individuals by fitting a model of such differential risk to observations on infection patterns. This has the advantage that in the process of estimating transmission probabilities by fitting transmission models, each new estimation and each new model development would contribute to the clarification of where data and theory are consistent or inconsistent. Each new application of a model to data would provide insight as to what observational or experimental data could be gathered to help us complete and clarify our image of the transmission system. Fitting models without appropriate statistical theory, however, will not get us where we need to go. Only as transmission system modelling and modern statistical methods come together in the analysis of epidemiological data will a science of transmission system analysis emerge.

The epidemiologist, the statistician, and the mathematical modeller of transmission too often live in quite distant worlds. As we address the statistics of chronic infections, those worlds are coming together.

Response from Sheila Gore

I welcome Professor Farewell's five commented and well chosen examples on covariate coding and variable selection. It is instructive to link the first on lagged covariates with the fourth on inter-visit times to note that careful attention must be given to lag duration so that explanatory value is not unduly sacrificed in avoidance of agonal perturbation of marker values. The first report of the MRC-Inserm Concorde trial (Aboulker and Swart 1993) endorses Farewell's reservations about the use of surrogate markers: despite zidovudine's apparent impact on CD4 lymphocyte count, patients randomized to early versus deferred zidovudine obtained advantage neither in terms of delayed progression to AIDS nor to death. Triallists would do well to concentrate greater effort on modelling, and hence understanding, how zidovudine affects patients' CD4 count (McNeil 1993) than on CD4 as a surrogate for clinical endpoints, Longini's remarks on staged models for HIV disease notwithstanding.

Dr. Koopman argues forcefully for a science of transmission system analysis, in which designs for data collection are informed by the transmission models under consideration, so that parameters are better estimable and model criticism becomes possible. Studies of HIV transmission from infected index to a sole heterosexual contact, by contrast, have limited scope for criticism. Koopman and Dietz also highlight the importance of contact pattern for the design and evaluation of vaccine strategies. Importantly, a dual scientific approach is envisaged by Koopman to 'data relevant parameters': model reparametrization in conformity with existing data but also redesign of data collection to accord with efficient parametrization.

References

Aboulker, J-P., and Swart, A.M. (1993) 'Preliminary analysis of the Concorde trial', *Lancet* **341**, 889–890.

McNeil, A.J. (1993) *Statistical Methods in AIDS Progression Studies with an Analysis of the Edinburgh City Hospital Cohort*, PhD thesis, Cambridge University.

Piece-wise Constant Models to Estimate Age- and Time-specific Incidence of Toxoplasmosis from Age- and Time-specific Seroprevalence Data

A.E. Ades and D.J. Nokes

1 Introduction

Consider an infectious disease which results in no mortality or morbidity, and which generates lifelong specific antibody. Let $q(a,t)$ be the probability that an individual at age a and time t is seronegative. It is well-known that the relation between seroprevalence and incidence $h(a,t)$ is:

$$q(a,t) = \exp(-\int_0^a h(z, t - a + z)dz); \qquad (1.1)$$

see for example Becker (1989). However, while there have been numerous attempts to derive incidence estimates from age-specific *or* time-specific seroprevalence data, few if any have modelled the effects of age and time simultaneously. This paper presents some further developments of piecewise constant incidence models described in earlier work (Ades and Nokes 1993).

The data is based on 3785 blood samples sent for routine virological examination in Sheffield Public Health Laboratory, England, in mid year 1969, 1973, 1976, 1979, 1981, 1985, 1988, 1989, and 1990, from patients aged from 2 to 100 (Walker and Nokes 1992). Observations were aggregated into 171 groups, each representing a 5-year age band in a single survey year. Children under 2 years of age were excluded, as maternal antibody passes across the placenta and could persist into the second year of life. Details of laboratory methods, and of possible biases in the data may be found in earlier papers (Ades and Nokes 1993, Walker and Nokes 1992).

Toxoplasmosis is a common infection caused by the protozoan *Toxoplasma gondii*, transmitted in the form of oocysts from soil contaminated with cat faeces, or via tissue cysts in under-cooked meat (Remington 1990). Because a primary maternal infection in pregnancy may be transmitted to the foetus, occasionally resulting in severe disease, incidence in the childbearing period has been of central concern.

2 Methods

Generalising the piece-wise constant age-related incidence models suggested by Becker (1989), we partition the age and time domains into blocks, and assume incidence μ_i attaching to a person in age band i and incidence θ_j attaching to time band j. A set of models can then be considered:

$$
\begin{aligned}
\text{CONSTANT INCIDENCE:} \quad & h(a,t) = \mu \\
\text{AGE-DEPENDENCE ONLY:} \quad & h(a,t) = \mu_i \\
\text{TIME-DEPENDENCE ONLY:} \quad & h(a,t) = \theta_j \\
\text{AGE AND TIME, ADDITIVE:} \quad & h(a,t) = \mu_i + \theta_j \\
\text{AGE AND TIME, MULTIPLICATIVE:} \quad & h(a,t) = \exp(\mu_i + \theta_j)
\end{aligned}
$$

It may be preferable to impose a non-negative incidence constraint on the first four models:

$$\mu_i + \theta_j \geq 0 \quad \text{for all } i,j$$

Non-negativity is inherent in the multiplicative model.

Consider an individual k of age a at time t. Let A_{ik} be the time k has so far spent in age band i, T_{jk} the time spent in time band j, and X_{ijk} the time simultaneously spent in both. Then, substituting in (1.1), the probability that k is seronegative is:

$$\text{ADDITIVE:} \quad q_k = \exp(-(\sum_i \mu_i A_{ik} + \sum_j \theta_j T_{jk})) \qquad (2.1)$$

$$\text{MULTIPLICATIVE:} \quad q_k = \exp\left(-(\sum_{ij} X_{ijk} \exp(\mu_i + \theta_j))\right) \qquad (2.2)$$

The age domain was divided into 5 bands: 2-10, 10-20, 20-30, 30 to 50 and > 50. Time was segmented into 7 intervals: pre 1930, 1930-40, 1940-50, 1950-60, 1960-70, 1970-80, 1980-90. The cut-points were chosen in advance to give approximately equal time at risk of infection within each segment. Note that the oldest patients from the earliest survey were born in 1870, while the youngest patients in the latest survey were born in 1989. In order to explain the seroprevalence observed between 1969 and 1990, it is necessary to model incidence over a 121 year period.

The proportion of seronegatives was considered as a binomially distributed outcome variable in generalised linear or non-linear models. Using subroutines from a standard library for optimisation with derivatives, values of incidence parameters were sought which maximised the likelihood (Ades and Nokes 1993). Likelihood ratio χ^2 tests were used to compare nested models. Profile likelihood confidence intervals for predicted incidence were calculated by the same subroutines.

3 Results

The Age-only model was a poor fit compared to the Time-only model (Table 1), but there was strong evidence that incidence is both time-dependent after accounting for age ($\chi_6^2 = 52.4$), and age-dependent after accounting for time ($\chi_4^2 = 23.1$). There was little difference between models with and without non-negativity constraints, and the data failed to distinguish between additive and multiplicative formulations of the age-time relationship.

	χ^2	*df*
CONSTANT	229.5	170
AGE ONLY - Unconstrained	207.5	166
- Non-negative incidence	207.5	
TIME ONLY - Unconstrained	178.4	164
- Non-negative incidence	178.4	
AGE AND TIME - ADDITIVE - Unconstrained	155.1	160
AGE AND TIME - Non-negative incidence	158.3	
AGE AND TIME - MULTIPLICATIVE	156.6	160

Table 1. Residual log-likelihood χ^2 deviance in piecewise constant models.

Incidence estimates from multiplicative and additive models present a consistent picture. There was a marked fall in incidence after 1950 (Table 2). Incidence is highest in the 2-10 and 10-20 age bands, falling to an estimated zero incidence at age 20 onwards (Table 3). Confidence intervals for predicted age-specific incidence in 1980-90 generated by the additive and multiplicative models are very similar.

Failure to include both age and time terms in the incidence model not only produces a poor fit, but also yields biased incidence estimates. This is particularly clear when the age-and-time models, which estimate a near-zero incidence over age 20, are compared to the poorly fitting age-only model, which predicts a dramatically high incidence in those over age 30 (Table 3).

4 Discussion

Piece-wise constant models can be used to explore how incidence varies in age and time while making few assumptions. Results pointed to a rapid

TIME SEGMENT	TIME ONLY	AGE and TIME Additive	AGE and TIME Multiplicative
1870–1930	1.05	1.59	2.55
1930–1940	1.17	1.86	1.43
1940–1950	1.48	2.06	1.59
1950–1960	0.10	0.57	0.51
1960–1970	0.79	0.62	0.50
1970–1980	0.43	0.57	0.52
1980–1990	0.38	0.57	0.40

Table 2. Estimated incidence (percent per year) in 10-20 year-olds as a function of time, non-negative incidence models. The same pattern would be predicted in all age bands.

AGE SEGMENT	AGE ONLY	AGE and TIME Additive	AGE and TIME Multiplicative
2-10	0.58	0.63 (0.33–1.02)	0.59 (0.22-1.11)
10-20	0.89	0.57 (0.00–1.06)	0.40 (0.00–1.22)
20-30	0	0 (0.00–0.32)	0 (0.00–0.32)
30-50	1.01	0 (0.00–0.27)	0 (0.00–0.27)
> 50	1.13	0 (0.00–0.68)	0.14 (0.00–0.59)

Table 3. Estimated incidence, percent per year (95% profile likelihood confidence intervals), in 1980-1990 as a function of age, non-negative incidence models. The same pattern would be predicted over all time periods.

fall in incidence after 1950, possibly due to increased consumption of frozen meat. The peak incidence in childhood and adolescence was unexpected, but is consistent with some new findings on ocular toxoplasmosis following post-natally acquired infection (Glasner *et al.* 1992).

Such models may also be useful for short-term incidence prediction. Confidence intervals on predicted incidence reported here are very similar to those produced by a range of parametric models studied in earlier work (Ades and Nokes 1993). Further, although zero incidence in those over 20 is not plausible, the confidence intervals on incidence are consistent with results from recent UK studies of seroconversion and prevalence of specific IgM (Ades 1992).

References

Ades, A.E. (1992) 'Methods for estimating the incidence of primary infection in pregnancy: a reappraisal of toxoplasmosis and cytomegalovirus data', *Epidemiol. Infect.* **108**, 367–375.

Ades, A.E. and Nokes, D.J. (1993) 'Modelling age- and time-specific incidence from seroprevalence: toxoplasmosis', *Am. J. Epidemiol.* **137**, 1022–34.

Becker, N.G. (1989) *Analysis of Infectious Disease Data*, Chapman and Hall, London.

Glasner, P.D., Silveira, C., Kruszon-Moran, D., Martins, M.C., Burnier, M., *et al.* (1992) 'An unusually high prevalence of ocular toxoplasmosis in southern Brazil', *Am. J. Ophthalmol.* **114**, 136–44.

Remington, J.S. and Desmonts, G. (1990) 'Toxoplasmosis'. In *Infectious Diseases of the Fetus and Newborn*, J.S. Remington and J.O. Klein (eds.), W.B. Saunders, Philadelphia, PA, 90–195.

Walker, J., Nokes, D.J., and Jennings, R. (1992) 'Longitudinal study of toxoplasma seroprevalence in South Yorkshire', *Epidemiol. Infect.* **108**, 99–106.

Discussion

VAN DRUTEN** In the Netherlands seroprevalence data on toxomplasmosis infection (using the IFA-test) tend to reach a maximum at the older ages of say 60%. The hypothesis is that this level reflects a dynamic equilibrium between seroreversion and seroconversion (due to infection) in the older ages. Ades finds little or no rise in infections in the older age classes. Is it possible that this is due to a violation of the model assumption that one remains seropositive throughout life after *Toxoplasma* infection?

REPLY There is no evidence that antibody declines to a level where it cannot be detected by the latex agglutination test used in Sheffield. However, in principle, the plateau in seroprevalence in older groups could be due to loss of detectable antibody. Indeed, it may not be possible to distinguish a decline in incidence with age from a loss of antibody. For this reason it might be equally plausible to assume that the maximum 60% toxoplasmosis seroprevalence reached in the Netherlands is the result of low incidence in older people, rather than seroreversion.

New Methodology for AIDS Back Calculation

D. De Angelis and W.R. Gilks

Back-calculation methods have been widely used to reconstruct the past history of the HIV epidemic and to provide short-term predictions of AIDS incidence, on the basis of reported AIDS cases, knowledge of the incubation period distribution and assumptions on the shape of the HIV infection curve.

Within the back-calculation framework, a great variety of different model assumptions and modelling approaches have been employed at each stage of the process (infection, incubation and reporting). Considerable uncertainty exists about the appropriate form for each stage. For example only information on first half of the incubation distribution is available, and knowledge of the effect and extent of AIDS prophylaxis and treatment is still limited. Furthermore, the history of HIV incidence can only be inferred indirectly.

The complexity of the total model has prevented a formal treatment of uncertainty in model formulation and parameter estimation. For example, parameters of the incubation distribution are usually fixed. Further complexities are added through use of other sources of data, such as seroprevalence estimates (and their inherent imprecision). Informal sensitivity analyses and bootstrapping have provided partial answers to the effects of uncertainty on AIDS projections, but a formal treatment of uncertainty demands a new approach to estimation. In particular, a Bayesian framework is indicated, since informative prior distributions on some parameters would allow useful compromises between assuming complete ignorance about their values, and fixing them absolutely.

We describe the basics of AIDS back calculation, reviewing model assumptions and generalisations. We motivate our approach to model building, and propose estimation through Markov chain Monte Carlo (MCMC). We show some results for the epidemic in England and Wales.

Discussion

ARCA Would it not make more sense to use death as the end point from which to conduct back-calculation?

SOLOMON Deaths due to AIDS and HIV infection are generally less well reported than AIDS diagnoses, so that there is more complete and reliable data for AIDS diagnoses.

RAAB When the back-calculation procedure is used to predict future cases, it is the cost absorbing nature of the disease that is of most interest. As death is the end point of association of a patient with health-care services, if the end point was to be taken different from AIDS diagnoses, then it should be moved further toward the point of infection rather than away.

Imperfect HIV Vaccines, the Consequences for Epidemic Control and Clinical Trials

S.M. Blower and A.R. McLean

We develop a transmission model to examine three facets of prophylactic vaccine failure: take (the vaccine may only work in a fraction of those who are vaccinated), degree (the vaccine may only reduce and not eliminate the probability of infection upon exposure), and duration (the vaccine may only confer protection for a limited time period).

We demonstrate:

1. how to derive a summary measure of vaccine imperfection;

2. how to calculate the critical vaccination coverage that is required to eradicate an HIV epidemic;

3. how to assess the potential impact of different types of imperfect prophylactic vaccines (i.e. vaccines that fail in different way) in both clinical trials and mass vaccination campaigns.

We present analytic and scenario results, the latter being based upon parameter values that are derived from the HIV epidemic in gay men in San Francisco, California. For further details see McLean and Blower (1993).

References

McLean, A.R., and Blower, S.M. (1993) 'Imperfect vaccines and herd immunity to HIV', *Proc. Roy. Soc. Lond. B* **253**, 9.

Discussion

GARNETT To what extent do the results of Blower and McLean depend on their assumption of an exponential decay in loss of vaccine-induced immunity?

REPLY The initial HIV vaccine model that we have presented is based upon reasonable biological assumptions and is also based upon what is known about the mechanism of action of prophylactic vaccines for other diseases. The data that are available from (non-HIV) clinical trials with long follow-up periods, although fairly limited, suggest generally that vaccine-induced immunity is either life-long or tends to decay exponentially. The data that are available from non-human primate studies of candidate HIV prophylactic vaccines indicate that for these vaccines loss of immunity appears to be both rapid and exponentially distributed. As further HIV data accumulate, if it appears that loss of immunity is not exponentially distributed, we will investigate the sensitivity of our results to different distributional assumptions.

KOOPMAN The effect of vaccine-induced immunity that has a half-life of 35yrs may be reduced in Blower and McLean's model by the lack of age-structure within their model. Sexual behaviour and hence exposure are known to change with age, and especially to decrease beyond the age of about 30yrs, so that ignoring this pattern may result in under-estimation of the impact of such a vaccine.

REPLY We wish to stress that many studies of sexual behaviour have indicated that there appears to be a great deal of difference in aging and its effects on sexual behaviour in heterosexuals and homosexuals; the link between aging and sexual behaviour appears to be fairly clearly established for heterosexuals, but the effect of aging on homosexual behaviour remains unclear. The model that we have presented for examining the effects of HIV vaccines only includes homosexual men. One of us has analysed several large sexual behaviour surveys that have been conducted in Europe and North America, and these analyses reveal that (1) considerable heterogeneity in sexual behaviour can be found in all age classes, and (2) it is extremely difficult to untangle whether any apparent 'age' effect is really a cohort effect, a period effect or a 'real' age effect. On the basis of these analyses and the results from many other similar studies we formulated a model which lacks age-structure. We stress that any specific scenario that we presented (i.e. for a vaccine that has a half-life of 35yrs) is merely to illustrate qualitative aspects of the results. We also presented analytical results where we derived an overall measure of vaccine imperfection with any duration of vaccine-induced immunity.

LONGINI Some of the concepts raised by Blower and McLean can be encapsulated in the terms efficacy and effectiveness: the former term relates to the protection conferred to the individual vaccinated (including the notions of take, protection and duration), and the latter refers to the effect of the vaccine in the community, as in the model investigated by Blower and McLean.

REPLY We agree that some of the concepts that we have raised can be encapsulated to some degree in the terms efficacy and effectiveness. However, unfortunately, the literature is now confused by several different definitions of these terms; furthermore many of these definitions are time-dependent, for example, the efficacy of an imperfect vaccine will change over time. Therefore, we formulated some new terminology because we wished (1) to examine three facets of prophylactic vaccine failure (take, degree and duration) independently and not subsume them all under the single terms efficacy and effectiveness, and (2) to derive a summary measure of vaccine imperfection that was time independent and hence could be used to calculate the critical vaccination coverage that is necessary for HIV eradication.

Feasibility of Prophylactic HIV Vaccine Trials: Some Statistical Issues

M. Elizabeth Halloran, Ira M. Longini Jr., C.J. Struchiner and Michael Haber

Introduction

In 1915, Greenwood and Yule (1915) articulated that a valid vaccine efficacy study requires equal exposure to infection in the vaccinated and unvaccinated groups. One issue in planning prophylactic HIV vaccine trials is that people who are randomized to a blinded, placebo trial may have themselves tested to see if they have a positive HIV antibody response. If the test is positive, they might believe that they have received the vaccine. Then, depending on their belief about the protective effects of the vaccine, they may increase their sexual activity, thus increasing their exposure to infection. This increased exposure to infection in the vaccinated population could bias the estimate of the biological efficacy of the vaccine to protect against infection if it is not included in the analysis.

Pre-infection evaluation

Exposure to infection versus susceptibility

To study the relative contribution of unequal exposure to infection and differential susceptibility to the estimate of vaccine efficacy, we formulate a simple model that explicitly includes both susceptibility and exposure to infection. Post-infection change in the probability or rate of developing disease that might be induced by a prophylactic vaccine is discussed below.

A simple model for the hazard of infection of a susceptible i at time t with covariate vector z_i is

$$h_i(t) = \lambda_i(t)e^{\beta z_i}\theta_i(t),$$

where $\lambda_i(t)$ is the rate of contacts, in this case sexual acts, of susceptible i at time t, $e^{\beta z_i}$ is the transmission probability per contact with an infective that depends on the covariate vector z_i and parameter vector β, and $\theta_i(t)$ is the probability that a sexual partner of person i is infective. This assumes that all infectives are equally infectious, that there is just one type of contact, and that each contact is independent of the previous contact, at least in terms of whether the contact is infectious or not. We could make the rate of infection dependent on the covariates of the infectives, or make $h_i(t)$ a weighted average of the rates of infection from two or more types of contacts, such as anal versus oral sex.

Assume we are concerned with just one covariate, vaccination status. Let $z_i = 0$ if a person is unvaccinated, and $z_i = 1$ if a person is vaccinated. Let e^{β_0} and $e^{\beta_0+\beta_1}$ be, respectively, the probability of transmission to an unvaccinated and a vaccinated susceptible from an infective. The relative residual susceptibility in the unvaccinated group is e^{β_1}, and a parameter measuring the biological efficacy of the vaccine in reducing susceptibility to infection in an individual would be $VE = 1 - e^{\beta_1}$. In principle, e^{β_1} could vary between 0 and 1. Either everyone could have the same benefit from the vaccine, so that e^{β_1} is the same for everyone, or e^{β_1} could vary among individuals. Here we assume that e^{β_1} is the same for everyone. Smith *et al.* (1984) also discussed the possibility that some people would be completely protected by the vaccine while others would not be protected at all.

The hazard of infection, or incidence, or force of infection, of a susceptible i could be increased either by increasing the rate of contacts $\lambda_i(t)$, by choosing contacts from a pool with a higher prevalence of infection $\theta_i(t)$, or by increasing the proportion of type of contacts that have a higher transmission probability. These produce a higher hazard of infection for reasons that have nothing to do with the biological efficacy of the vaccine, but rather with the exposure to infection. We call this change in exposure to infection induced by the intervention the *exposure efficacy* (Halloran *et al.* 1994b). In particular, in this case the increase in exposure is due to a change in behaviour, so we call it *behaviour* efficacy.

If everyone in the vaccinated group were to increase the rate of sexual contacts by a factor of e^a, then $1 - e^a$ would be a measure of the exposure efficacy, assuming all other things are equal. If $e^a = 1.5$, then the exposure efficacy is negative. If a proportion h of the vaccinated group increases the rate of contacts, but a portion $(1 - h)$ does not, then $1 - [he^a + (1 - h)] = h(1 - e^a)$ gives a measure of the average exposure efficacy of the vaccine.

Choice of outcome parameters

Assume that for each person we are able to know or to estimate the total number of potentially infectious contacts during the study period. Let $C_0(t)$ and $C_1(t)$ be the total number of potentially infective contacts made with susceptibles in the vaccinated and unvaccinated groups up to time t, respectively, and $d_0(t)$ and $d_1(t)$ be the number of infections in the two groups. Then, the maximum likelihood estimators are

$$e^{\hat{\beta}_0} = \frac{d_0(t)}{C_0(t)} \quad , \text{ and } \quad e^{\hat{\beta}_1} = \frac{d_1(t)/C_1(t)}{d_0(t)/C_0(t)}.$$

Thus, if we have detailed information about the number of contacts and whether they are infective, and when infection occurs, we could estimate vaccine efficacy based on the relative transmission probabilities. This is closely related to using the secondary attack rate to evaluate vaccine efficacy (Kendrick and Eldering 1939, Orenstein *et al.* 1988).

Assume that before vaccination, all $\lambda_i(t) = \lambda$, and $\theta_i(t) = \theta$. It can easily be seen that if h_0 and h_1 are the hazards of infection in the unvaccinated and the vaccinated, then $h_1/h_0 = e^{\beta_1}$ under these simple assumptions. The Cox regression coefficient from the proportional hazards model would be an estimator of e^{β_1}. Rhodes *et al.* (1994) have shown this formally using counting processes. Using the relative hazards to estimate efficacy would give $VE = 1 - e^{\beta_1}$. The only data we need for this estimate are the times, or even the order of the infections.

In the design of prophylactic HIV vaccine trials, discussion has centred on whether to conduct small, detailed studies or large simple trials. Meier (1990) drew attention to similarities with the polio vaccine trials, in which high public expectations of a quick result, and the highly variable, but generally low incidence of disease lead to the choice of the large simple trials. If we were interested in estimating relative transmission probabilities, then we would need detailed information on the sexual behaviour of people. This would likely be restricted to smaller trials. Use of the hazard ratios to estimate VE would be possible in fairly large trials. In contrast to polio, active follow-up is required. HIV study participants probably will be tested every three to six months for evidence of infection. This will make even large scale, simple trials more complex than the polio vaccine trials.

The advantage of gathering information on the sexual contacts, and potential exposure to infection is that if people unblind themselves and increase their exposure to infection due to belief in the protective effects of the vaccine, it will be possible to include this in the analysis. The denominator $C_1(t)$ of the estimator of the transmission probability in the vaccinated group increases as the number of infections in the numerator $d_1(t)$ increases. If people increase their rate of contacts when the relative hazard of infection is used to estimate VE, and this is not taken into account, then this could bias the estimate. If everyone increases the contact rate by a factor e^a, the estimated vaccine estimate would be $1 - e^{\beta_1 + a}$.

Table 1 compares expected vaccine efficacy estimates obtained from transmission probabilities and hazards for different levels of relative residual susceptibility ($e^{\beta_1} = 0.50$ and $e^{\beta_1} = 0.05$) and different amounts of change in exposure to infection. The baseline hazard in the unvaccinated is $\lambda = 0.05$ infections per year, which corresponds to several different combinations of parameters. The tables were computed for 10 years of follow-up. The increase in contacts in the vaccinated group varies from no change to factors e^a of 1.5,

2.0, and 5.0. The fraction h of the vaccinated group changing behaviour is 0.5 or 1.0.

Vaccine efficacy based on the transmission probabilities when the number of infective contacts can be estimated remains unbiased even when everyone increases their rate of sexual contacts by a factor of five. The vaccine efficacy estimator based on relative hazards is easily biased by the increased rate of contacts in the vaccinated group. When $e^{\beta_1} = 0.5$ and $e^a = 2$, the expected measure of vaccine efficacy is $1 - (0.5)(0.2) = 0$. It even becomes negative when the increase in rate of contact is higher. When the vaccine is highly efficacious, in this case $1 - e^{\beta_1} = 0.95$, the estimators are less biased than at low efficacy.

Combinations of small and large trials could be considered. In place of detailed sexual histories, participants could supply post-randomization information on whether they tested themselves, changed their behaviour, and by how much. Another approach would be to use a small detailed study as a validation sample for a larger study (Robins 1992). Following the arguments presented above, valid and reliable risk factors need to be divided into risk factors for exposure to infection (partner choice, type of sex act, barrier protection, etc.) and risk factors for host susceptibility. In order to emphasize the difference as well as to emphasize that actual exposure to infection is seldom measured, the word *surrogate* for exposure to infection could be used instead of the term risk factor.

Post-infection evaluation

Prophylactic HIV vaccines may alter the post-infection natural history by changing the infectivity or by altering the rate of CD4 decline or the incubation period for AIDS. Evaluating whether a vaccine reduces infectivity by studying the relative transmission probability from vaccinated and unvaccinated persons will be extremely difficult, for all the same reasons that estimation of the transmission probability is difficult, and in addition only a small sample size is likely to be available. If there are 5000 people in each arm of a vaccine trial in a population with baseline incidence of infection of 0.05 per year, then after one year, there would be only 250 infections expected in the unvaccinated group, and fewer than that in the vaccinated group if the vaccine has an effect on infection. If some other correlate of infectivity, such as virus in the semen or blood, could be found, it would facilitate the study of relative residual infectivity (Halloran *et al.* 1994a). Considerations of relative infectivity have been raised with regards to other vaccines, such as malaria (Halloran *et al.* 1989), pertussis (Fine and Clarkson 1987), and varicella vaccine virus (Tsolia *et al.* 1990). The problem of study design to estimate relative infectivity still requires systematic research.

Increase in contacts (e^a)	Fraction increasing contacts (h)	$1 - e^{\beta_1} = 0.50$ Estimated VE based on		$1 - e^{\beta_1} = 0.95$ Estimated VE based on	
		TP	hazards	TP	hazards
no change	0	0.50	0.50	0.95	0.95
1.5	0.5	0.50	0.38	0.95	0.94
	1.0	0.50	0.25	0.95	0.93
2.0	0.5	0.50	0.28	0.95	0.93
	1.0	0.50	0.00	0.95	0.90
5.0	0.5	0.50	-0.04	0.95	0.85
	1.0	0.50	-1.50	0.95	0.75

Table 1. Comparison of expected vaccine efficacy estimates using transmission probabilities (TP) and hazard ratios under different assumptions about increased exposure to infection

Another aspect of vaccine efficacy can be defined with respect to the probability or rate of developing disease conditional on having been infected. The former could be called the relative pathogenicity (Halloran *et al.* 1994a). The latter was used as the vaccine efficacy definition for BCG vaccine in the context of a mathematical model of tuberculosis by ReVelle *et al.* (1967). Since the median incubation period is of the order of ten years, however, rate of CD4 decline (Longini *et al.* 1991) might be more useful as an outcome measure.

In this paper, we have discussed the importance of separating exposure to infection from susceptibility when evaluating the pre-infection effect of prophylactic HIV vaccines, as well as a few considerations of post-infection evaluation. Many other problems of analysis and interpretation are introduced by allowing for heterogeneities in susceptibility (Greenwood and Yule 1915), infectivity (Longini *et al.* 1989, Kim and Lagakos 1990, Shiboski and Jewell 1992), vaccine effects (Svensson 1991, Halloran *et al.* 1992, Brunet *et al.* 1993, Longini *et al.* 1993), and mixing patterns (Koopman *et al.* 1991). Blinded and unblinded studies could also have different consequences for the effect of behaviour change on parameter estimates in the presence of heterogeneous response to the vaccine (Halloran *et al.* 1994b). Many lessons can be learned for trials of prophylactic HIV vaccines from extensive historical experience with other vaccines.

Acknowledgments

M.E. Halloran, I.M. Longini, and M.J. Haber were partially supported by NIAID grant 1-R01-AI32042-01. C.J. Struchiner was partially supported by the Brazilian Research Council (CNPq).

References

Brunet, R.C., Struchiner, C.J and Halloran, M.E. (1993) 'On the distribution of vaccine protection under heterogeneous response', *Math. Biosc.* **116**, 111-125.

Fine, P.E.M. and Clarkson, J.A. (1987) 'Reflections on the efficacy of pertussis vaccines', *Rev. Inf. Dis.* **9**, 866–883.

Greenwood, M. and Yule, U.G. (1915) 'The statistics of anti-typhoid and anti-cholera inoculations, and the interpretation of such statistics in general', *Proc. Roy. Soc. Med.* **8**, 113–194.

Halloran, M.E., Struchiner, C.J. and Spielman, A. (1989) 'Modelling malaria vaccines II: Population effects of stage-specific malaria vaccines dependent on natural boosting', *Math. Biosc.* **94**, 115–149.

Halloran, M.E., Haber, M.J. and Longini, I.M. (1992) 'Interpretation and estimation of vaccine efficacy under heterogeneity', *Am. J. Epidemiol.* **136**, 328–343.

Halloran, M.E., Struchiner, C.J. and Watelet, L. (1994a) 'Epidemiologic effects of vaccines with complex effects in an age-structured population', *Math. Biosc.* **121**, 193–225.

Halloran, M.E., Longini, I.M., Struchiner, C.J., Haber, M.J. and Brunet, R.C. (1994b) 'Exposure efficacy and change in contact rates in evaluating HIV vaccines in the field', *Stat. Med.* **13**, 357–377.

Kendrick, P. and Eldering, G. (1939) 'A study in active immunization against pertussis', *Am. J. Hyg., Sect. B* **38**, 133.

Kim, M.Y. and Lagakos, S.W. (1990) 'Estimating the infectivity of HIV from partner studies', *AEP* **1**, 117–128.

Koopman, J.S., Longini, I.M., Jacquez, J.A., Simon, C.P., Ostrow, D.G., Martin, W.R. and Woodcock, D.M. (1991) 'Assessing risk factors for transmission of infection', *Am. J. Epidemiol.* **133**, 1199–1209.

Longini, I.M., Clark, W.S., Haber, M. J. and Horsburgh, R. (1989) 'The stages of HIV infection: waiting times and infection transmission probabilities', *Lecture Notes in Biomathematics* **83**, 111–137.

Longini, I.M., Clark, W.S., Gardner, L.I. and Brundage, J.F. (1991) 'The dynamics of CD4$^+$ T-lymphocyte decline in HIV-infected individuals: a Markov modeling approach', *J. Acquir. Immun. Defic. Syndr.* **4**, 1141–1147.

Longini, I.M., Halloran, M.E. and Haber, M.J. (1993) 'Estimation of vaccine efficacy from epidemics of acute infectious agents under vaccine-related heterogeneity', *Math. Biosc.* **117**, 271–281.

Meier, P. (1990) 'Polio trial: an early efficient clinical trial', *Stat. Med.* **9**, 13–16.

Orenstein, W.A., Bernier, R.H. and Hinman, A.R. (1988) 'Assessing vaccine efficacy in the field: further observations', *Epidemiol. Rev.* **10**, 212–241.

ReVelle, C.S., Lynn, W.R. and Feldman, F. (1967) 'Mathematical models for the economic allocation of tuberculosis control activities in developing nations', *Am. Rev. Resp. Dis.* **96**, 893–909.

Rhodes, P.H., Halloran, M.E. and Longini, I.M. (1994) 'Counting process models for differentiating exposure to infection and susceptibility'. Technical Report No. 94–1, Division of Biostatistics, Emory University School of Public Health, Atlanta, GA.

Robins, J. (1992) 'Estimation of exposure effects in the presence of missing or mismeasured data (abstract)', *Am. J. Epidemiol.* **136**, 1035.

Shiboski, S.C. and Jewell, N.P. (1992) 'Statistical analysis of the time-dependence on HIV-iinfectivity based on partner study data', *JASA* **87**, 360–372.

Smith, P.G., Rodrigues, L.C. and Fine, P.E.M. (1984) 'Assessment of the protective efficacy of vaccines against common diseases using case-control and cohort studies', *Int. J. Epidemiol.* **13**, 87–93.

Svensson, Å. (1991) 'Analyzing effects of vaccines', *Math. Biosc.* **107**, 407–412.

Tsolia, M., Gershon, A.A., Steinberg, S.P. *et al.* (1990) 'Live attenuated varicella vaccine: evidence that the virus is attenuated and the importance of skin lesions in transmission of varicella-zoster virus', *J. Pediatrics.* **116**, 184–189.

The Design of Immunisation Programmes against Hepatitis B Virus in Developing Countries

W.J. Edmunds, G.F. Medley and D.J. Nokes

Hepatitis B virus (HBV) is one of the most common viral infections in many parts of the world. There are an estimated 300 million carriers of the virus worldwide, each of whom has a high probability of suffering chronic liver disease. There is a safe and effective vaccine against HBV which does not interfere with other vaccines commonly given in childhood and would therefore appear to be ideally suited to mass cohort immunisation. However the vaccine is expensive compared to other Expanded Programme of Immunisation vaccines and there is evidence that vaccine induced immunity declines with time. As the epidemiology of HBV is complex (see below) the outcome of mass immunisation is difficult to predict. The aim of this work is to use a mathematical model of the transmission of HBV to aid the design of vaccination programmes in developing countries.

The epidemiology of HBV has a number of interesting features which complicate the dynamics of infection. Infection with HBV can lead to long-term carriage of the virus. Furthermore the propensity for individuals to develop this chronic carrier state is related to the age at infection in a highly non-linear manner. The probability of developing the chronic carrier state is highest amongst infants (approximately 0.9), then rapidly declines, and levels off in late childhood so that older children and adults have approximately a 1 in 10 chance of becoming carriers if infected. The epidemiological study of HBV is further complicated by its modes of transmission. It is well known that in developed countries HBV shares the same transmission routes as HIV, ie the virus can be transmitted by blood or blood products, by sexual contact or from infected mother to infant at or around the time of birth. However in developing countries HBV is also transmitted via close contact particularly amongst children. Although the mechanisms of this 'horizontal' transmission are poorly understood, it is the most common route by which HBV is transmitted in the developing world. The relative importance of the different modes of transmission is reflected in the rate or force of infection. In developing countries HBV is primarily a childhood infection, however the pattern of the force of infection differs from other close contact diseases in that it is typically highest amongst infants and young children, declines steadily throughout childhood and may rise again slightly in adults (probably due to sexual transmission). To investigate the effect of these features on the dynamics of HBV transmission and the implications for control of the virus a model of the transmission of HBV was constructed.

The predominant mode of transmission in developing countries is horizontal. Thus the model is based on the age-structured models of the common childhood infections in developing countries (McLean and Anderson 1988) and extended to include a carrier class with an age-dependent probability of becoming a carrier. We sub-divide the population into 5 epidemiological classes: susceptibles, latents, acutes (the initial highly infectious stage of infection), carriers and immunes. Immunity, by natural infection or vaccination is initially assumed to be lifelong (we later relax this assumption to investigate the effect of declining vaccine induced immunity). We assume that there is no additional mortality associated with infection by HBV. The model consists of a set of coupled PDEs which were solved numerically by the Euler method. The force of infection $\lambda(a,t)$ is defined as

$$\lambda(a,t) = \frac{\int_0^\infty \beta(a,a')\left(Y(a',t) + \alpha C(a',t)\right)\,da'}{\int_0^\infty N(a',t)\,da'}$$

where $\beta(a,a')$ is the transmission coefficient, $N(a',t)$ is the population size and α represents the relative infectiousness of carriers (C) compared to acutes (Y). This ratio of infectiousness was estimated from perinatal transmission studies to be approximately 0.16. The age-dependent force of infection was estimated from age serological profiles by maximum likelihood (Grenfell and Anderson 1985). By assuming that the force of infection is constant over discrete age classes one can estimate a matrix of transmission coefficients (the WAIFW matrix) (Anderson and May 1985). The probability of an individual, infected at age a, developing the carrier state ($p(a)$) has been described by the expression

$$p(a) = \exp(-ra^s)$$

where r and s were estimated from field data by maximum likelihood (Edmunds *et al.* 1993). Other parameters such as the duration of the latent and infectious periods were estimated independently from a variety of published sources (Edmunds *et al.* 1995a).

The model, which was found broadly to capture the observed patterns of infection in developing countries, was subsequently used to assess the effectiveness of different vaccination strategies (Edmunds *et al.* 1995b). Carriers suffer the major morbidity and mortality associated with HBV infection. We thus used the reduction in the prevalence of carriers as a measure of the success of different control strategies.

The model results suggest that due to the age-dependent nature of developing the carrier state and the form of the age-dependent force of infection, vaccination should be targeted at the youngest age group (infants under the age of 1yr). Mass immunisation of this age group has a disproportionately large impact on the prevalence of carriers in the population, whereas any delay in immunisation to older age groups has a markedly reduced impact on the prevalence of chronic carriers for a particular level of coverage. High levels of vaccine coverage are predicted to achieve elimination of HBV, though due to the long infectious period of carriers, mass immunisation must be maintained for very long periods of time at high levels of coverage. If the primary aim of a vaccination programme is the reduction in the prevalence of carriers, then the loss of vaccine induced immunity is predicted to be of little importance. This may be of considerable significance where resources are limited, since booster doses of vaccine (which are expensive and impractical) are not required. However, if the elimination of HBV is the primary aim, then the loss of vaccine induced immunity renders this goal practically impossible in hyper-endemic areas. The loss of vaccine induced immunity coupled with the effect of herd immunity leads to an increase in the average age at infection. Consequently, the predominant mode of transmission might shift from horizontal to sexual and a pattern of infection similar to developed countries might arise.

References

Anderson, R.M. and May, R.M. (1985) 'Age-related changes in the rate of disease transmission: implication for the design of vaccination programmes', *J. Hyg. (Camb.)* **94**, 365–436.

Edmunds, W.J., Medley, G.F., Nokes, D.J., Hall, A. and Whittle, H. (1993) 'The influence of age on the development of Hepatitis-B carrier state', *Proc. Roy. Soc. Lond. B* **253**, 197–201.

Edmunds, W.J., Medley, G.F., Nokes, D.J., Whittle, H. and Hall, A.J. (1995a) 'Epidemiological patterns of Hepatitis-B virus (HBV) in highly endemic areas', *Epidem. Infect.*, submitted.

Edmunds, W.J., Medley, G.F. and Nokes, D.J. (1995b) 'The transmission dynamics and control of Hepatitis-B virus in a developing country', *Stats. Med.*, submitted.

Grenfell, B.T. and Anderson, R.M. (1985) 'The estimation of age-related rates of infection from case notifications and serological data', *J. Hyg. (Camb.)* **95**, 419–36.

Sobeslavsky, O. (1980) 'Prevalence of markers of Hepatitis-B infection in various countries: a WHO collaborative study', *Bull. WHO* **58**, 621–8.

Discussion

DIETZ What evidence is there to suggest that the data on the age-related rate of change of hepatitis B virus should not be interpreted in terms of time-dependent changes?

REPLY The force of infection appears to have a common pattern in all the hyper-endemic areas studied even though the data were from very diverse communities. This suggests that the observed trends in the force of infection are due to common causes. It is possible that the apparent decline in the force of infection with age is due to common temporal factors such as population growth. However, there is no evidence to suggest that increasing population density increases the force of infection for HBV (Sobeslavsky 1980), and it is difficult to envisage alternative time-dependent factors common to all areas studied.

The Effect of Different Mixing Patterns on Vaccination Programs

David Greenhalgh and Klaus Dietz

Introduction

This paper is concerned with evaluation of vaccination programs for viral diseases such as measles, mumps, rubella and hepatitis A. For such diseases an individual starts off susceptible, at some stage catches the disease and after a short infectious period becomes permanently immune. Vaccines for measles, mumps and rubella are currently in use and vaccines for hepatitis A are not yet widely available but are currently undergoing testing. The aim of this paper is to look at the evaluation of vaccination programs and their sensitivity to different mixing assumptions.

Mathematical models which accurately describe the spread of a disease must take into account the age-structure of the population amongst whom the disease is spreading. Anderson and May (1985) describe an age-structured mathematical model using partial differential equations, which is the basis of the one which we shall use. Age-structured data for these diseases is available in the form of case reports, or more reliably age-serological profiles. Anderson and May divide the population into discrete age classes and use computer simulation methods to evaluate different vaccination programs for measles, mumps and rubella.

Method

The *force of infection at time t*, $\lambda(a, t)$, is defined as the probability per unit time that a susceptible individual of age a will become infected. We follow Keiding's non-parametric maximum likelihood method to estimate the force of infection assuming that the disease has settled down to its long-term equilibrium value. We use age-structured serological profiles for hepatitis A in Bulgaria given by Keiding (1991). Our data is of the form $(Z_1, \delta_1), (Z_2, \delta_2), \ldots, (Z_n, \delta_n)$ ordered according to age, where Z_i is the age of individual i and

$$\delta_i = \begin{cases} 1 & \text{if individual } i \text{ is immune} \\ 0 & \text{otherwise.} \end{cases}$$

Define

$$H(i) = \sum_{j=1}^{i} \delta_j,$$

the cumulative number in the sample up to age Z_i who have experienced the disease. We take the left continuous derivative of the convex hull of $H(i)$ to give an estimate of the proportion of people of age Z_i who have experienced the disease. This is a step function so we must produce a smoothed estimate. We then estimate the force of infection using a minor modification of Keiding's kernel density estimation method.

The age-dependent transmission coefficient $\beta(a, a')$ is defined as the per capita rate at which a susceptible individual of age a comes into contact with and infects an infected individual of age a'. Individuals are grouped into n age classes such as pre-school children, school-children, young adults and older adults. The transmission coefficient is then given by a square matrix of n^2 effective contact rates. We can write down a relationship between the force of infection and the matrix of transmission coefficients. However this gives a set of n^2 equations in n unknowns and to proceed further more assumptions must be made about the form of this matrix.

Mixing

The classical assumption is of homogeneous mixing, that everyone mixes at the same rate. This has been proved unrealistic for measles. The next simplest assumption is proportional mixing (Dietz and Schenzle 1985), which means that the contact rate between groups i and j is $b_i b_j$ where $b_1, b_2, \ldots, b_n$ are constants. An extreme assumption is associative mixing where individuals mix only with their own age groups. A realistic mixing matrix might well be somewhere between proportional and associative mixing. Another alternative is symmetric mixing (the matrix of effective contact rates is symmetric). In the latter case assumptions must be made on biological grounds to reduce the number of unknowns from n^2 to n.

A key epidemiological parameter is R_0, the basic reproductive ratio. This is defined as the expected number of secondary cases produced by a single infected individual entering a completely susceptible population. If R_0 exceeds one the infection will spread, otherwise it will die out. If we are using a vaccination program ϕ we can evaluate the corresponding reporduction ratio R_ϕ, say. For an age-structured model R_ϕ is given as the largest eigenvalue of a certain matrix (Greenhalgh 1990).

Once we have estimated the matrix of transmission coefficients we can proceed to evaluate vaccination programs. A given vaccination program, ϕ will just eradicate the disease if R_ϕ is one.

We describe some theoretical results on the effect of different mixing assumptions on eradication vaccination programs. We are particularly interested in one stage and two stage vaccination policies which vaccinate fixed proportions of individuals at pre-specified ages as they are commonly used in practice. For a given age-serological profile and vaccination program ϕ, associative mixing maximises the value of R_ϕ. Hence more vaccination effort must be applied with associative mixing than with any other mixing assumption. We can also obtain lower bounds for R_ϕ (Greenhalgh and Dietz 1994).

Numerical results

Finally the methods discussed here are applied to age-structured serological data on hepatitis A in Bulgaria. Numerical evaluations of the proportions necessary to be vaccinated to eradicate hepatitis A using one stage and two stage vaccination policies are discussed under different mixing assumptions. Because hepatitis A is spread by an oral-faecal transmission route its epidemiological pattern is different from that of diseases spread by aerial transmission such as measles, mumps and rubella.

References

Anderson, R.M. and May, R.M. (1985) 'Age-related changes in the rate of disease transmission: implication for the design of vaccination programmes', *J. Hyg. Camb.* **94**, 365–436.

Dietz, K. and Schenzle, D. (1985) 'Proportionate mixing for age-dependent infection transmissions', *J. Math. Biol.* **22**, 117–120.

Greenhalgh, D. (1990) 'Vaccination campaigns for common childhood diseases', *Math. Biosci.* **100**, 201–240.

Greenhalgh, D. and Dietz, K. (1994) 'Some bounds on estimates for reproductive rations derived from the age-specific force of infection', *Math. Biosci.*, to appear.

Keiding, N. (1991) 'Age-specific incidence and prevalence: a statistical perspective', *J. Roy. Statist. Soc. A* **154**, 371–412.

Discussion

HADELER How can the disease persist with completely associative mixing as there would be no transmission between age groups?

REPLY The disease can persist with associative mixing as we are using a discrete age-class model and so for example three year olds can mix with four year olds. This sustains the infection. In the limit for the model with infinitely many age-classes the mixing matrix would become a delta function and associative mixing could not sustain the disease.

MORRIS Would it not be possible to eradicate the disease under associative mixing by making a block vaccination of a complete age class? As this block of vaccinated individuals aged the disease would eventually be eradicated?

REPLY Yes, block vaccination of 0–5 year olds for at least five years and then no more vaccination would eradicate the disease, at least in the youngest age-class 0–5 years. However this is a different issue from the one addressed in the paper as we were considering a vaccination campaign applied uniformly and constantly. In practice associative mixing would not be exactly realistic and this policy would break down because the disease would be transmitted between age classes.

ADES The age-related force of infection shown by Greenhalgh seemed to have some evidence of time-dependent changes, especially as the force of infection has been analyzed by Schenzle and colleagues (1979) and they concluded that there was a time-dependent trend.

REPLY The model assumes that the age-related force of infection for hepatitis A in Bulgaria does not change with time. I am unsure how realistic this is as it would depend on how the sanitary and socio-economic conditions, including water supplies, have changed with time. Frösner *et al.* (1979) look at the change in the force of infection over time in seven European countries. This decreases as sanitary conditions improve but the decrease is more marked in northern European countries countries such as Norway and Switzerland than southern European countries such as Greece.

If the force of infection varied with time this would lead to inaccuracies in our estimate of the force of infection. I do not feel that this is the reason for the plot which shows the force of infection decreasing to zero at about ninety years of age. This is unreliable due to the fact that most cases of the disease occur at low ages and only a few cases at extremely high ages. It is this latter fact which causes a decrease to zero at ninety years of age.

REPLY The answer depends on the timescale of the changes which you were proposing. If the virus were inactive a short period after being placed in the environment then this would not make a difference and a mass action term would still be suitable. If the infectious material stayed in the environment for a long time remaining infectious then a proportional mixing term might be more appropriate as it might then be appropriate to assume that individuals come into contact with this environment at a constant rate depending on their ages.

References

Frösner, G., Papavangelou, G., Butler, R., Iwarson, S., Lindholm, A., Courouce-Pauty, A., Haas, H. and Deinhardt F. (1979) 'Antibody against hepatitis A in seven European countries', *Am. J. Epidemiol.* 110, 63–69.

Schenzle, D., Dietz, K. and Frösner, G. (1979) 'Hepatitis A antibodies in European countries II: Mathematical analysis of cross-sectional surveys', *Am. J. Epidemiol.* 110, 70–76.

Vaccination in Age Structured Populations I: The Reproduction Number

K.P. Hadeler and J. Müller

1 Introduction

There is a vast and well-developed theory for the spread of infectious diseases in randomly mixing populations and in populations structured by age. In general we have the following situation. There is an uninfected stationary state. For certain parameter specifications, i.e. in the case of low transmission rate, fast recovery, or high mortality, this uninfected state is stable. If, say, the transmission rate is increased then there is a bifurcation, the uninfected state loses its stability, and a stable infected state comes into existence. The conditions for stability of the uninfected situation or for the bifurcation, respectively, are usually formulated as threshold conditions. In simple cases the threshold condition is given in such a way that certain quantities describing transmission of the disease, multiplication of parasites etc. exceed other terms describing recovery, death of infected etc. In many cases the quotient of these terms is formed, and the threshold condition assumes the form that a certain quantity is compared to the number one. This quantity has often been interpreted as the basic reproduction number R_0, i.e. as the number of cases that will be produced by one 'typical' infected individual in a totally susceptible population during its infected period. From this interpretation it is obvious, that the condition for stability should be the inequality $R_0 < 1$. It should be underlined that this interpretation of R_0 is not a definition as long as the notion of a typical individual or the underlying averaging procedure has not been specified. Until recently this had been done only for some simple cases of randomly mixing populations.

On the other hand, from the analytic treatment of the bifurcation phenomenon it is evident that stability and bifurcation are connected to some eigenvalue of some related linear operator (or matrix) being negative or positive, respectively. Only quite recently Heesterbeek (1992) has shown that indeed the basic reproduction number can be defined in the context of this operator and its critical eigenvalue (Perron root). Without studying a possible stochastic interpretation he has shown that in many cases so far treated in

This work has been supported by a grant from SIMS and NIDA

the literature this analytically defined R_0 agrees with the expression defined *ad hoc*.

If the population is subject to a vaccination campaign, we have a different situation. We cannot simply consider the non-vaccinated part of the population as the 'totally susceptible' population requested in the definition of the basic reproduction number since the vaccinated individuals participate in the mixing and contact processes. On the other hand we can compute analytically the threshold condition for the spread of an infectious disease in a population which has undergone vaccination. Later we can try to define a reproduction number for vaccinated populations.

The aim of a vaccination has to be specified. First the terminology has to be established. If a person is 'vaccinated', i.e., if a vaccine is applied to the person, then either the status of the person is unchanged (unsuccessful 'vaccination') or the susceptibility of the person is reduced. There can be various side effects, e.g., when the person gets infected then the illness is less severe or the duration of the illness or the infected period is shortened. We shall not consider these side effects of the vaccination. In our terminology a vaccination moves an individual from the susceptible state to a vaccinated state. Whereas the age-dependent susceptibility of a susceptible individual is $\beta(a)$, the susceptibility of a vaccinated individual is $\tilde{\beta}(a) < \beta(a)$. In the extreme case of complete immunity we have $\tilde{\beta}(a) = 0$. Any application of vaccine which does not lead to this transition is not considered a vaccination.

Of course the person to whom a vaccine has been applied is interested to know whether this application has been successful. Even if it is known that the application of the vaccine leads to a vaccination with a certain probability p, the individual wants to know whether the application of the vaccine has been successful or not.

From the point of the medical service the situation is somewhat different. Although one tries to protect every individual, the main goal is to prevent an outbreak of an epidemic or to eliminate the disease. This is done by reducing the reproduction number to a value below one. If an elimination seems unlikely one might think of reducing the prevalence or the incidence. Also in this case reduction of the reproduction number may be a good policy. At least in many simple models of the mass action type reducing the reproduction number is equivalent to lowering the level of prevalence.

The reproduction number is reduced by vaccination. Each application of vaccine is related to costs. These costs include expenses for calling patients, advertising vaccinations etc. and are surely age-dependent. Any unsuccessful application of vaccine to a susceptible causes similar expenses, as does application of vaccine to an immune or infected person. Hence for the vaccination campaign it is important whether immunized individuals (by having been infected or vaccinated) carry markers (as in smallpox) or are not easily distinguished from susceptibles (as in polio).

One of the main ideas of the present papers is to count only transitions into the vaccinated state as vaccinations, and to collect all unsuccessful and unnecessary applications of vaccine into cost functionals. Therefore we can keep the dynamic model simple and we can easily compute the reproduction rate.

As in previous publications (cf. Hadeler 1992) we consider demographic models in the form of homogeneous equations. The case of constant population size is included as a special case, though, and Part II of this paper (Optimal Strategies) is restricted to that case. It is expected that the optimality results can be extended to the general case in future research. The concept of homogeneous models as applied to human populations is appropriate for various reasons. First of all, practically all demographic models applied to human populations (Lexis, Leslie, Sharpe-Lotka or McKendrick models) are homogeneous, i.e., they couple recruitment to the state of the population. Furthermore, even in cases where the actual infective period (as in rubella or measles) is extremely short in comparison to life expectancy or the generation cycle time, vaccination campaigns related to the same diseases have longlasting effects. Homogeneous models may appear more complicated than 'stationary models (models with constant recruitment or constant population size) at first glance, but they are not. Homogeneous models are in fact easier to understand in situations with differential mortality (where the concept of constant population size breaks down). Finally, the stationary model can be easily recovered by introducing the assumption that fertility and mortality are balanced by the requirement of zero net population growth.

The 'stationary' solutions of homogeneous systems are exponential solutions, usually called persistent solutions. A persistent solution describes exponential growth (or decay) of the total population whereas the population structure, expressed in proportions of age, sex or other classes, remains constant. Typically we find exponential solutions describing uninfected populations, populations subject to vaccination campaigns, and infected populations. There is no bifurcation or transition from the totally susceptible to the vaccinated solution. Once the vaccination strategy is applied, the vaccinated solution just replaces the totally susceptible solution. On the other hand, there is a transition via a bifurcation from the vaccinated to the infected solution once the vaccination has not been sufficiently successful.

In loose terms, a persistent solution is defined as stable if, after a perturbation, the previous proportions are reestablished, with possibly altered total population size. Similarly to the stationary case, this concept of stability is related to a spectral problem. One has to form the linearization at the exponential solution, compute the eigenvalues of that problem, and compare to the exponent $\hat{\lambda}$ of the persistent solution (cf. Hadeler 1992). The persistent solution is linearly stable if the differences $\lambda - \hat{\lambda}$ (with $\lambda \neq \hat{\lambda}$, multiplicities counted) have negative real parts. Comparing the real parts to $\hat{\lambda}$ rather than to 0 can be understood as taking into account the 'dilution' of the infected in the growing population.

2 Model description

The variables of the model are

u susceptibles
w vaccinated (immune)
v infected.

The infected (infectious) are considered as a separate compartment in order to include diseases with long lasting or even lifelong infectivity. A limit problem with the infectious period going to zero could be studied, as suggested in Dietz and Schenzle (1985), but would not cover many important diseases. Although it may be somewhat confusing that the vaccinated are not denoted by the letter v, the notation is consistent because the vaccinated play the role of recovered in the standard SIR-model.

The parameters are

$\mu(a)$ age dependent mortality
$b(a)$ age dependent fertility
$\tilde{\mu}(a)$ mortality of infected
$\tilde{b}(a)$ fertility of infected
$\delta(a)$ differential mortality $(= \tilde{\mu}(a) - \mu(a))$
$\alpha(a)$ recovery rate
$\gamma(a)$ loss of immunity

It can be argued that α should depend on the time since infection and γ on the time since vaccination rather than on chronological age. That assumption would lead to a complicated model (two more independent variables) which lies outside the scope of the present study.

$k(a)$ contact distribution

In the present treatment of the vaccination problem the transmission coefficient is assumed as a product of the infectivity depending on the ages of the infected present in the population and on susceptibility depending on the age of the susceptible exposed to the infectivity.

$\beta(a)$ susceptibility of susceptibles
$\tilde{\beta}(a)$ susceptibility of vaccinated
$\Delta(a)$ differential susceptibility $(= \beta(a) - \tilde{\beta}(a))$
$\psi(a)$ age dependent vaccination rate

We do not introduce a separate parameter for vaccination at birth since in practice this effect can be seen as vaccination with high probability at a very early age.

L maximum age

The special case $L = \infty$ is formally used in many demographic models.

The model consists of three partial differential equations

$$
\begin{aligned}
u_t + u_a &= -\mu(a)u - \psi(a)u + \gamma(a)w - \beta(a)uV/N, \\
w_t + w_a &= -\mu(a)w + \psi(a)u + \alpha(a)v - \gamma(a)w - \tilde{\beta}(a)wV/N, \quad (2.1) \\
v_t + v_a &= -\tilde{\mu}(a)v - \alpha(a)v + (\beta(a) + \tilde{\beta}(a)w)V/N
\end{aligned}
$$

(where $u_t = \frac{\partial}{\partial t}u(t, a)$, etc.) together with appropriate boundary conditions

$$
\begin{aligned}
u(t, 0) &= \int_0^L [b(a)(u(t, a) + w(t, a)) + \tilde{b}(a)v(t, a)]\, da, \\
w(t, 0) &= 0, \quad (2.2) \\
v(t, 0) &= 0 \, .
\end{aligned}
$$

Here

$$
N(t) = \int_0^L [u(t, a) + w(t, a) + v(t, a)]\, da \quad (2.3)
$$

is the total population size, and

$$
V(t) = \int_0^L k(a)v(t, a)\, da \quad (2.4)
$$

is the number of contacts with infected of one susceptible, here assumed as independent of the age of the susceptible.

Models of a similar form have been proposed by several authors but mostly have not been investigated in detail. Probably one of the first was Dietz (1975) who proposed the stationary model with the appropriate form of the vaccination term used here and a special kernel k and the distinction of immunization by vaccination and by infection. He also proposed to study jointly the costs of the disease and the vaccination. Anderson and May (1982) consider a class of similar models, also presented in Anderson and May (1991), Section 7.2. Dietz and Schenzle (1975) have studied a model with proportionate mixing and constant population size, without differential mortality, with complete immunization. On the other hand their model is more general in the sense that the recovery rate and the infectivity depend on the time since infection. Greenhalgh (1990) studies a slightly different model (without differential mortality and without loss of immunity, but with general mixing patterns; for some of the results separability of the mixing kernel is assumed). The present model and related models just mentioned cover some typical cases, without too many special features. There are many vaccination scenarios which are not incorporated in these models, for example, one can study vaccination against sexually transmitted disease (for the case of heterosexual populations see, e.g., Hadeler and Müller (1993) or a disease like polio where several very distinct vaccines are used in different populations (Eichner 1992, Eichner *et al.* 1995). Immunization against macroparasites (Anderson and May 1991) is again a different problem.

As abbreviations we introduce

$$M(a) = \int_o^a \mu(s)ds, \qquad P(a) = \exp\{-M(a)\}. \tag{2.5}$$

The system (2.1–2.4) is homogeneous of degree 1. Hence the interesting objects are persistent solutions, i.e., exponential solutions with constant population structure.

3 Model analysis

First we consider the uninfected and non-vaccinated population which is governed by the equations (McKendrick model)

$$u_t + u_a = -\mu(a)u, \tag{3.1}$$

$$u(t,0) = \int_0^L b(a)u(t,a)\,da. \tag{3.2}$$

The persistent solution is obtained from the eigenvalue problem

$$\lambda u + u_a = -\mu(a)u, \tag{3.3}$$

$$u(0) = \int_0^L b(a)u(a)\,da, \tag{3.4}$$

as

$$u(t,a) = \hat{u}(a)\exp\{\hat{\lambda}t\}, \tag{3.5}$$

where

$$\hat{u}(a) = P(a)\exp\{-\hat{\lambda}a\} \tag{3.6}$$

is the stable age distribution, and the exponent $\hat{\lambda}$ is obtained from the characteristic equation

$$\int_0^L b(a)P(a)e^{-\hat{\lambda}a}da = 1. \tag{3.7}$$

Thus the exponential solution of the system (2.1–2.4) describing a totally susceptible population is

$$(\hat{u}(a), 0, 0)^T \exp\{\hat{\lambda}t\}. \tag{3.8}$$

Next consider the persistent solution describing a vaccinated state. It has the form

$$(\bar{u}(a), \bar{w}(a), \bar{v}(a))^T e^{\hat{\lambda}t} \tag{3.9}$$

where

$$
\begin{aligned}
\bar{u}(a) &= P(a)e^{-\hat{\lambda}a} \cdot D(a), \\
\bar{w}(a) &= P(a)e^{-\hat{\lambda}a} - \bar{u}(a), \\
\bar{v}(a) &= 0, \tag{3.10} \\
\bar{N} &= \int_0^L (\bar{u}(a) + \bar{w}(a))\, da \tag{3.11}
\end{aligned}
$$

and

$$
\begin{aligned}
D(a) &= e^{-\int_o^a (\gamma + \psi)d\tau} + \int_0^a e^{-\int_s^a (\gamma + \psi)d\tau}\gamma(s)\, ds \\
&= 1 - \int_0^a e^{-\int_s^a (\gamma + \psi)d\tau}\psi(s)\, ds \tag{3.12}
\end{aligned}
$$

From (3.12) one sees that u is an increasing function of γ and a decreasing function of ψ, as it should be according to the biological interpretation.

In order to investigate the effects of vaccination strategies on the uninfected solution one could try to compute the infected solution explicitly. This would provide information about the stationary prevalence in the presence of vaccination. However, the rather complicated calculations do not give much insight. Therefore we linearize at the vaccinated state and determine the threshold condition as well as the reproduction number.

The following steps are applied to obtain the reproduction number. First linearize the system (2.1–2.4) at the vaccinated state, then integrate over age to obtain an implicit equation for V.

The linearized system reads

$$
\begin{aligned}
u_t + u_a &= -\mu(a)u - \psi(a)u + \gamma(a)w - \beta(a)\bar{u}V/\bar{N}, \\
w_t + w_a &= -\mu(a)w + \psi(a)u + \alpha(a)v - \gamma(a)w - \tilde{\beta}(a)\bar{w}V/\bar{N}, \tag{3.13} \\
v_t + v_a &= -\tilde{\mu}(a)v - \alpha(a)v + (\beta(a)\bar{u} + \tilde{\beta}(a)\bar{w})V/\bar{N},
\end{aligned}
$$

$$
\begin{aligned}
u(t, 0) &= \int_0^L [b(a)(u(t, a) + w(t, a)) + \tilde{b}(a)v(t, a)]\, da, \\
w(t, a) &= 0, \tag{3.14} \\
v(t, 0) &= 0.
\end{aligned}
$$

We look for exponential solutions to this problem, i.e., formally we replace the derivatives u_t by λu, etc. It turns out that the problem separates. The most important equation is the equation for v, which can be written

$$v_a = -(\tilde{\mu}(a) + \alpha(a) + \lambda)v + (\beta(a)\bar{u} + \tilde{\beta}(a)\bar{w})V/\bar{N}. \qquad (3.15)$$

This equation is the key relation for the discussion of stability. From this equation we derive a characteristic equation. For the moment we assume that V is known. Then we integrate (3.15) and use the boundary condition $v(0) = 0$. We obtain an expression for $v(a)$, depending on V,

$$v(a) = \int_0^a e^{-\int_s^a (\tilde{\mu}+\alpha+\lambda)d\tau} P(s)e^{-\hat{\lambda}s}[\beta(s)D(s) + \tilde{\beta}(s)(1 - D(s))]ds V/\bar{N}.$$

This equation can be more conveniently written as

$$v(a) = P(a)e^{-\lambda a} \int_0^a e^{-\int_s^a (\delta+\alpha+\lambda-\hat{\lambda})d\tau}[\beta(s)D(s) + \tilde{\beta}(s)(1 - D(s))]ds V/\bar{N}.$$

Since V is nothing other than the weighted integral of v, we can multiply by $k(a)$, integrate with respect to a, and divide by V.

Using the explicit expression for $\bar{N}$ from (3.6), we obtain a characteristic equation for the eigenvalue λ,

$$S(\lambda) = 1, \qquad (3.16)$$

where

$$S(\lambda) = \frac{\int\limits_0^L k(a)P(a)e^{-\lambda a} \int\limits_0^a e^{-\int_s^a (\delta+\alpha+\lambda-\hat{\lambda})d\tau}[\beta(s)D(s) + \tilde{\beta}(s)(1 - D(s))]\, ds\, da}{\int\limits_0^L P(a)e^{-\lambda a}\, da}.$$

$$(3.17)$$

Notice that the eigenvalue $\hat{\lambda}$ is already determined by the demographic parameters and equation (3.7). The right hand side can also be written in the form

$$\frac{\int_0^L \left[\beta(a)D(a) + \tilde{\beta}(a)(1 - D(a))\right] P(a) \int_a^L k(s)e^{-\hat{\lambda}s-\int_a^s (\tilde{\mu}+\alpha+\lambda-\hat{\lambda})}\, ds\, da}{\int_0^L P(a)e^{-\hat{\lambda}a}\, da}.$$

$$(3.18)$$

Since $0 \leq D(s) \leq 1$, the kernel in (3.17) is nonnegative for real λ. As a function for real λ, it is strictly decreasing. It goes to zero for λ going to $+\infty$, and it goes to $+\infty$ for decreasing λ. Therefore the characteristic equation (3.16) has a unique real root λ_0. Let $\lambda = x + iy$ be another root. From $1 = S(\lambda) = |S(x + iy)| \leq S(x)$ it follows that $Re\lambda \leq \lambda_0$. Hence λ_0 is the leading root. From the general theory of homogeneous equations (see

Hadeler (1992) for a review of the finite dimensional case) it follows that λ_0 has to be compared with the exponent of growth $\hat{\lambda}$. Therefore we have the following stability criterion.

Theorem 1 *The uninfected state is linearly stable if $\lambda_0 < \hat{\lambda}$ and it is linearly unstable if $\lambda_0 > \hat{\lambda}$.*

From the explicit formula (3.17–3.18) we observe the following features (which are biologically evident but give some credibility to the model).

λ_0 increases

     if k is increased,

     if β or $\tilde{\beta}$ is increased,

     if γ is increased.

λ_0 decreases

     if α is increased,

     if $\tilde{\mu}$ is increased,

     and, most important, if ψ is increased.

Notice that the coefficient $\tilde{b}$ does not influence λ_0. In fact, it should be underlined that λ_0 is not directly related to the exponent of exponential growth of an infected solution.

Now we consider the case of constant population size, $\hat{\lambda} = 0$. This assumption says that in the uninfected state there is balanced population growth. The uninfected population is in static equilibrium,

$$\int_0^L b(a)P(a)\,da = 1. \tag{3.19}$$

Thus zero is the critical value for λ_0. Hence the critical quantity is

$$R(\psi) = \frac{\int_0^L k(a)P(a)\int_0^a e^{-\int_s^a (\delta + \alpha)\,d\tau}[\beta(s)D(s) + \tilde{\beta}(s)(1 - D(s))]ds\,da}{\int_0^L P(a)\,ds}.$$
$$\tag{3.20}$$

We define the number $R(\psi)$ as the *reproduction number in the presence of the vaccination strategy* ψ.

If no vaccination is applied ($\psi = 0$) then $R(0) = R_0$, where R_0 is the *basic reproduction number*. By what has been said earlier, vaccination leads to a decrease of R, in particular $R(\psi) \leq R_0$ for any ψ.

For subsequent applications it is convenient to write $R(\psi)$ in a different form. In (3.20) we exchange the order of integrations. Then

$$R(\psi) = \int_0^L [\beta(a)D(a) + \tilde{\beta}(a)(1 - D(a))] \int_a^L k(s)P(s)e^{-\int_a^s (\delta + \alpha)d\tau}\,ds\,da/N \tag{3.21}$$

where (from now on)

$$N = \int_0^L P(a)\,da. \tag{3.22}$$

This expression can also be seen as the life expectancy of a newborn individual.

Since $\psi \equiv 0$ implies $D(a) \equiv 1$, we find the basic reproduction number $R_0 = R(0)$ as

$$R_0 = \int_0^L \beta(a) \int_a^L k(s)P(s)e^{-\int_a^s (\delta+\alpha)d\tau}\,ds\,da/N, \tag{3.23}$$

and the representation

$$R(\psi) = R_0 - F(\psi)/N, \tag{3.24}$$

where

$$F(\psi) = \int_0^L (\beta(a) - \tilde{\beta}(a)) \int_a^L k(s)P(s)e^{\int_s^a (\delta+\alpha)\,d\tau}\,ds \int_0^a e^{-\int_\sigma^a (\gamma+\psi)\,d\tau}\psi(\sigma)\,d\sigma\,da \tag{3.25}$$

or, using the previously defined differential susceptibility,

$$F(\psi) = \int_0^L \Delta(a) \int_a^L k(s)P(s)e^{\int_s^a (\delta+\alpha)\,d\tau}\,ds \int_0^a e^{-\int_\sigma^a (\gamma+\psi)\,d\tau}\psi(\sigma)\,d\sigma\,da. \tag{3.26}$$

Theorem 2 *The quantity $F(\psi)$ is (up to the factor N) the reduction in the reproduction number that can be achieved by applying the vaccination strategy ψ.*

It is interesting to observe that this quantity depends on the differential susceptibility $\Delta(a)$ and not on $\beta(a)$, $\tilde{\beta}(a)$ separately.

Any actual vaccination campaign must aim at making $F(\psi)$ large and thus possibly reducing $R(\psi)$ to values below 1. Whether this is possible, depends, apart from economic and social side conditions (so far not incorporated into the model) on the differential susceptibility $\Delta(a)$ and the loss of immunity $\gamma(a)$.

There are three rather different situations. In the first situation we have $R_0 < 1$. Then R can be further reduced (e.g., to make it considerably less than one), but in principle vaccination is not necessary. In the second situation we have $\tilde{R}_0 > 1$ where

$$\tilde{R}_0 = \int_0^L \tilde{\beta}(a) \int_a^L k(s)P(s)e^{-\int_a^s (\delta+\alpha)d\tau}\,ds\,da/N,$$

is the reproduction rate in a totally vaccinated population. Then the disease can spread in a totally vaccinated population, and thus vaccination seems useless. Nevertheless vaccination can be used to give partial protection to individuals. The third, and most interesting situation occurs when $\tilde{R}_0 < 1 < R_0$. In that case certain strategies will reduce $R(\psi)$ to values below one and thus will lead to the elimination of the disease. The problem of how to choose optimal strategies will be covered in the second part of this paper.

We close with the explicit result for the constant coefficient case. Then we can integrate the model equations with respect to age and obtain a set of ordinary differential equations of the following form (the number k is now incorporated into β, $\tilde{\beta}$).

$$
\begin{aligned}
\dot{u} &= b(u+w) + \tilde{b}v - \mu u - \psi u + \gamma w - \frac{\beta u v}{u+w+v}, \\
\dot{w} &= \psi u - \mu w - \gamma w + \alpha v - \frac{\tilde{\beta}wv}{u+w+v}, \\
\dot{v} &= -\tilde{\mu}v - \alpha v + \frac{\beta u + \tilde{\beta}w}{u+w+v}v.
\end{aligned}
\tag{3.27}
$$

The uninfected vaccinated exponential solution is

$$
(b+\gamma, \psi, 0)^T \exp\{(b-\mu)t\}.
$$

The critical eigenvalue of the Jacobian is

$$
\lambda_0 = \frac{\beta(b+\gamma) + \tilde{\beta}\psi}{b+\gamma+\psi}.
$$

In the case of balanced population growth, $b = \mu$, the basic reproduction rate is $R_0 = \beta/(\tilde{\mu}+\alpha)$ and $N = 1/\mu$,

$$
R(\psi) = R_0 - (\beta - \tilde{\beta}) \cdot \frac{1}{\tilde{\mu}+\alpha} \cdot \frac{\psi}{\mu+\gamma+\psi} \cdot \frac{1}{\mu} \cdot \frac{1}{N}.
$$

We keep the denominator N in this expression in accordance with the general formula (3.24).

References

Anderson, R.M. and May, R.M. (1982) 'Directly Transmitted Infectious Diseases: Control by Vaccination', *Science* **215**, 1053–1060.

Anderson, R.M. and May, R.M. (1991) *Infectious Diseases of Humans, Dynamics and Control*, Oxford University Press, Oxford.

Dietz, K. (1975) 'Transmission and control of Arbovirus diseases'. In *Epidemiology*, D. Ludwig and K.L. Cooke (eds,), SIAM, Philadelphia, PA, 104–121.

Dietz, K. and Schenzle, D. (1985) 'Proportionate mixing for age-dependent infection transmissions', *J. Math. Biol.* **22**, 117–120.

Eichner, M. (1992) *Epidemiologische Modelle zur Ausrottung der Kinderlähmung*, Dissertation Tübingen.

Eichner, M., Hadeler, K.P. and Dietz, K. (1995) 'Stochastic models for the eradication of poliomyelitis; minimum population size of polio virus persistence'. In *Models for Infectious Human Diseases: Their Structure and Relation to Data*, V. Isham and G. Medley (eds.), Cambridge University Press, Cambridge.

Greenhalgh, D. (1990) 'Vaccination campaigns for common childhood diseases', *Math. Biosc.* **100**, 201–240.

Hadeler, K.P. (1992) 'Periodic solutions of homogeneous equations', *J. Diff. Eq.* **95**, 183–202.

Hadeler, K.P. and Müller, J. (1993) 'Vaccination strategies for sexually transmitted diseases'. In *Proc. 3rd Internat. Conf. on Mathematical Population Dynamics*, Pau (France), 1992, O. Arino, D. Axelrod and M. Kimmel (eds.).

Hadeler, K.P., Müller, J. (1995) 'Vaccination in age structured populations II: Optimal strategies'. In *Models for Infectious Human diseases: Their Structure and relation to Data*, V. Isham and G. Medley (eds.), Cambridge University Press, Cambridge.

Heesterbeek, H. (1992) R_0, Dissertation, University of Leiden.

Vaccination in Age Structured Populations II: Optimal Strategies

K.P. Hadeler and J. Müller

1 Introduction

In the first part of this paper a model for vaccination in an age structured population was presented.

We consider the situation where the population is in demographic equilibrium. A vaccination strategy ψ converts susceptibles of age a into (partly) immunes of age a (Dietz 1974). We underline also that the vaccination strategy is stationary. When a cohort arrives at age a, the (still) existing susceptibles are converted into vaccinated. Let R_ψ be the reproduction number in the presence of the vaccination strategy ψ. Let $R_0 = R(0)$ be the basic reproduction number and let $\tilde{R}_0$ be the reproduction number in the situation where all individuals are vaccinated. In the first part it has been shown that the reproduction number is given by

$$R(\psi) = R_0 - F(\psi)/N \tag{1.1}$$

where

$$F(\psi) = \int_0^L \Delta(a) \int_a^L k(s) P(s) e^{\int_s^a (\delta + \alpha)\, d\tau}\, ds \int_0^a e^{-\int_\sigma^a (\gamma + \psi)\, d\tau} \psi(\sigma)\, d\sigma\, da, \tag{1.2}$$

and

$$N = \int_0^L P(a)\, da. \tag{1.3}$$

The functions

$$\delta(a) = \tilde{\mu}(a) - \mu(a), \qquad \Delta(a) = \beta(a) - \tilde{\beta}(a)$$

are the differential mortality and the differential susceptibility.

The aim of the vaccination strategy ψ is to make $F(\psi)$ large and thus decrease $R(\psi)$. In practice the application of vaccination strategies is limited by costs. The costs include expenses for the application of the vaccine, compliance of the different age classes and necessary advertisement campaign, etc. We assume that the expenses of one vaccination at age a are given by a positive number $\kappa(a)$, and that otherwise the total costs depend linearly on

This work has been supported by a grant from SIMS and NIDA

the number of vaccinations. This assumption is not unrealistic since any basic expenses getting the campaign started represent an additive constant which does not play a role in the optimization process. We repeat that vaccination always means a transition from the susceptible state u to the vaccinated (partly immune) state w. Applications of vaccine which do not lead to a vaccination are incorporated into the cost function $\kappa(a)$. If, e.g., the costs for application of the vaccine is $\kappa_0(a)$ and only a proportion p of applications is successful then $\kappa(a) = \kappa_0(a)/p$. Thus the expenses are high if the vaccine is not very effective. It is tacitly assumed that vaccine applications can be rapidly repeated, at correspondingly high costs.

As pointed out earlier there is an essential difference between the case where susceptibles can be recognized and the other case where susceptibles, vaccinated and infected cannot be distinguished. Thus we have

Scenario I: Only susceptibles are vaccinated.

Scenario II: Vaccination is applied to susceptibles, immunes, and infected.

Assume the costs of the vaccination strategy ψ are $C(\psi)$. Then we can define several optimization problems.

P1. Achieve a prescribed goal at minimal costs, i.e., prescribe a level R_* for $R(\psi)$ and minimize $C(\psi)$ under the side condition $R(\psi) \leq R_*$.

P2. Achieve an optimum at given expenses, e.g., prescribe the maximal expenses $\bar{\kappa}$ and minimize $R(\psi)$ under the side condition that $C(\psi) \leq \bar{\kappa}$.

P3. The naive optimum: Minimize the quotient $(R_0 - R(\psi))/C(\psi)$.

2 Scenario I: vaccination of susceptibles only

Here susceptibles can be distinguished from immunes. The total cost of the vaccination strategy is $C(\psi) = \int_0^L \kappa(a)\psi(a)\bar{u}(a)\,da$, so that

$$C(\psi) = \int_0^L \kappa(a)P(a)\psi(a)D(a)da, \tag{2.1}$$

where

$$\begin{aligned}
D(a) &= e^{-\int_0^a (\gamma+\psi)\,d\tau} + \int_0^a e^{-\int_s^a (\gamma+\psi)d\tau}\gamma(s)\,ds \\
&= 1 - \int_0^a e^{-\int_s^a (\gamma+\psi)d\tau}\psi(s)\,ds
\end{aligned}$$

(see equations (3.9–3.12) of paper I, with $\lambda = 0$). First we consider the case where immunity lasts,

$$\gamma(a) \equiv 0. \tag{2.2}$$

Then the functionals $F(\psi)$, $C(\psi)$ simplify to

$$F(\psi) = \int_0^L \Delta(a) \int_a^L k(s)P(s)e^{\int_s^a (\delta+\alpha)\,d\tau}\,ds \cdot \int_0^a e^{-\int_\sigma^a \psi\,d\tau}\psi(\sigma)\,d\sigma\,da, \tag{2.3}$$

$$C(\psi) = \int_0^L \kappa(a)P(a)\psi(a)e^{-\int_0^a \psi\,d\tau}\,da. \tag{2.4}$$

In this formulation both functionals are nonlinear. Therefore we apply a transformation (which is similar to the transition from a hazard function to a density)

$$\phi(a) = -\frac{d}{da}e^{-\int_0^a \psi(s)\,ds} = \psi(a)e^{-\int_0^a \psi(s)\,ds}, \qquad (2.5)$$

or, conversely,

$$\psi(a) = \frac{\phi(a)}{1 - \int_0^a \phi(s)ds}. \qquad (2.6)$$

We denote $F(\psi) = \tilde{F}(\phi)$, $C(\psi) = \tilde{C}(\phi)$. In a first step the substitution leads to

$$\tilde{F}(\phi) = \int_0^L \Delta(a) \int_a^L k(s)P(s)e^{-\int_a^s(\delta+\alpha)\,d\tau} \int_0^a \phi(\sigma)\,d\sigma\,da. \qquad (2.7)$$

If we exchange the order of integrations, we arrive at

$$\tilde{F}(\phi) \;=\; \int_0^L K(a)\phi(a)\,da, \qquad (2.8)$$

$$\tilde{C}(\phi) \;=\; \int_0^L B(a)\phi(a)\,da, \qquad (2.9)$$

$$Q(\phi) \;=\; \int_0^L \phi(a)\,da, \qquad (2.10)$$

where the kernels are given by

$$K(a) \;=\; \int_0^L \Delta(\sigma) \int_\sigma^L k(s)P(s)e^{-\int_\sigma^s(\delta+\alpha)\,d\tau}\,ds\,d\sigma \qquad (2.11)$$
$$B(a) \;=\; \kappa(a)P(a). \qquad (2.12)$$

We define

$$\rho = (R_0 - R_*)N. \qquad (2.13)$$

Again consider Problems P1, P2, P3, now for the function ϕ. In view of (9) we require that $\phi(x)$ is nonnegative and that the integral does not exceed 1, i.e., $Q(\phi) \le 1$. Then these problems assume the following form.

P1. Find the minimum of $\tilde{C}(\phi)$ under $\tilde{F}(\phi) \ge \rho$, $\phi \ge 0$, $Q(\phi) \le 1$.

P2. Find the maximum of $\tilde{F}(\phi)$ under $\tilde{C}(\phi) \le \bar{\kappa}$, $\phi \ge 0$, $Q(\phi) \le 1$.

P3. Find the maximum of $\tilde{F}(\phi)/\tilde{C}(\phi)$ under $\phi \ge 0$, $Q(\phi) \le 1$.

First consider **P1**. We assume that the goal can be achieved, i.e., $\tilde{R} < R_*$. The minimum problem is linear, and thus established tools can be applied. We shall use the necessary conditions of the Kuhn–Tucker theorem (saddle point theorem) for restricted convex (here: linear) optimization problems. The classical formulation of the Kuhn–Tucker theorem (see, e.g., Stoer and Witzgall (1970, chapter 6) for a detailed exposition) has been given for problems in finite dimensions. We shall not introduce a formal analytic setting for the problem to make the application of the theorem rigorous. At present we want to gain insight into the problem and explain why it is sufficient to look for relatively simple types of vaccination strategies. A rigorous proof, following a somewhat different approach, will be given in a forthcoming paper by J. Müller. Of course the present approach is valid for finite dimensional discretizations of the problem (Lexis models) and thus covers the cases of practical importance.

We introduce the Lagrange function

$$H(\phi, \xi, \eta) \equiv \tilde{C}(\phi) - \eta[\rho - \tilde{F}(\phi)] - \xi[Q(\phi) - 1] \qquad (2.14)$$

where ξ, η are nonnegative real numbers. The Kuhn–Tucker conditions read

$$B(a) - \eta K(a) - \xi \ \geq \ 0 \quad \text{for} \quad 0 \leq a \leq L, \qquad (2.15)$$
$$Q(\phi) \ \leq \ 1, \qquad (2.16)$$
$$\tilde{F}(\phi)) \ \geq \ \rho, \qquad (2.17)$$
$$\tilde{C}(\phi) - \eta \tilde{F}(\phi) - \xi Q(\phi) \ = \ 0, \qquad (2.18)$$
$$\eta(\rho - \tilde{F}(\phi)) \ = \ 0, \qquad (2.19)$$
$$\xi(Q(\phi) - 1) \ = \ 0. \qquad (2.20)$$

There are several cases.

Case 1: $Q(\phi) < 1$.
Then $\xi = 0$, and $B(a) \geq \eta K(a)$ with $\eta \geq 0$. From (15d) it follows that $\tilde{C}(\phi) = \tilde{F}(\phi)$. Invoking the explicit expressions for $\tilde{C}(\phi)$, $\tilde{F}(\phi)$ from (12), we find

$$\frac{B(a)}{K(a)} \geq \frac{\int_0^L B(a)\phi(a)\,da}{\int_0^L K(a)\phi(a)\,da}. \qquad (2.21)$$

The right hand side is the weighted arithmetic mean (with weight ϕ) of the left hand side, and it is smaller than all the quantities averaged. Thus necessarily, in a generic situation, ϕ is a delta function concentrated at the minimum of the function $B(a)/K(a)$.

Remark. The word 'generic' is used in the following sense. For arbitrary positive continuous functions $B(a)$ and $K(a)$ nothing can be said about the set where the quotient assumes its minimum. However, for almost all functions the minimum is assumed at a single point. This argument can be made mathematically rigorous by fixing a topology (say, the uniform topology), then there is an open dense set where the quotient assumes its minimum at a single point. Hence generically the quotient assumes its minimum at a single point. In our case some of the coefficient functions are special, e.g., the function $K(a)$ is monotone. The argument is still valid if we accept general functions κ.

We return to the function ψ. Formally $\psi(a) = c\delta_A(a)$ with some fixed age A and some constant c. Then

$$\int_0^a \psi\,d\tau = \begin{cases} 0 & \text{for } a < A, \\ c & \text{for } a > A, \end{cases}$$

and

$$e^{-\int_0^a \psi d\tau} = \begin{cases} 1 & \text{for } a < A, \\ e^{-c} & \text{for } a > A, \end{cases}$$

$$\phi(a) = \psi(a)e^{-\int_0^a \psi\, d\tau} = -\frac{d}{da}e^{-\int_0^a \psi\, d\tau} = (1 - e^{-c})\delta_A(a),$$

and thus

$$C(\psi) = B(A)(1 - e^{-c}), \tag{2.22}$$

$$F(\psi) = K(A)(1 - e^{-c}). \tag{2.23}$$

Case 2: $Q(\phi) = 1$.
Then ξ need not vanish, $\xi = C(\phi) - \eta F(\phi)$,

$$B(a) - \eta K(a) \geq \frac{\int_0^L [B(a) - \eta K(a)]\phi(a)\, da}{\int_0^L \phi(a)\, da}.$$

For fixed η the right hand side is the weighted average of the left hand side. Hence, in a generic situation (η fixed) the weight is a delta function concentrated at the minimum of the left hand side. But here η is an unknown parameter. This parameter can be chosen, in a generic situation, in such a way as to make the function $B(a) - \eta K(a)$ assume its minimum at exactly two points. Hence, in a generic situation, ϕ is a convex combination of two delta functions, and η is chosen in such a way that $B(a) - \eta K(a)$ assumes its minimum at two points A_1, A_2. Thus $\psi(a) = c\delta_{A_1}(a) + c_1\delta_{A_2}(a)$. As before we find

$$\phi(a) = \delta_{A_1}(a)(1 - e^{-c}) + \delta_{A_2}(a)(e^{-c} - e^{-c-c_1}).$$

Since we know $Q(\phi) = 1$ we have formally $c_1 = \infty$ and thus

$$C(\psi) = B(A_1)(1 - e^{-c}) + B(A_2)e^{-c}, \tag{2.24}$$

$$F(\psi) = K(A_1)(1 - e^{-c}) + K(A_2)e^{-c}. \tag{2.25}$$

Result 1 *In a generic situation the optimal vaccination strategy in Problem P1 is either a one-age strategy with vaccination at exactly one age A, or it is a two age strategy where part of the population is vaccinated at an age A_1 and at a later age A_2 all then remaining susceptibles are vaccinated.*

The phenomenon that certain optimization problems show optimal distributions in the form of a sum of two point masses is known otherwise. In the context of epidemic models it has been found by Kaplan (1991) in connection with a worst case analysis of epidemic spread. These continuous problems bear some similarity to discrete optimization problems known as knapsack problems or bin packing problems (see, e.g., Foulds (1981) or Parker and Rardin (1988)).

Now we determine the optimal vaccination ages for the two types of strategies. Notice that $K(a)$ is a decreasing function of a and that $\rho < K(0)$.

Since K decreases to 0, there is a first value of A such that $K(A) = \rho$. Call this value A_*. Then the optimal one-age strategy is obtained by minimizing the quotient $B(A)/K(A)$ in the interval $[0, A_*]$. Let $\bar{A}$ be the optimal age. Then the corresponding c is obtained from the equation $e^{-c} = 1 - \rho/K(\bar{A})$, and the corresponding total costs are

$$C = B(\bar{A})/K(\bar{A})\rho.$$

Now consider two-age strategies. For given A_1, A_2 we find the appropriate c as

$$e^{-c} = \frac{K(A_1) - \rho}{K(A_1) - K(A_2)}.$$

Since $e^{-c} \in (0,1)$, we have necessarily $A_1 \in [0, A_*]$, $A_2 \in [A_*, L]$. Then the expenses are

$$C(A_1, A_2) = \frac{\rho - K(A_2)}{K(A_1) - K(A_2)}B(A_1) + \frac{K(A_1) - \rho}{K(A_1) - K(A_2)}B(A_2). \tag{2.26}$$

Hence the expenses are a convex combination of $B(A_1)$, $B(A_2)$. This expression can also be written as

$$C(A_1, A_2) = B(A_1) - \frac{B(A_1) - B(A_2)}{K(A_1) - K(A_2)}[K(A_1) - \rho], \tag{2.27}$$

$$C(A_1, A_2) = B(A_2) + \frac{B(A_1) - B(A_2)}{K(A_1) - K(A_2)}[\rho - K(A_2)], \tag{2.28}$$

or

$$C(A_1, A_2) = (1 - \sigma)\frac{B(A_1)}{K(A_1)}\rho + \sigma\frac{B(A_2)}{K(A_2)}\rho \tag{2.29}$$

with

$$\sigma = \frac{K(A_1)K(A_2)}{K(A_1) - K(A_2)} \cdot \frac{K(A_1) - \rho}{\rho K(A_1)} \in (0,1).$$

Hence we have the following result on Problem 1.

Result 2 *Determine A_* from $K(A_*) = \rho$. Determine the minimum of the quotient $B(A)/K(A)$ for $0 \leq A \leq L$. Suppose the minimum is assumed in $\hat{A}$. If $\hat{A} \in (0, A_*]$ then there is an optimal strategy which is a one-age strategy with age $\hat{A}$.*

If $\hat{A} \in (A_*, L]$ then the optimal two-age strategy is found by minimizing the expression $C(A_1, A_2)$ on $A_1 \in [0, A_*]$, $A_2 \in [A_*, L]$. As it is obvious from the representation (2.27,2.28) the minimum is found by determining the extremes of the quotient $(B(A_1) - B(A_2))/(K(A_1) - K(A_2))$ (it depends on the qualitative properties of the function $B(A)$ whether the maximum or the minimum of the quotient has to be chosen).

A verbal explanation of the result seems appropriate. For simplicity we assume $\tilde{\beta} = 0$ (complete protection). If everybody were vaccinated at birth

108 Hadeler and Müller

then $R(\psi) = 0$. That strategy would vaccinate many unnecessarily. The age A_* is that age, at which vaccination of the whole age class would lead exactly to the requested reduction from R_0 to R_*. Since at that age, application of vaccine is possibly too expensive, one would rather apply vaccine at some earlier age. A candidate for an optimum age is that age that minimizes $B(a)/K(a)$. Assume the quotient assumes its minimum over $a \in [0, L]$ at $\hat{A}$. If $\hat{A} \in [0, A_*]$ then an optimal one age strategy has been found. If $\hat{A} > A_*$ then one tends to choose a one age strategy at that age at which the quotient assumes its minimum over $[0, A_*]$. But in this case there is a better strategy, namely a two age strategy where indeed some individuals are vaccinated before A_* (namely at A_1) but all others (then remaining) at a later age A_2 when expenses per vaccination are low.

Problem P2 seems slightly more complicated. Again we define a Lagrange function

$$H_2(\phi, u, v) = \tilde{F}(\phi) - \eta[\tilde{C}(\phi) - \bar{\kappa}] - \xi[Q(\phi) - 1]$$

where ξ, η are nonnegative reals. The necessary conditions read

$$B(a) - \eta K(a) - \xi \geq 0, \tag{2.30}$$
$$\tilde{C}(\phi) \leq \bar{\kappa}, \qquad Q(\phi) \leq 1, \tag{2.31}$$
$$\tilde{F}(\phi) - \eta\tilde{C}(\phi) - \xi Q(\phi) = 0, \tag{2.32}$$
$$\xi(Q(\phi) - 1) = 0, \qquad \eta(\tilde{C}(\phi) - \bar{\kappa}) = 0. \tag{2.33}$$

There are essentially four cases.
Case 1: $Q(\phi) < 1$, $\tilde{C}(\phi) < \bar{\kappa}$.
Then necessarily $\xi = 0$, $\eta = 0$, $\tilde{F}(\phi) = 0$ which leads immediately to a contradiction.
Case 2: $Q(\phi) = 1$, $\tilde{C}(\phi) < \bar{\kappa}$.
This leads to $\eta = 0$ and $\xi = \tilde{F}(\phi)/Q(\phi)$. Thus an optimal ϕ satisfies $\phi \geq 0$, $Q(\phi) = 1$, and $B(a) \geq \tilde{F}(\phi)$ for all a with $\tilde{F}(\phi)$ maximal. Hence, in a generic situation, ϕ is concentrated at one point, and ψ is a one-age strategy.
Case 3: $Q(\phi) < 1$, $\tilde{C}(\phi) = \bar{\kappa}$.
Then $\xi = 0$, and $\eta = \tilde{F}(\phi)/\tilde{C}(\phi)$, and

$$\frac{K(a)}{B(a)} \geq \frac{\int_0^L K(a)\phi(a)da}{\int_0^L B(a)\phi(a)da} \quad \text{for} \quad 0 \leq a \leq L,$$

which leads to one-age strategies.
Case 4: $Q(\phi) = 1$, $\tilde{C}(\phi) = \bar{\kappa}$.
Then

$$B(a) - \eta K(a) \geq \int_0^L (B(a) - \eta K(a))da \quad \text{for} \quad 0 \leq a \leq L$$

which again leads to a two-age strategy.

We can use the tools which have been developed for Problem 1. The essential cases are Cases 2,3,4. Notice that, in contrast to the function $K(a)$, the functions $\kappa(a)$ and $B(a)$ need not be monotone.

Cases 2,3.

For a one-age strategy we have equations (2.22–2.23). Hence necessarily $B(A)(1 - e^{-c}) = \bar{\kappa}$ and thus $B(A) \geq \bar{\kappa}$. Also

$$F(\psi) = \kappa K(A)/B(A). \tag{2.34}$$

Put $\mathcal{M}_{\bar{\kappa}} = \{a : 0 \leq a \leq L, B(a) \geq \bar{\kappa}\}$. Maximize (2.34) on $\mathcal{M}_{\bar{\kappa}}$. Let a maximum be assumed at $\bar{A}$. Then determine c from the equation $(1 - e^{-c}) = \bar{\kappa}/B(\bar{A}) \in (0, 1]$ and $F(\psi) = K(\bar{A})(1 - e^{-c})$.

Case 4

For two-age strategies we have (2.24–2.25). We find e^{-c} from the equation

$$\bar{\kappa} = B(A_1)(1 - e^{-c}) + B(A_2)e^{-c}.$$

This value may not be feasible. The set of feasible pairs is

$$\mathcal{N}_{\bar{\kappa}} =$$
$$\{(A_1, A_2) : 0 \leq A_1 \leq A_2 \leq L, 0 \leq (\bar{\kappa} - B(A_1))/(B(A_2) - B(A_1)) \leq 1\}.$$

On this set one considers the function

$$F(\psi) = K(A_1)\frac{B(A_2) - \bar{\kappa}}{B(A_2) - B(A_1)} + K(A_2)\frac{\bar{\kappa} - B(A_2)}{B(A_2) - B(A_1)}. \tag{2.35}$$

Hence we have the following result on Problem 2.

Result 3 *For the solution of Problem 2 first determine the two sets $\mathcal{M}_{\bar{\kappa}}$ and $\mathcal{N}_{\bar{\kappa}}$ and maximize the two expressions (2.34), (2.35), respectively.*

Without any monotonicity assumptions on $\kappa(a)$ it will be impossible to get a more detailed description.

We do not discuss Problem 3 which seems of lesser interest.

3 Scenario II: vaccination regardless of epidemiological status

Again we have problems P1, P2, P3. One might think that, similarly to the infection term in a structured population model, the vaccination term should be modeled by some nonlinear term describing the 'vaccination kinetics', in particular saturation effects. However, this approach does not seem appropriate. On the contrary, the equations for the time evolution remain unchanged since, by definition, the rate ψ counts effective vaccinations. The noneffective vaccinations have to be considered in the cost functional. To find the appropriate form of the functional, assume that a vaccination strategy ψ is indiscriminately applied to susceptibles, vaccinated, and infected. Then the total treatments at age a are $\psi(a)(u(a) + w(a) + v(a))$, but only $\psi(a)u(a)$ lead to immunization of susceptibles. Hence the cost functional is

$$C(\psi) = \int_0^L \kappa(a)P(a)\psi(a)\,da = \int_0^L B(a)\psi(a)\,da. \tag{3.1}$$

First consider Problem 1. Prescribe a level R_* for $R(\psi)$ which should be achieved at least, $R(\psi) = R_0 - F(\psi)/N \leq R_*$, i.e., we require

$$F(\psi) \geq N(R_0 - R_*) = \rho. \tag{3.2}$$

From (3) we find by integration

$$F(\psi) = \int_0^L \Delta(a) \int_a^L k(s)P(s)e^{-\int_s^a (\delta+\alpha)\,d\tau}\,ds(1 - e^{-\int_o^a \psi\,d\sigma})\,da \tag{3.3}$$

from where we see that F is concave in ψ. We have to minimize the linear functional C under the convex side conditions $\rho - F(\psi) \leq 0$ and $\psi \geq 0$. Again define a Lagrange functional

$$H_3(\psi, \xi) \equiv C(\psi) + \xi(\rho - F(\psi)) \tag{26}$$

with ξ nonnegative.

The Kuhn-Tucker conditions read

$$C'(\psi) - \xi F'(\psi) \ \geq \ 0, \tag{3.4}$$
$$F(\psi) \ \geq \ \rho, \tag{3.5}$$
$$C'(\psi)\psi - \xi F'(\psi)\psi \ = \ 0, \tag{3.6}$$
$$\xi(\rho - F(\psi)) \ = \ 0. \tag{3.7}$$

Case 1: $F(\psi) > \rho$, $\xi > 0$.
This leads immediately to a contradiction.

Case 2: $F(\psi) = \rho$, $\xi > 0$.
To the conditions $C'(\psi) - \xi F'(\psi) \geq 0$, $C'(\psi)\psi - uF'(\psi)\psi = 0$, we can apply the same argument as in Scenario I, Problem 1, Case 1. If we eliminate ξ, the conditions say $C'(\psi)(a)/F'(\psi)(a) \geq C'(\psi)\psi/F'(\psi)\psi$. Thus we have an arithmetic mean which is below all the values it is averaging. In a generic situation, this is possible only if ψ is a one-age strategy. But here the kernel of F' is depending itself on the function ψ. Hence, taking this freedom into account, we should look rather for two-age strategies.

Remark. In contrast to Scenario I, Problem 1, Case 2, where the existence of one additional parameter, in a generic situation, leads to a two-age strategy by a rigorous argument, the present argument is not rigorous. Nevertheless the family of one- and two-age strategies that will be discussed now looks very convincing.

For a one-age strategy at age A we find the same expression as in (2.22-2.23). This is not surprising since for a one-age strategy scenarios I and II are equivalent.

For a two-age strategy $\psi(a) = c_1\delta_{A_1}(a) + c_2\delta_{A_2}(a)$ with $A_1 < A_2$ we obtain, quite differently from (2.24–2.25), the expressions

$$C(\psi) = B(A_1)(1 - e^{-c_1}) + B(A_2)(1 - e^{-c_2}), \qquad (3.8)$$
$$F(\psi) = K(A_1)(1 - e^{-c_1}) + K(A_2)e^{-c_1}(1 - e^{-c_2}). \qquad (3.9)$$

Consider the problem of minimizing $C(\psi)$ under the side condition $F(\psi) \geq \rho$. This problem requires some elementary calculations. Denote $K(A_i) = K_i$, $B(A_i) = B_i$, $1 - e^{-c_i} = \xi_i$, for $i = 1, 2$. Then $B_1\xi_1 + B_2\xi_2$ has to be minimized under the conditions $K_1\xi_1 + K_2(1 - \xi_1)\xi_2 \geq \rho$ and $0 \leq \xi_i \leq 1$. Thus the feasible set is bounded by straight lines and the graph of the hyperbola $\xi_2 = \varphi(\xi_1) \equiv (\rho - K_1\xi_1)/(K_2(1 - \xi_1))$. The graph of the hyperbola is concave and it intersects the ξ_1-axis somewhere in $(0,1)$ and the ξ_2-axis somewhere in $(0, \infty)$. There are two cases. If $\varphi(0) < 1$ then the minimum is attained for either $\xi_1 = 0$ or $\xi_2 = 0$ and we are back at a one-age strategy. If $\varphi(0) > 1$ then the minimum is either attained at a point with $\xi_2 = 0$ (one-age strategy) or at a point with $\xi_2 = 1$ corresponding to a two-age strategy where at the second age the whole age class is vaccinated.

From this argument the next result follows.

Result 4 *In Scenario II, Problem 1, the optimal strategy can be found as follows. Define A_* as the solution of the equation $K(A) = \rho$. Minimize the quotient $B(a)/K(a)$ in $[0, L]$. Let the minimum be attained at $\hat{A}$. If $\hat{A} \leq A_*$ then $A = \hat{A}$, $1 - e^{-c} = \rho/K(\hat{A})$ defines an optimal one-age strategy. If $\hat{A} > A_*$ then there is an optimal two-age strategy which can be found by minimizing*

$$C(\psi) = B(A_1)\frac{\rho - K(A_2)}{K(A_1) - K(A_2)} + B(A_2). \qquad (3.10)$$

Notice the difference from (2.26–2.29). At present we shall not discuss Problem P2 with Scenario II.

Next we discuss the case where immunity can be lost, i.e., the case $\gamma > 0$. We just give an outline of the approach and the results. For simplicity we assume that γ is a positive constant. We also assume constant expenses, $\kappa \equiv 1$, and $L = \infty$, and that $\mu(a)$ has a positive lower bound.

We define the operator S which associates with each vaccination strategy ψ (in the space $L_1[0, \infty)$) the remaining susceptible population. For a given vaccination strategy $\psi(a)$, which lies in the space L_1,

$$S[\psi](a) = P(a)D(a).$$

This makes sense from a biological point of view because *the infectious agent 'sees' $S[\psi]$ and not ψ*. On the space of strategies we define a new metric by $d(\psi_1, \psi_2) = \|S[\psi_1] - S[\psi_2]\|_1$. Now the space Ψ of strategies is the closure of the positive cone of L_1 with this metric. It can be shown, that Ψ is compact and that the set $S[\Psi]$ (the set of susceptible populations left by strategies ψ) is compact and convex. Now problem P2 can be formulated as follows.

P2 Prescribe costs $\bar{\kappa}$, assume $\bar{\kappa} \leq S[0](0) + \int_0^\infty \gamma S[0](\tau)\, d\tau$, and find a $\psi \in \Psi$ with costs not greater than $\bar{\kappa}$ and minimal reproduction number. It turns out

that at the optimum the costs are equal to $\bar{\kappa}$. Now the cost functional and the reproduction number are both linear in $S[\psi]$.:

$$R(\psi) = \int_0^\infty k(a) \int_0^a e^{-\int_\tau^a \bar{\mu} + \alpha\, d\sigma} \frac{S[\psi]}{N} \beta(\tau)\, d\tau\, da,$$

$$C(\psi) = S[0](0) + \int_0^\infty \gamma S[0](\tau)\, d\tau - \int_0^\infty (\mu + \gamma) S[\psi](\tau)\, d\tau.$$

So the level sets $M_\eta = \{S[\psi] : \psi \in \Psi,\ C(\psi) = \eta\}$ are convex and compact, and, in a generic situation, the optimum is assumed at an extremal point (vertex) of $M_{\bar{\kappa}}$. A strategy for which $S[\psi]$ is an extremal point of $M_{\bar{\kappa}}$ is called an extremal strategy for costs $\bar{\kappa}$. A rather lengthy argument shows that the extremal strategies for costs $\bar{\kappa}$ can be found in the following way.

Choose $\mathcal{A}$ as an arbitrary closed subset of $[0, L]$. Vaccinate all individuals in the age classes $a \in \mathcal{A}$. If costs are too high then this strategy is not feasible. If costs are $\bar{\kappa}$ then an extremal strategy has been found. If costs are less than $\bar{\kappa}$ choose an additional one age strategy where possibly only a part of the population has to be vaccinated, so that the expenses $\bar{\kappa}$ are reached.

This set is still far too big to find explicit optimal strategies. Therefore we look for monotonicity conditions which ensure that extremal strategies have connected support (cover an age interval).

Monotonicity condition.
Let

$$r(a) = \frac{\beta(a)}{N} \int_a^\infty e^{-\int_a^\tau \bar{\mu} + \alpha\, d\tau'} k(\tau)\, d\tau,$$

and

$$G(a) = \int_a^\infty e^{-\int_a^\tau \mu + \gamma\, d\tau'} r(\tau)\, d\tau.$$

Then $\psi = c\delta_a$ with $G(\psi) = v$ yields

$$R(\psi) = R(0) - vG(a)$$

Result 5 *Assume there is a nonnegative a_0 such that $dG(a)/da > 0$ for $a < a_0$, $dG(a)/da < 0$ for $a > a_0$, and $\frac{d}{da}[r(a)/(\mu(a) + \gamma)] > 0$ for $a < a_0$ Then there exists a unique optimal vaccination strategy. This strategy has the form that in one closed age interval everybody is vaccinated. The interval* *may shrink to a point and in that case perhaps only a part of the population needs to be vaccinated.*

The function $G(a)$ describes the effect of one single vaccination at age a. Caused by the monotonicity conditions this effect has one maximum at age a_0 and it decreases monotonely with the distance $|a - a_0|$. Therefore a good strategy will choose a vaccination age as close to a_0 as possible. Thus the support of the best strategy must be connected, it is an interval.

We give a verbal description of the strategy. There is an age interval $[A_1, A_2]$ with optimally chosen A_1 and A_2. Everybody who reaches the age A_1 will be vaccinated. Everybody who loses immunity during the age interval $[A_1, A_2]$ is revaccinated. Individuals of older age who lose immunity will not be vaccinated again.

Thus even in this case there is an indication that cohort vaccination is close to optimal. Scenario I with $\gamma > 0$ is realistic only when the loss of immunity can be observed. Scenario II will be studied in a forthcoming paper.

References

Foulds, L.R. (1981) *Optimization Techniques*, Springer Verlag.

Hadeler, K.P., and Müller, J. (1995) 'Vaccination in age-structured populations I: The reproduction number', this volume.

Kaplan, E.H. (1991) 'Mean-max bounds for worst-case endemic mixing models', *Math. Biosc.* **105**, 97–109.

Parker, R.G., and Rardin, R.L. (1988) *Discrete Optimization*, Academic Press.

Stoer, J., and Witzgall, Chr. (1970) *Convexity and Optimization in Finite Dimension I*, Springer Verlag.

Discussion

PETO Within age-class, mixing can generate transmission dynamics such that virus may continue to circulate within age classes younger than that which the model of Hadeler and Muller suggests to be optimal for vaccination. By removing the possibility of heterogeneities in contact between different age classes, do the results produced by the model ignore this possibility?

REPLY Our assumption of (weighted) proportionate mixing rules out mixing patterns which are close to 'within age-class'. The general case is much harder since R_0 can be given only implicitly (see the paper by Greenhalgh quoted in Part I).

HASIBEDER I would like to add two comments to Karl Hadeler's talk:

(1) One problem dealt with is that of determining an optimal vaccination pattern which yields a maximal reduction of the basic reproduction number R_0 at prescribed costs. The optimal solution obviously is useful if

R_0 becomes less than 1 and consequently the infection is eliminated. But if, for any possible vaccination strategy, R_0 remains greater than 1, i.e. the infection cannot be eliminated at the prescribed costs, one would regard that vaccination pattern as optimal which reduces the prevalence in the whole population (or some weighted average of the prevalences in the various age cohorts) to a minimum.

Dye and Hasibeder (1986) showed, though for a vector-transmitted infection and without considering vaccination, that an increase of R_0 due to heterogeneity can coincide with a decrease of the prevalence. For this reason I suspect that Hadeler's optimal vaccination pattern is not necessarily in general always that strategy which also reduces the prevalence to a minimum.

(2) At the end of his talk, Karl Hadeler posed the question whether we still should use the term 'critical vaccination level' (which reduces R_0 exactly to 1) if, as in his paper, different proportions have to be vaccinated at different ages: I think that certainly we should, but the concept of the 'critical vaccination level' has to be generalized from being a simple number.

When the definition of R_0 was extended to heterogeneous populations, R_0 became the spectral radius of some operator, and the 'primary case' in its interpretation had to be replaced with the 'typical infected individual' which is characterized by some density (Diekmann, Heesterbeek and Metz 1990). Similarly the 'critical vaccination level' for a heterogeneous population has to be viewed as some vector, if there is a finite number of homogeneous subpopulations, or as some function of age, if the model deals with an age-structured population.

REPLY

(1) For many epidemic dynamics there is monotone dependence between R_0 and prevalence. Even in this situation the minimum problems for prevalence should be investigated too.

(2) In a general setting, there is a separating surface in the parameter space.

References

Diekmann, O., Heesterbeek, J.A.P. and Metz, J.A.J. (1990) 'On the definition and computation of the basic reproduction ratio in models for infectious diseases in heterogeneous populations', *J. Math. Biol.* **28**, 365–382.

Dye, C. and Hasibeder, G. (1986) 'Population dynamics of mosquito-borne disease: effects of flies which bite some people more frequently than others', *Trans. Roy. Soc. Trop. Med. Hyg.* **80**, 69–77.

Part 2
Dynamics of immunity

Evolutionary Dynamics of HIV Infections

Martin Nowak

1 Introduction

The human immunodeficiency virus (HIV) is the aetiological agent of the acquired immunodeficiency syndrome (AIDS). Despite intensive research during the past 9 years since the discovery of the virus, the epidemic continues to spread in the human population. Analysis of epidemiological data reveals a depressing picture for the worst afflicted regions such as sub-Saharan Africa, with increasing amounts of infection in the heterosexual population. In these regions it is likely that AIDS may result in population decline within a few decades if present trends continue (Anderson *et al.* 1991, Anderson and May 1991).

The course of HIV infections can be separated into three stages.

1. Acute clinical illness during primary HIV infection occurs in 50-70% of infected patients, starts generally 2-4 weeks after infection and lasts from 1-2 weeks (Tindall and Cooper 1991). The clinical manifestations are varied and include fever, neuropatic and dermatological symptoms. Virus can be isolated from infected blood cells, cell free plasma, cerebrospinal fluid and bone marrow cells. The high replication and widespread distribution of virus is followed by strong immunological responses, which result in a decrease of viral antigens to almost undetectable levels and a resolution of clinical symptoms.

2. The second, chronic, phase (8-10 years on average) is characterized by low levels of HIV expression and only small pathological changes. Patients are generally asymptomatic. CD4 cell concentrations are constant or slowly decreasing.

3. The final phase is characterized by the development of AIDS. CD4 cell levels are low. Virus levels – both in terms of infected cells and free virus in the plasma – are about 100 times larger than in the asymptomatic stage (Ho *et al.* 1989, Coombs *et al.* 1989). The clinical symptoms are varied and characterised by opportunistic infections. (For a mathematical model of the interaction between HIV and other pathogens see McLean and Nowak (1992)). The life expectation of AIDS patients in the absence of chemotherapeutic interaction is about one year.

What controls the three phases is a central but unanswered question. There is extensive variability in the rate of progression to disease; it is not understood why some people develop AIDS within 2 years after HIV infection, while others are still asymptomatic after 15 years.

HIV displays extensive genetic and antigenic variation during the course of an infection (Balfe *et al.* 1990, Fisher *et al.* 1988, Meyerhans *et al.* 1989, Phillips *et al.* 1991, Saag *et al.* 1988, Simmonds *et al.* 1990). This large variability of HIV has formed the basis of recent mathematical theories that aim to understand the mechanism of disease progression in patients infected with HIV (Nowak, May and Anderson 1990, Nowak and May 1991, Nowak *et al.* 1991, Nowak 1992). The essential assumptions are (1) that HIV mutates rapidly during the course of an individual infection and can generate new antigenic variants that essentially escape current immunological attack, (2) that each such 'escape mutant' evokes, and is controlled (mainly) by, a strain-specific immune response, and (3) that populations of immune cells (CD4 cells) that mount strain-specific and cross-reactive immune responses against HIV are killed – directly or indirectly – by all strains of HIV, and consequently are depleted in HIV infected patients.

With these main assumptions, our 'diversity threshold' theory becomes an intuitive and simple concept. We may assume that the infection occurs with a rather heterogeneous inocculum of virus (this seems to be correct for all natural routes of transmission, such as sexual contact, needle sharing, blood transfusion or mother-child transmission). During the earliest stages of infection we expect strong selection for the fastest growing variants. This would result in a fairly homogeneous population at seroconversion.

Subsequently the immune response to HIV is likely to result in escape mutants, and thence in proliferating virus diversification. We expect variation to accumulate in those epitopes that are recognised by relevant immune responses. Such increasing antigenic diversity makes it more and more difficult for the immune system to downregulate the various mutants simultaneously. The cause is the asymetric interaction between immunological and viral diversity. Each virus strain can impair all immune responses by cutting off their CD4 help, but individual strain-specific immune responses can only attack specific virus strains. In more heterogeneous virus populations the ratio between immune-response-induced killing of virus and virus-induced killing of immune cells is shifted in favour of the virus. This may lead to a complete breakdown of the immune system and uncontrolled virus replication (as seen in AIDS patients).

We call this phenomenon 'diversity threshold', because in the simplest mathematical model there is a critical number of antigenically distinct variants that can be controlled simultaneously by the immune system. In more realistic and more complicated versions of the model this 'diversity threshold' condition takes a more general form, and indicates the point when the immune system fails to control the virus population. These complications arise, for example, when one acknowledges that different virus strains have different replication rates or immunological properties, or that the basic parameters of the model are not constant but change during the course of infection (such as increasing virus replication rates, resulting from increasing CD4 cell activation).

Once the immune response has been overcome, there is no longer selection for variation. Again, as in the earlier stages, we may expect selection for the fastest growing strains. This effect may lead to a very low diversity in AIDS patients at advanced stages of the diseases.

The new idea arising from this work is that an evolutionary mechanism– on a very fast time scale (years) – is responsible for viral pathogenesis. The evolutionary dynamics of the HIV population (based on mutation and natural selection) leads to the development of AIDS.

2 The basic antigenic drift equations for HIV

We use the following set of ordinary differential equations to describe the replication dynamics of n different strains of HIV together with their specific immune responses

$$\frac{dv_i}{dt} = v_i(r - px_i) \qquad i = 1, .., n \tag{2.1}$$

$$\frac{dx_i}{dt} = kv_i - uvx_i \qquad i = 1, .., n . \tag{2.2}$$

The variables v_i and x_i denote, respectively, the densities of virus strain i and of specific immune cells directed at strain i. In this simple model we assume that the virus replication rate is constant for all strains and given by the parameter r. The specific immune response against strain i is represented by the term, pv_ix_i. The production of immune cells, x_i, is assumed to be proportional to the density of strain i, i.e. given by kv_i. Immune cell function is impaired by viral action. This is represented by the term uvx_i. In this simple homogeneous model the parameters, r, p, k and u are the same for all viral strains. We use the notation $v = \sum v_i$ and $x = \sum x_i$.

For the total densities of virus and immune cells we obtain (by summing equations (2.1) and (2.2) over all strains i)

$$\frac{dv}{dt} = v\left(r - p\sum_i x_iv_i/v\right) \tag{2.3}$$

$$\frac{dx}{dt} = kv - uxv . \tag{2.4}$$

The diversity threshold can be derived as follows: Strain i can be controlled by the immune system (i.e. $dv_i/dt < 0$) if $r < px_i$. All strains $(i = 1,..,n)$ can be controlled simultaneously if $nr < px$. From (2.4) we see that x converges to k/u. Hence if

$$n > \frac{pk}{ru} \tag{2.5}$$

then the virus population will eventually escape from control by the immune system and replicate to high levels. This is the diversity threshold. Alternatively condition (2.5) can be derived directly from (2.3) by assuming that $v_i = v/n$.

Next we assume that the replication rate, r, the virulence, u, and the two immunological parameters, p and k, are different for different strains of virus. Thus each virus strain is characterized by its own 4 parameters, r_i, p_i, k_i and u_i. This reflects the large biological variability among HIV isolates from the same infected patients. The basic equations now have the form

$$\frac{dv_i}{dt} = v_i(r_i - p_i x_i) \qquad i = 1,..,n \tag{2.6}$$

$$\frac{dx_i}{dt} = k_i v_i - x_i \sum_{j=1}^{n} u_j v_j \qquad i = 1,..,n . \tag{2.7}$$

We have shown (Nowak and May 1992) that the diversity threshold now takes the form

$$\sum_{i=1}^{n} \frac{r_i u_i}{p_i k_i} > 1 . \tag{2.8}$$

This is necessary and sufficient for eventual virus escape. If $\sum_{i=1}^{n} \frac{r_i u_i}{p_i k_i} < 1$ then the total virus population cannot escape from the immune response, but individual virus strains do not have frequencies that converge to zero. Thus there is coexistence among different virus strains below the diversity threshold. This is very different from the original notion of quasispecies dynamics. If $\sum_{i=1}^{n} \frac{r_i u_i}{p_i k_i} > 1$ then the virus population will eventually escape from the immune response. Now there is competition between individual virus strains, i.e. some virus strains will dominate the population, while others will have frequencies that converge to zero. Interestingly the ensemble of virus strains that is selected is the fastest growing of all possible ensembles.

3   Cross reactive immune responses

Further realism can be added by including cross reactive immune responses that are directed against several strains simultaneously. We subdivide the immune response to HIV into strain specific and cross reactive responses.

This leads to the equations

$$\frac{dv_i}{dt} = v_i(r - sz - px_i) \qquad i = 1,..,n \tag{3.1}$$

$$\frac{dx_i}{dt} = kv_i - uvx_i \qquad i = 1,...,n \tag{3.2}$$

$$\frac{dz}{dt} = k'v - uvz. \tag{3.3}$$

To keep the mathematics simple we model the whole range of more or less cross reactive immune responses by taking into account only the two extreme cases. The terms sz and px_i represent cross-reactive and specific immune responses, respectively; z is the number of immune cells activated against conserved regions, x_i is the number of immune cells specifically against a particular strain and $x = \sum x_i$ denotes the total density of these 'specific' immune cells. The killing of immune cells by viral mechanisms is denoted by the terms uvx_i and uvz. The densities of specific and cross-reactive immune cells converge towards the levels, $\hat{x} = k/u$ and $\hat{z} = k'/u$.

There are three different parameter regions according to the magnitude of specific and cross-reactive immune responses.

1. The cross-reactive immune response is by itself able to suppress viral growth (i.e. $r < s\hat{z}$). There will be a rise in viral abundance following the initial infection, but once the cross-reactive immune response has been mounted the initial strain and all subsequently-evolved ones will be suppressed by this generalised response. In this case antigenic variation cannot prevent the virus population from being cleared by the immune response.

2. The replicative capacity of a single strain can outrun both the specific and cross-reactive immune responses (i.e. $r > s\hat{z} + \hat{x}$). The immune system is not able to cope with any single strain. The initial viraemia is not suppressed by the immune response, there is no incubation period, no delay until the onset of disease. Antigenic variation is not neccessary for the virus to escape from immune control. This seems to be the case for some acutely lethal variants of the simian immunodeficiency virus, the closest relative of HIV.

3. Between these two extremes lies the interesting region of dynamical behaviour, with its viral diversity threshold. This situation corresponds to individual viral strains having replication rates that can outrun the cross-reactive immune response, but not the combined effect of cross-reactive and specific immune responses (i.e. $p\hat{x} > r - s\hat{z} > 0$). Only the continuous generation of new resistant strains enables the virus population to survive immunological attack. In this parameter region we observe the diversity threshold. The critical number of strains that can be suppressed by the immune system is obtained as

$$n_c = \frac{pk}{ru - sk'}. \tag{3.4}$$

The cross-reactive immune response in our model is responsible for the fact that the initial strains grow to higher levels than the succeeding escape mutants. Therefore we obtain a peak of initial viraemia followed by a period with low virus abundance. Roughly speaking, the higher the effect of the cross-reactive response the higher the difference between the initial peak and the average virus density in the silent phase. A stronger cross-reactive immune response is correlated with lower viral abundance in the incubation period and with an increased length of this period.

4   Discussion

The interaction between HIV and the cells of the immune system is of extraordinary complexity. Thus our simple mathematical models can only be poor reflections of reality. They are not designed to capture many detailed aspects, but only a few which seem to be essential. The basic assumptions are that the immune system mounts strain-specific responses against HIV and that the virus impairs immune responses in a general, non-specific way. This is the intuitive explanation for the occurence of the diversity threshold phenomenon (which is not an *a priori* assumption of the theory). If all strains have the same biological parameters, then simply the total number of strains determines whether or not the virus population will eventually escape (see (2.5)). For the more realistic model with different parameters for different strains, we have a more complex condition (3.4) which determines eventual virus escape. Here fast replicating strains, highly cythopatic strains, or strains that are not very well recognised by the immune system have a disproportionately larger effect. (Nelson and Perelson (1992) have discussed a mechanism by which slowly replicating strains of HIV can more efficiently escape from immune responses.)

The theory presented here describes virus mutation and variability as essential for survival of the virus population in the presence of immune responses, and for the subsequent development of immunodeficiency disease. Each HIV infection represents a (unique) evolution of a series of different HIV variants. This evolutionary process leads eventually to the development of AIDS after a long and variable incubation period, during which the balance between viral cytopathicity and the immune response is slowly shifted by increasing viral diversity. During the asymptomatic period the immune system itself drives diversification of the virus population by continuous selection for new escape mutants. The accumulation of diversity is the cause of immunodeficiency disease. As the virus population breaches the diversity threshold the immune system becomes unable to control the virus. The consequence is extensive HIV replication, increasing virus load and rapidly decreasing CD4 numbers as AIDS is developed. Finally when severe immunodeficiency is established there is no longer a strong immune response to HIV that would drive diversification. The fastest replicating strains will outgrow other variants. Antigenic diversity may decrease in AIDS patients.

First experimental support for the suggested pattern of population diversity comes from a study of two male homosexual patients who were followed since their infection in 1985 (Nowak *et al.* 1991). Genetic variation of a certain part (the so called V3 loop) of the HIV envelope protein was measured at sequential time points in both patients. The V3 loop is a region of about 30 amino acids and seems to be a major site of antibody and killer cell attack. The V3 loop is also involved in the process of infecting cells. Thus mutation in V3 may result both in antigenic variation (escape from immune responses) and changes in reproduction rates. In both patients the genetic diversity is extremely low at the beginning of the infection. In one patient all V3 loops were identical (sample size: 11), in the other patient there were 6 identical V3 loops out of 7 samples. Subsequently the genetic diversity increased during the asymptomatic phase in both patients. One patient developed AIDS after 55 months. This was followed by a decline in viral diversity.

The presented coevolutionary process of the HIV population and the human immune system during the course of an individual infection is unique with respect to the time scale. The emergence of new escape mutants can occur within weeks and the immune system may require a similar time to respond. We are confronted with the complex interaction between two highly variable biological structures: (1) the HIV population under the pressure of the immune response and (2) the immune system exposed to mutating HIV antigens.

The agreement between a number of model predictions and experimental observations is encouraging at the moment. These are (1) an early peak in virus levels (primary HIV-1 infection) following infection; (2) a long and variable incubation period with low viral abundance for much of the period; (3) an increase of viral levels in the final phase of infection as the failing immune system fails to control viral population growth (the appearance of the disease AIDS); (4) coevolution and coexistence of many viral mutants in one infected person; (5) increasing population diversity during the asymptomatic phase and (6) a positive correlation between the presence of high replicative viral strains and the rate of progression to disease (AIDS).

The theoretical analysis suggests that antigenic variation of HIV not only enables the virus population to remain persistent in the presence of a strong immune response but can also be responsible for disease progression. HIV infections are evolutionary processes on the time scale of a few years. The evolution of the HIV population within an infected patient may lead to the final outbreak of disease. While experimental evidence is accumulating that genetic (and antigenic) diversity increases during HIV infections, the relative importance of this effect compared to other effects that may drive disease progression has to be established. It would be important to look for a correlation between viral diversity and pathogenicity in primate lentivirus infections (see Shpaer and Mullins 1993).

Acknowledgements

I would like to thank Robert May for many interesting discussions. The author is a Wellcome Trust Senior Research Fellow and an E.P. Abraham Junior Research Fellow of Keble College, Oxford.

References

Anderson, R.M., May, R.M., Boily, M.C., Garnett, G.P. and Rowley, J.T. (1991) 'The spread of HIV-1 in Africa', *Nature* **352**, 581–9.

Anderson, R.M. and May R.M. (1991) *Infectious Diseases of Humans*, Oxford University Press, Oxford.

Balfe, P., Simmonds, P., Ludlam, C.A., Bishop, J.O. and Leigh-Brown, A.J. (1990), 'Concurrent evolution of HIV-1 in patients infected from the same source', *J. Virol.* **64**, 6221.

Coombs, R.W., Collier, A.C., and Allain, J.P. (1989) 'Plasma viremia in HIV infection', *N. Eng. J. Med.* **321**, 1626–31.

Fisher, A.G., Ensoli, B., Looney, D., Rose, A., Gallo, R.C., Saag, M.S., Shaw, G.M., Hahn, B.H. and Wong-Staal, F. (1988) 'Biologically diverse molecular variants within a single HIV-1 isolate', *Nature* **334**, 444–7

Ho, D.D., Mougdil, T. and Alam, M. (1989) 'Quantitation of HIV-1 in the blood of infected persons', *N. Eng. J. Med.* **321**, 1621–25.

McLean, A.R. and Nowak, M.A. (1992) 'The interaction between HIV and other pathogens', *J. Theor. Biol.* **155**, 69–102.

Meyerhans, A., Cheynier, R., Albert, J., Seth, M., Kwok, S., Sninsky, J., Morfeldt-Manson, L., Asjö, B. and Wain-Hobson, S. (1989) 'Temporal fluctuations in HIV population *in vivo* are not reflected by sequential HIV isolations', *Cell* **58**, 901–910.

Nelson, G.W. and Perelson, A.S. (1992) 'A mechanism of immune escape by slow replicating HIV strains', *J AIDS* **5**, 82–93.

Nowak, M.A., May, R.M. and Anderson, R.M. (1990) 'The evolutionary dynamics of HIV-1 population and the development of immunodeficiency disease', *AIDS* **4**, 1095.

Nowak, M.A. and May, R.M. (1991) 'Mathematical biology of HIV infections: antigenic variation and diversity threshold', *Math. Biosci.* **106**, 1–21.

Nowak, M.A., Anderson, R.M., McLean, A.R., Wolfs, T., Goudsmit, J. and May, R.M. (1991) 'Antigenic diversity thresholds and the development of AIDS', *Science* **254**, 963–9.

Nowak, M.A. (1992) 'Variability of HIV infections', *J. Theor. Biol.* **155**, 1–20.

Nowak, M.A. and May, R.M. (1992) 'Competition and coexistence in HIV infections', *J. Theor. Biol.* **159**, 329–342.

Phillips, R.E., Rowland-Jones, S., Nixon, D.F., Gotch, F.M., Edwards, J.P., Ogunlesi, A.O., Elvin, J.G., Rothbard, J.A., Bangham, C.R.M., Rizza, C.R. and McMichael, A.J. (1991) 'HIV genetic variation that can escape cytotoxic T cell recognition', *Nature* **354**, 453–459.

Saag, M.S., Hahn, B.H., Gibbons, J., Li, Y., Parks, E.S., Parks, W.P. and Shaw, G.M. (1988) 'Extensive variation of HIV-1 *in vivo*', *Nature* **334**, 440–444.

Shpear, E.G. and Mullins, J.I. (1993) 'Rates of amino acid change in the envelope protein corellate with pathogenicity of primate lentiviruses', *J. Mol. Evol.* **37**, 57–65.

Simmonds, P., Balfe, P., Peutherer, J.F., Ludlam, C.A., Bishop, J.O. and Leigh-Brown, A.J. (1990) 'Analysis of sequence diversity in hypervariable regions of the external glycoprotein of HIV-1', *J. Virol.* **64**, 5840.

Tindall, B. and Cooper, D.A. (1991) 'Primary HIV infection', *AIDS* **5**, 1–14.

Discussion

AGUR There are some new data relating to the heterogeneity in spatial distribution of HIV within the patient during the incubation period. In particular, the lymph nodes seem to harbour more virus during the asymptomatic period of incubation so the reduction in quantity of circulating virus in peripheral blood may not mean that total virus is reduced.

REPLY It has always been recognised that HIV infections are mainly a disease of the lymph system (as already the original name of HIV – Lymph adenotrophic virus, LAV, suggests). More recently exact molecular techniques have allowed the quantification of the virus load in the peripheral blood and the lymph system. It is indeed a very important and to my knowledge open question, as to how the virus load in the peripheral blood is at related to total virus load.

HADELER** Nowak's model for HIV vs. the immune system is a set of ordinary differential equations coupled to a stochastic process which determines the (increasing) number of variables. Nowak has presented a mathematical analysis of the ordinary differential equations and computer simulations of the entire system which lead to a well-founded possible explanation for what happens after a HIV infection. Even less serious mathematicians, in the terminology of Nowak, may ask how the system, apart from the verbal description, can be defined. I suggest that the system should be defined as a multi-type stochastic process where the number of types is itself a random variable. The question is whether results (existence, asymptotic behaviour etc.) for such multi-type processes are available or envisaged and how the behaviour of the system depends on the choice of the process which governs the number of types.

REPLY We have derived a number of our results just by analysing the deterministic part of the model. We have also looked at some simple stochastic models that would serve as approximations. It would indeed be an excellent project for more (or less) serious mathematicians to investigate the multi-type stochastic process (in the terminology of Hadeler). But I believe the important biological conclusions of our model are robust.

DE BOER I would have expected that, as AIDS develops due to the collapse of the immune system, the diversity of viral types would reflect that during the period immediately preceding AIDS development. Once the mechanism whereby HIV is controlled is removed, I see no reason why diversity should reduce.

REPLY The immune system may be the main driving force to maintain and increase diversity of HIV during the asymptomatic phase. Once the immune response has disappeared in AIDS patients there is no longer selection for variation. All strains could in principle grow to higher levels, but some may grow fastest and therefore outcompete the others in terms of relative frequency.

Statistical Models for Analysis of Longitudinal CD4 Data

J.M.G. Taylor, W.G. Cumberland, J.P. Sy and R.T. Mitsuyasu

1 Introduction

The importance of CD4 T-cells in AIDS and HIV infection has long been recognized. Measurements of the CD4 number, obtained from the peripheral blood, give an indication of the amount of immune suppression, with lower numbers indicating more severe immune deficiency. They have been shown to be of great prognostic significance for predicting clinical outcomes (Fahey *et al.* 1990); they are useful in patient care for monitoring an individual's health; they are used in epidemiological studies and in some countries they are used in determining the availability of health care resources and even are incorporated into the definition of AIDS. CD4 T-cell numbers are also used in determining the eligibility criteria and as stratification variables in randomised clinical trials.

In a previous paper (Taylor *et al.* 1994) we considered various statistical models which attempted to describe the variation in the patterns of decline of CD4 T-cell numbers in HIV infected subjects. These models were fitted to data from the Los Angeles portion of the Multicenter AIDS cohort study (MACS). One of the aims in this analysis is to investigate whether individuals maintain a fixed rate of decline of CD4 after allowing for the variability of the measurements, that is whether a subject who is following a certain path in their CD4 measurements will remain on that path in the future. One possibility is that individuals do maintain a fixed slope indefinitely, another possibility is that the future slope is unrelated to the past slope. We develop a family of models in which these two scenarios are special cases. The family of models also include the possibility that individuals tend to maintain a fixed slope for short periods of time, but not indefinitely. We find that the model which best describes the data is the one in which the future slope is unrelated to the past slope, that is the derivatives of CD4 do not track. This finding has some implications, in particular it says that previous CD4 values add little information to the prediction of future CD4 values if the current value is known. We will discuss later other implications of this finding to the design of clinical trials and to understanding factors responsible for patterns of decline in CD4.

There are some caveats associated with these conclusions. In particular a limitation of the MACS data is that measurements were only taken at 6 month intervals (or 3 month intervals in some cases); thus, we cannot make any conclusions about whether the derivative tracks for time periods shorter than 3 months. To investigate this issue in Section 3.2 we analyse a cohort in which the time interval between measurements is less than 3 months. A second caveat is that a majority of subjects in the MACS were healthy, although HIV antibody positive, with relatively high CD4 values. It is conceivable that for individuals in the later stages of disease progression the derivatives of CD4 do track whereas in the early stages there is no derivative tracking, or vice-versa. To investigate this issue in Section 3.3 we separately analyse subgroups of the MACS data, defined by having high or low CD4 values. A third concern regarding our conclusions is the notoriously variable nature of the CD4 number measurements. One might question whether it is possible to infer anything about the tendency of individuals to maintain a fixed slope from such noisy data. Although we did perform some simulations which support our conclusion that it is possible to investigate derivative tracking from such noisy data, the concerns may still remain. In an analysis presented in Section 3.1 we repeat the analysis of the MACS using CD4 percent rather than CD4 number. CD4 percent is usually thought to be less variable than CD4 number and has equal prognostic significance for the development of AIDS.

Many other authors have considered longitudinal models for serial CD4 measurements (Berman 1990, DeGruttola *et al.* 1991, Lange *et al.* 1992, Longini *et al.* 1989). The two which are closest in spirit to our approach are those of DeGruttola and Lange. They each assumed a random effects model in which each person had their own fixed intercept and slope. One of the main motivations for our work was to investigate the assumption in these two papers that each individual has his or her own linear trajectory of CD4 on which they remain forever.

2 Statistical models

The statistical models we consider have the general form

$$Y_i(t_{ij}) = a_i + b_i t_{ij} + W_i(t_{ij}) + \varepsilon_{ij}, \tag{1}$$

where $Y_i(t_{ij})$ is the measurement on subject i at time t_{ij}, where $t_{ij} = 0$ is the time of HIV infection. The model fitting we perform allows for unequal numbers of observations per subject and irregular time intervals between successive measurements. In equation (1) the ε_{ij} term represents independent noise, which is a combination of technical variation and the natural within person variability which is seen on a daily basis even in a healthy control group. The terms a_i and b_i represent person specific random effects, so that each person has their own underlying intercept (a_i) and rate of decline of CD4 (b_i). It is assumed that a_i, b_i are jointly normally distributed

$$\begin{pmatrix} a_i \\ b_i \end{pmatrix} \sim N\left(\begin{pmatrix} a \\ b \end{pmatrix} \begin{pmatrix} \sigma_a^2 & \rho\,\sigma_a\sigma_b \\ & \sigma_b^2 \end{pmatrix} \right).$$

The term $W_i(t_{ij})$ is a stochastic process which allows deviation from a fixed path, implied by $a_i + b_i t_{ij}$, in addition to independent noise. The expression $a_i + b_i t_{ij} + W_i(t_{ij})$ could be thought of as the 'true' underlying CD4, and thus the observed measurement equals the 'true' value plus independent error. A possible interpretation of the 'true' CD4 is as the average of many independent measurements of CD4 taken over a short period of time. It is the term W which is the crucial aspect of our work and allows us to assess the degree of derivative tracking. For $W_i(t_{ij})$ we assume an integrated Ornstein-Uhlenbeck process, which is a continuous time version of an integrated auto-regressive time series process of order 1. We motivate this choice of $W_i(t_{ij})$ by considering the following discrete time model in which the derivatives are allowed to 'track' for short periods of time. Let $\beta_{t,i}$ be the slope for person i at time t, and $E(\beta_{t,i})$ be the expected slope for that person, then an AR(1) process for the derivatives is

$$\beta_{t+\Delta t,i} - E(\beta_{t+\Delta t,i}) = e^{-\alpha\Delta t}\left(\beta_{t,i} - E(\beta_{t,i})\right) + e$$

where $\mathrm{Var}(e) = \sigma^2 \Delta t$. In this model, there is an elastic pull back toward each person's mean slope. The strength of the pull depends on the magnitude of α. The term e represents perturbation of this elastic pull, with the magnitude of the perturbation determined by σ^2. A model in which the derivatives track for long periods of time can be obtained with a small α and σ^2, alternatively a model in which both α and σ^2 are large has the current derivative essentially unrelated to the earlier derivative; i.e. the derivatives do not track. The limit of the above auto-regressive process for the derivatives as $\Delta t \to 0$ is an Ornstein-Uhlenbeck (OU) process (Cumberland and Sykes 1982). We are primarily interested in the process itself, not its derivative. If the derivative is an OU process, then the process itself is an integrated OU process. Let $Z(t)$ be an OU process then $Z(t)$ is Gaussian and Markov, and for large t, $Z(t)$ is stationary with

$$\mathrm{Cov}\left(Z(s), Z(t)\right) = \frac{\sigma^2}{2\alpha} e^{-\alpha|t-s|}.$$

Let $W(t) = \int_0^t Z(u)\, du$ be an integrated OU process (IOU), then $W(t)$ is Gaussian and hence

$$\mathrm{Var}\left(W(t)\right) = \frac{\sigma^2}{2\alpha^3}(\alpha t + e^{-\alpha t} - 1)$$

and

$$\text{Cov}\left(W(s), W(t)\right) = \frac{\sigma^2}{2\alpha^3}\left(2\alpha \min(s, t) + e^{-\alpha t} + e^{-\alpha s} - 1 - e^{-\alpha|t-s|}\right). \quad (2)$$

It is interesting to note that scaled Brownian motion is a special case of $W(t)$ in which α is infinitely large and σ^2/α^2 is constant. Another appealing aspect of the IOU model is that the limiting case as $\alpha \to 0$ is a special case of a random effects model. In particular in this case it can be shown that the covariance structures of the two models

$$Y_{it} = a_i + b_i t + \varepsilon_{it}$$

and

$$Y_{it} = a_i + bt + W_{it} + \varepsilon_{it}$$

are the same provided $\sigma_{ab} = 0$ and $\sigma_b^2 = \sigma^2/2\alpha$.

Equations (1) and (2) specify the mean and covariance structure of the multivariate normal vector of observations. Parameter estimates are obtained by maximising the likelihood using a Fisher-Scoring algorithm written in SAS-IML and standard errors are obtained from the second derivative of the log-likelihood. Profile likelihood confidence intervals are obtained for α.

One feature of an IOU process is that it is not stationary and an implicit time zero is needed for each person. In one of our data analyses in Section 3 there is no natural time zero, and in another time zero is not exactly known. This problem can be overcome by analysing differences, for example, we analyse for person i the set of values

$$D_i(t_{ij}) = Y_i(t_{ij}) - Y_i(t_{i1}), \quad j = 2, 3, \ldots$$

with an appropriate adjustment to the covariance structure of the D.

3   Data analysis

For all the datasets described in this section we fit the following five models

$$\begin{aligned}
Y_i(t_{ij}) &= a_i + b_i t_{ij} + \epsilon_{ij} & (3) \\
Y_i(t_{ij}) &= a_i + bt_{ij} + W_i(t_{ij}) + \epsilon_{ij} & (4) \\
Y_i(t_{ij}) &= a_i + bt_{ij} + B_i(t_{ij}) + \epsilon_{ij} & (5) \\
Y_i(t_{ij}) &= a_i + b_i t_{ij} + W_i(t_{ij}) + \epsilon_{ij} & (6) \\
Y_i(t_{ij}) &= a_i + b_i t_{ij} + B_i(t_{ij}) + \epsilon_{ij} & (7)
\end{aligned}$$

where $W_i(t_{ij})$ is an IOU process and $B_i(t_{ij})$ is Brownian motion, which is a special case of $W_i(t_{ij})$ with $\alpha = \infty$.

Although it is a popular statistical model, it seems implausible *a priori* that model (3) is realistic. It is unlikely that the within-individual residuals from a linear fit are not serially correlated, because any departure from the assumed linearity would tend to induce serial correlation.

Model	Log-likelihood	Number of Parameters	a	b	σ_b	α	95% confidence interval for α
3	1073.5	6	0.640	-0.040	0.032	—	—
4	1089.5	6	0.644	-0.039	—	2.7	$(0.9, \infty)$
5	1089.0	5	0.643	-0.039	—	∞	—
6	1089.8	8	0.643	-0.039	0.016	13.9	$(1.0, \infty)$
7	1089.8	7	0.643	-0.039	0.016	∞	—

Table 1. Model fits for MACS seroconverters, arc-sine CD4 percent

3.1 CD4 percentage in the Los Angeles MACS

The Los Angeles MACS is a cohort study of 1637 gay and bisexual men recruited in Los Angeles in 1984/85. Further details of the cohort are given in Taylor *et al.* (1994) and references therein. Two separate datasets are considered in the study: the seroconverter cohort and the seroprevalent cohort. The response variable $Y_i(t_{ij})$ is the arc-sine square root of the CD4 T-cell percentage. This transformation, which is variance stabilising for binomial proportions, was chosen empirically because it achieved homogeneity of within subject variance, and approximate Gaussian distributions.

The seroconverter cohort

The seroconverter cohort consisted of 87 people who were observed to change from HIV negative to HIV positive within a window of time, usually less than nine months. There are a total of 724 measurements with each subject having between 1 and 18 measurements usually spaced at 3 month intervals. Data after December 1989 were excluded to reduce the influence of effective therapy on the results, and data in the first six months after seroconversion were excluded because CD4 is known to drop sharply in that period. Table 1 shows some of the parameter estimates from the fits. We see that the simple random effects model (equation (3)) gives the least satisfactory fit to the observations and the other four models are all roughly equivalent. Low values of α are excluded from the confidence intervals, indicating that a pattern in which each individual is on his own fixed slope for an extended period of time is not supported by the data. An interpretation of α is that the correlation between the derivatives Δt apart in time is $\exp(-\alpha\Delta t)$; thus the correlation between slopes 6 months and one year apart is 0.47 and 0.22 if $\alpha = 1.5$, and 0.14 and 0.02 if $\alpha = 4$.

Table 1 also shows the number of parameters in the various models. We can see that there is no particular advantage to model 3 in terms of fewer parameters. In fact, model 5 has fewer parameters and a higher likelihood, so solely on grounds of parsimony it is preferred.

Model	Log-likelihood	b	σ_b	α	95% confidence Interval for α
3	4859.4	-0.039	0.035	—	—
4	4901.2	-0.039	—	2.8	(1.5, 15)
5	4899.2	-0.039	—	∞	—
6	4901.2	-0.039	0	2.8	(1.5, ∞)
7	4899.8	-0.039	0.013	∞	—

Table 2. Model fits for MACS seroprevalent, arc-sine CD4 percent

The seroprevalent cohort

The seroprevalent cohort consists of 809 subjects who were HIV positive at entry into the study. Individuals had up to 13 measurements usually spaced at approximately 6 month intervals, for a total of 4636 measurements. All observations after December 1987 were excluded because the use of AZT in the cohort increased significantly after this date, and was used infrequently before then. For this data set differences from the baseline measurement were analysed. Table 2 shows the parameter estimates from the fits of the five models. Again, we see that the models which include the IOU term or Brownian motion give a much better fit than the random effects model (eqn. (3)). Also, again, the data are not consistent with small values of α.

3.2   CD4 number in ACTG016 and 019

The subjects in this data set consist of the placebo group Los Angeles participants in two AZT v placebo randomised clinical trials. The results and design of these trials have been described elsewhere (Fischl *et al.* 1990, Volberding *et al.* 1990); but briefly the participants in the trials were AIDS-free HIV seropositive. For ACTG016 the subjects were mildly symptomatic, the recruitment period began in October 1987 and the study closed in August 1989. For ACTG019 the subjects were asymptomatic at entry, the recruitment period began in September 1987 and the study closed and the randomisation code was broken for subjects with initial CD4 less than 500 in August 1989. For ACTG016 there was at least one baseline measurement plus follow-up measurements which were scheduled at 4, 8, 12, 16, 24, 40, 52 and 64 weeks. For ACTG019 the scheduled follow-up measurements were at 8, 16, 32, 48 and 64 weeks. The actual visit dates, except for missed visits, were generally within one week for the scheduled time for the first six months and within four weeks after that. In addition, many participants also had several intermediate measurements. There were a total of 46 participants in the placebo group

Model	Log-likelihood	b	σ_b	α	95% confidence Interval for α
3	-12.30	-0.066	0.046	—	—
4	-10.64	-0.059	—	56.3	$(0, \infty)$
5	-10.65	-0.059	—	∞	—
6	-10.64	-0.059	0	56.3	$(0, \infty)$
7	-10.65	-0.059	0	∞	—

Table 3. Model fits for ACTG016/019 data, fourth root CD4 number

with CD4 T-cell measurements performed in UCLA laboratories. Nineteen of these patients were in ACTG016 and twenty seven were in ACTG019. The total number of measurements per person ranged from 1 to 13 and the total number of observations was 290. As we have done previously (Taylor *et al.* 1992), we fitted the models to the fourth root of CD4 T-cell number. This transformation was chosen because it was preferable to other power transformations in achieving approximate Gaussian distributions and homogeneity of within subject variability. Table 3 shows the results of fitting the five models. Again we see that models 4, 5, 6 and 7 are preferred to model 3. However, the difference in log-likelihood is small, and because of the low sample size there is no precision associated with the estimate of α, although a very high value of 56 is the estimate which gives the best fit.

3.3   High and low CD4 number in the Los Angeles MACS

The analysis in our previous paper (Taylor *et al.* 1994) had considered the CD4 number in both the seroconverter and seroprevalent cohort of the Los Angeles MACS data. In this section we divide those data into two halves and analyse each separately. The separation is based on the average of the CD4 number for each participant over their complete follow up.

The seroconverter cohort

For the seroconverter cohort if the average is larger than 500 they are denoted as the high CD4 group and if it is lower than 500 they are the low CD4 group. Table 4 gives the results of the five models for both the high CD4 group and the low CD4 group. For the high CD4 group there is very little difference between the log-likelihood for the five models. Thus, these data could be consistent with the theory that individuals maintain a fixed trajectory, however the best fitting model is equation 6 for which the estimated α is infinite. This together with the very wide confidence interval for α does not support the

Model	Log-likelihood	a	b	σ_b	α	95% confidence Interval for α
A. High CD4						
3	-90.44	5.43	-0.179	0.177	—	
4	-91.05	5.42	-0.166	—	1.29	$(0, \infty)$
5	-91.58	5.42	-0.160	—	—	
6	-90.21	5.43	-0.177	0.158	∞	$(0, \infty)$
7	-90.21	5.43	-0.177	0.158	∞	—
Low CD4						
3	-134.72	4.88	-0.262	0.215	—	—
4	-114.54	4.90	-0.263	—	16.8	$(2.0, \infty)$
5	-114.57	4.90	-0.263	—	∞	—
6	-113.13	4.89	-0.259	0.120	12.6	$(1.6, \infty)$
7	-114.21	4.89	-0.259	0.122	∞	—

Table 4. Model fits for MACS seroconverter, fourth root CD4

theory that derivative tracking is the only, or necessarily the best explanation of the pattern of change of CD4.

For the low CD4 group, models 4, 5, 6 and 7 are preferred to model 3, and the confidence intervals for α exclude low values, again suggesting that the derivatives of CD4 do not track.

The seroprevalent cohort

For the seropositive cohort, the high CD4 group has an average of larger than 500 and the low CD4 group has an average of smaller than 500. Table 5 gives the results for both the high CD4 group and the low CD4 group. The log-likelihood values for model 3 are lower than for the other four models for both the high and the low CD4 group. The confidence intervals for α again exclude low values.

4   Conclusions and discussion

In this paper we have analysed several sets of data to examine the issue of whether individuals remain on a fixed trajectory in their path of CD4 values. Within the framework of the models we have considered, we find very little evidence that derivatives do track. If it were not for the presence of measurement error we would conclude that past CD4 measurements add almost no information to the knowledge about future CD4 values if the current CD4 value is known. However, because of the measurement error the past CD4 values are useful in helping to define the current CD4 value, and in this sense do add information about future CD4 values. It appears that CD4 data

Model	Log-likelihood	b	σ_b	α	95% confidence Interval for α
A. High CD4					
3	-563.69	-0.065	0.081	—	—
4	-556.36	-0.066	—	∞	$(1.7, \infty)$
5	-556.36	-0.066	—	∞	—
6	-556.36	-0.066	0	∞	$(1.7, \infty)$
7	-556.36	-0.066	0	∞	—
B. Low CD4					
3	-1117.75	-0.303	0.299	—	—
4	-1056.00	-0.292	—	3.6	$(1.9, \infty)$
5	-1056.91	-0.290	—	∞	—
6	-1056.00	-0.292	0	3.6	$(1.9, \infty)$
7	-1056.91	-0.290	0.040	∞	—

Table 5. Model fits for MACS seroprevalent, fourth root CD4

in an individual can be adequately described by a random intercept value at the time of infection, a fixed linear population rate of decline after infection plus scaled Brownian motion plus independent noise.

Our finding that the current CD4 value contains nearly all the information about future CD4 values is consistent with the findings of other authors (Tsiatis *et al.* 1992, Lin *et al.* 1993) regarding clinical progression. These authors show that the current CD4 count is the most predictive of survival and future opportunistic infections and that other aspects of the prior path of CD4 do not add significantly to the prediction.

It is interesting to play devil's advocate and question the quality and validity of the data and various assumptions which were made in the analysis. By its nature CD4 T-cell measurements are influenced by many uncontrollable sources of variation; the blood may be drawn at different times of day, the technicians who prepare the samples and operate the flow cytometer change with time, as do the reagents, and there have even been changes in the flow cytometers. Despite these problems, the CD4 measurements produced by the laboratories at UCLA have been shown to be less variable than those obtained in three other cities (Giorgi *et al.* 1990). So these data, despite their variability, are among the very best available for analysis.

Because of the variability in the data one may question whether it is justified to infer anything about the pattern of decline in individuals based on what might be quite small differences in the covariance structure of a multivariate normal distribution. We investigated this in a simulation study (Taylor *et al.* 1994) which was designed to mimic the MACS sero-converter cohort.

We simulated data either from a Brownian motion (BM) model (equation 5) or a random effects (RE) model (equation 3). One hundred data sets were simulated from each of the two models. Each data set was analysed twice assuming both equation 3 and equation 5. We found that for every one of the 200 data sets the fitted model with the correct covariance structure gave the higher likelihood. This result indicates that the sample size in the seroconverter cohort is large enough to be able to detect different covariance structures, and lends supports to the validity of interpreting parameters of a covariance structure in terms of the degree of derivative tracking. These and other simulation results described in Taylor *et al.* (1994) suggest that in this application we can separate the different components of variability described in (4)-(7).

The statistical models we used (equations (3)-(7) have various assumptions, for example, linearity of the mean structure, homogeneity of variance and multivariate normal distributions. The transformations we used, fourth root of CD4 number and arc-sine root for CD4 percent, were chosen to ensure that these assumptions were approximately satisfied. Despite this, violations of these assumptions due to outliers or person specific measurement error variability might cause the IOU or BM models to be favored over the random effects model (equation (3)), even though in the underlying process individuals do tend to maintain the same slope. This is possible although the very considerable difference in log-likelihood in nearly every case in Tables 1-5 between model (3) and the other four models suggests this is very unlikely.

We have shown that the CD4 measurements in a person are not well described by a model in which each person is on their own fixed straight line, and the measurement at any point in time is determined by the value on this line plus some noise. This finding may have some implications for the understanding of the biological mechanism responsible for the pattern of CD4 measurements. One possible model is an 'inherent susceptibility' model in which each person has their own fixed level of susceptibility. The most susceptible will have rapidly declining CD4 and develop disease quickly whereas the least susceptible will have essentially stable CD4 values. Possible non time varying factors which determine an individuals level of 'inherent susceptibility', are genetic factors or time invariant environmental factors, for example, some aspects of diet. This 'inherent susceptibility' model as the only mechanism determining the pattern of decline is not supported by the data. An alternative model, which is consistent with the data, is a 'random shocks' model. In such a model the mechanism responsible for the decline in CD4 is constantly changing, and could for example be due to varying environmental factors, or psychological factors, or varying immune factors.

Our findings may also have implications for the design of clinical trials in which CD4 measurements are obtained and the analysis to determine the efficacy of the treatment could be based on such summary measures of CD4 as, slope of regression line, last measurement, last minus first measurement, area under the curve, etc. Our results suggest that summary statistics which place more emphasis on the later measurements, rather than how the patients arrived at the last measurement, are likely to be better. However, other considerations, such as controlling between person variability and reducing the influence of measurement error by averaging may also be important.

Acknowledgements

This work was partially supported by NIH grants AI29196 and AI27660.

References

Berman, S.M. (1990) 'A stochastic model for the distribution of HIV latency time based on T4 counts', *Biometrika* **77**, 733–741

Cumberland, W.G. and Sykes, Z.M. (1982) 'Weak convergence of an autoregressive process used in modelling population growth', *J. Appl. Prob.* **19**, 45–455.

de Gruttola, V., Lange, N. and Dafni, U. (1991) 'Modelling the progression of HIV infection', *J. ASA* **86**, 569–577.

Fahey, J.L., Taylor, J.M.G., Detels, R. *et al.* (1990) 'The prognostic value of cellular and serologic markers in infection with human immunodeficiency virus type I', *N. Engl. J. Med.* **322**,166–172.

Fischl, M.A., Richman, D.D., Hansen, N. *et al.* (1990) 'The safety and efficacy of Zidovudine in the treatment of subjects with mildly symptomatic human immunodeficiency virus type I (HIV) infection', *Am. Intern. Med.* **112**, 727–737.

Giorgi, J.V., Cheng,H.-L., Margolick, J.B.*et al.* (1990) 'Quality control in the flow cytometric measurement of T-lymphocyte subsets: The Multicenter AIDS cohort study experience', *Clin. Immunol. Immunopathol.* **SS**, 173–186.

Lange, N., Carlin, B.P. and Gelfand, A.E. (1992) 'Hierarchical Bayes models for the progression of HIV infection using longitudinal CD4 T-cell numbers', *J. ASA* **87**, 615–626.

Lin, D.Y., Fischl, M.A. and Schoenfeld, D.A. (1993) 'Evaluating the role of CD4 lymphocyte counts as surrogate endpoints in human immunodeficiency clinical trials', *Stat. Med.* **12**, 835–842.

Longini, I.M., Clark, W.S., Byers, R.H. *et al.* (1989) 'Statistical analysis of the stages of HIV infection using a Markov model', *Stat. Med.* **8**, 831–843.

Taylor, J.M.G., Cumberland, W.G. and Sy, J.P. (1994) 'A stochastic model for analysis of longitudinal AIDS data', *J. ASA* **89**, 727–736.

Tsiatis, A.A., Dafni, U., de Gruttola V. *et al.* (1992) 'The relationship of CD4 counts over time to survival in patients with AIDS: Is CD4 a good surrogate marker'. In *AIDS Epidemiology: Methodological Issues*, Jewell, Dietz, Farewell (eds.) Birkhauser. Boston.

Volderding, P.A., Lagakos, S.W., Koch, M.A. *et al.* (1990) 'Safety and efficacy of Zidovudine in asymptomatic HIV infected individuals with less than 500 CD4+ cells/mm^3', *N. Engl. J. Med.* **322**, 941–949.

Discussion

SOLOMON I have two questions. First, I wondered if you have tried modelling possible seasonal effects in the data? Secondly, and more importantly, I understand that you have fitted models to the transformed CD4 cell counts, and I think that this raises the issue of what transformation is doing to underlying relationships in the data on the original scale. I wondered if you have investigated this? Analysis could be done either informally or formally – see Solomon and Cox (1992), 'Nonlinear component of variance models', *Biometrika* **79**, 1–11.

REPLY We did not observe any seasonal effects in CD4 numbers in the MACS data. We did observe quite large differences in the mean CD4 level over calendar time in a large seronegative control group. These changes were paralleled in the detrended mean CD4 levels in the seroprevalent MACS cohort. We believe that these non-seasonal effects are likely to be the result of changes in equipment, technicians and reagents. The MACS data which we analyzed was pre-cleaned to remove these variations.

Dr Solomon points out that Box–Cox transformations have subtle effects on the correlation structure of repeated measures data, which can be investigated using Taylor series methods. We have not done this. We choose the fourth root of the CD4 number primarily to stabilise the within-person variability and to symmetrise the distributions. We note that other authors have used square root or log, so fourth root seems to be a good average choice. We find that for the MACS seroconverters the assumption of linearity on the fourth root scale is well supported by the data, as an estimated quadratic coefficient is essentially zero. We also performed analysis of the MACS data on the log, square root and untransformed scales. We found essentially the same conclusions in the sense that the models which included the IOU term or Brownian motion gave better fits to the data than the random effects model.

Some Mathematical and Statistical Issues in Assessing the Evidence for Acquired Immunity to Schistosomiasis

A.J.C. Fulford, A.E. Butterworth,
D.W. Dunne, R.F. Sturrock and J.H. Ouma

1 Introduction

The problem of whether humans mount a protective immune response to schistosomiasis is both of basic, biological interest and important in the context of disease control. The immune response to this and other large parasites differs from that of microparasites, such as viruses and bacteria, and involves distinct branches of the immune system associated with IgE and eosinophils. The possibility of a protective immune response has consequences not just for vaccine development but also for the effectiveness of control programmes in general. Immune responses are altered by chemotherapy itself and may be involved in the schistosomicidal action of praziquantel, the main chemotherapeutic drug. The problem of demonstrating a protective response is closely related to that of quantifying the response, which would be essential for vaccine development.

In this paper we consider some mathematical, and especially statistical, problems that arise when assessing the evidence for immunity in man, illustrating these with data from our own studies in Kenya. We first briefly describe our studies in Kenya and outline the difficulty of interpreting simple age-intensity curves. The main part of the paper is divided into two sections, the first discussing two more sophisticated approaches to analysis of cross-sectional data and the second reviewing the analysis of treatment-reinfection studies.

2 Schistosomiasis studies in Kenya

For more than a decade studies have been undertaken on *Schistosoma mansoni* infection in the Machakos District of Kenya, as a collaboration between the Kenyan Medical Research Institute (KEMRI), the Division of Vector Borne Diseases (DVBD) of the Kenyan Ministry of Health and the University of Cambridge. We have focused on two localities, Kangundo and Kambu

(Butterworth *et al.* 1991, Fulford *et al.* 1991). Briefly, both are rural areas inhabited by the same tribe, the Wakamba. The areas are broadly similar, the major differences being that Kangundo is higher, cooler and less dry. Its population has been established in the area for several generations and is generally more affluent. Land in the Kambu area is more marginal and has only been settled in the last 2 or 3 decades. Many of its inhabitants were born outside the area. Streams are the main source of water for most inhabitants in both areas. Although Kambu is drier, its streams arise from springs fed by rains on the nearby Chyulu Hills and are consequently less prone to dry up. In both areas seasonal rains usually flush away the snails twice a year. The prevalence and intensity of *S. mansoni* infection is high in both areas but the infection appears to cause more hepatosplenomegaly in Kambu (Fulford *et al.* 1991). There is no *S. haematobium* in either area. Malaria and malnutrition are greater problems in the Kambu area than in Kangundo.

Our studies have been directed at two major objectives. The first was to optimise chemotherapy strategy for control of the disease. To this end we have considered the impact on whole communities (1500–2500 individuals) of various treatment strategies, often school-based. From these studies we have accumulated a large volume of stool egg count data from both school and community-wide surveys, before and after chemotherapy.

The other major objective has been to elucidate the human immunological response to the infection. In these investigations we have concentrated on smaller groups (80 to 150 individuals), selected from the same communities, studied in greater detail. These studies have followed a longitudinal, 'treatment-reinfection' format: individuals' egg outputs were measured prior to treatment and at 6 or 12 month intervals for 2 or 3 years after treatment, by which time reinfection had reached levels which required retreatment. Blood samples have been taken to assay antibody levels and other immunological variables and additional stool samples have been collected for more accurate estimation of egg output. The field operation for three such studies have now been completed: 'Study 129' (Butterworth, *et al.* 1988) and 'Study H' (Dunne *et al.* 1992) were based in the Kangundo area while 'Study I' (Roberts *et al.* 1993) was based in the Kambu area.

In each community studied we have also routinely recorded human water contact activity and snail observations at the potentially infective sites. Sites were carefully demarcated sections of stream and observations made according to a schedule balanced in its design. Water contact observations were made by specially trained local people who were able to identify all members of the community by sight. For each contact they observed between 9:00 am and 6:00 pm and within the boundaries of the site, they recorded the identity of the individual, duration and type of activity, degree of immersion and time of day.

3   Age-intensity profiles

Figure 1 shows the age intensity profiles of six communities from Machakos. They illustrate the typical pattern of a rise towards peak intensity around the teenage years and a decline thereafter. The extent to which the decline in adult years is due to reduced exposure or acquired immunity has long been debated (Warren 1973, Bradley and McCullough 1974). The problem comes into sharper focus when expressed mathematically. The mean of the simple immigration-death stochastic process is given by the solution of the equivalent differential equation. Writing $M(a)$ for the mean worm burden at age a and λ and μ for the force of infection and the rate of parasite death, the deterministic equation is:

$$\frac{dM(a)}{da} = \lambda - \mu M(a) \qquad (1)$$

It is not possible to count worms in humans: instead, intensity of infection is quantified by counting stool eggs in Kato smears. Equation (1) still holds for stool eggs if egg output is assumed to be proportional to worm burden (an assumption to be discussed later). The simple formulation, in which λ and μ are constant, is inadequate since it does not peak. Nor does the process peak if λ and μ are simple, continuous functions of $M(a)$: in order to peak the right hand side of equation (1), which starts positive, must pass through zero to become negative, but at zero the process reaches equilibrium. There are two modifications of λ and/or μ which can give rise to a peak: (i) λ and/or μ may be simple functions of host age (reflecting for instance behavioural or physiological changes) or (ii) they may be influenced by *previous* worm burdens (the most obvious physical basis for such memory being the immune response). Thus the same two explanations, behaviour and acquired immunity, are highlighted by the mathematical formulation. To these must be added age-related changes to any factor (not just behaviour) affecting the force of infection or the rate of parasite death.

Little is known about worm death. It is usually assumed to be constant but if it increases with host age it may cause the process to peak. The only way to estimate $\mu(a)$ is by first either estimating $\lambda(a)$, for example from reinfection studies (Fulford *et al.* 1994); or setting $\lambda(a)$ to zero, by stopping, or removing the host from, transmission (for instance Warren *et al.* 1974, Wilkins *et al.* 1984), and then solving for $\mu(a)$. Mollusciciding studies (e.g. Wilkins *et al.* 1984) indicate that μ is not strongly host-age dependent. It is also frequently assumed that acquired immunity would work by reducing λ (Anderson and May 1985) although this remains to be proven conclusively and baboon studies suggest that the immune response may cause a suppression of egg production, at least in the case of *S. haematobium* (Webbe *et al.* 1976).

Deterministic models of this sort do not include worm age: in equation

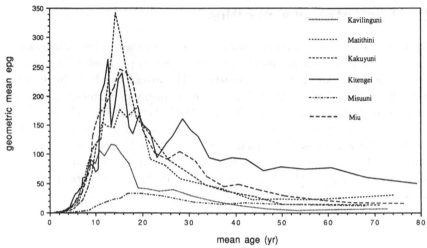

Figure 1. Age-intensity profiles for *S. mansoni* in six communities in Machakos District, Kenya. The first three communities, all from Kangundo Location, were surveyed as part of a study described by Butterworth *et al.* (1991). The other three, all from Ngwata Location, were surveyed in an identical manner for a later, as yet unpublished, study. Each community was stratified by age in such a way as to ensure that each stratum contained exactly 40 individuals. The mean values of these strata are plotted. Reproduced from Fulford *et al.* (1992).

(1) it is assumed that worm death is independent of worm age. Models which do include worm age are considerably more complicated and the mean of such stochastic models would not in general be given by the solution of their deterministic form. While it is conceivable that with more complicated models of worm death (i.e. not just a fixed life span or a constant hazard) the process might be made to peak, it seems improbable that this alone would be sufficient to explain the age-intensity profiles.

On the other hand, reinfection studies of communities in which the infection is well established indicate that the force of infection, λ, certainly does change with age (figure 2), although whether these changes are due to simple ageing effects in the host or to memory of previous infection is indeterminable. The host-ageing effect most often considered is that of behavioural change. Water contact is easy enough to observe (Dalton and Poole 1978, Wilkins *et al.* 1987, Dessein *et al.* 1988, Chandiwana and Woolhouse 1991) and it seems clear from most studies that adults do indeed have less contact than children (figure 3). Nevertheless, the difficulty in quantifying these (and other) changes leaves open the question as to whether they are sufficient to explain the decline in intensity seen in adults.

There are also other possible explanations. For example, egg output per worm pair may be host age-dependent, either due to suppression of fecundity

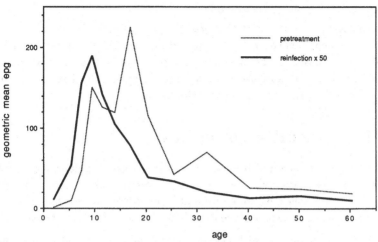

Figure 2. Reinfection and pretreatment intensities of *S. mansoni* (geometric mean epg) vs. age for Matithini community.

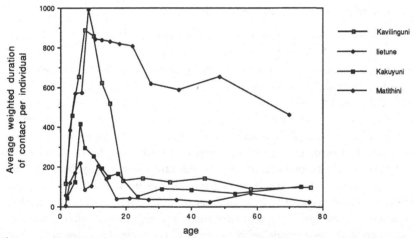

Figure 3. Mean weighted water contact scores vs age for four communities in the Kangundo area. Observations covered a two year period. N = approximately 70–80 individuals per point.

or to retention of eggs in the tissues. Eggs are diluted by the stool volume and this is almost certainly age-dependent (Bundy *et al.* 1987, Ouma 1987), although the difference in stool volume between adults and children is insufficient on its own to explain the difference in egg output. An alternative to stool egg count for estimating worm numbers would be very useful to check the possibilities of both host-age and worm-density dependence of egg output. In this respect the development of assays for circulating worm antigens (de

Jong *et al.* 1988) may prove valuable.

Alternatively, the shape of the age-intensity profile may be determined more by age-dependence of the immune response than by duration of immunological experience. For instance children may only be able to mount a protective immune response after a certain age, a fact that would have profound repercussions for vaccine development.

4   'Ecological' Approaches

Clearly, then, there is a multitude of alternative possible explanations for the decline in intensity in adulthood. This has led some researchers to turn to more subtle approaches, borrowed from ideas in ecology, to test for immunity. Two such have been discussed recently (Fulford *et al.* 1992, Woolhouse 1992):

1. Decline in dispersion with age (Anderson and Gordon 1982, Pacala and Dobson 1988).

2. Peak shift (Woolhouse *et al.* 1991): the age of peak intensity will be lower in communities of higher mean intensity.

Since we have discussed these in detail elsewhere (Fulford *et al.* 1992), we will only outline them here.

Both approaches present a problem with the measurement of the pertinent variable. The model from which the prediction of a decline in dispersion arises suggests that, in the absence of density dependence or immunological memory, the variance-mean relationship ought to be identical to that of the negative binomial distribution (Pacala and Dobson 1988). But this model does not take account of error in the measurement of parasite numbers, considerable in the case of schistosomiasis, since parasite numbers can only be estimated via egg output, or the fact that estimates of mean and variance may be correlated. Since any assumed variance-mean relationship needs to be checked it is simpler to work with the empirical relationship in the first place. If it can be assumed that the unmodelled component of the error is not age-dependent then, under the null hypothesis, the variance-mean relationship ought to be independent of age. Weighted curvilinear regression may then be used to test whether the relationship is age-dependent. In Kenya we find that the relationship (figure 4) is significantly age-dependent (Fulford *et al.* 1992).

There are also problems with locating the peak intensity, more so in the case of *S. mansoni* than *S. haematobium*. We were able to overcome the problem for *S. mansoni* by fitting quadratic curves to the age-intensity data. Woolhouse *et al.* (1991) found that the sharper peaks of *S. haematobium* profiles could be located accurately enough simply by using the data maxima. In both species a significant negative correlation is seen between intensity of infection and the age of peak intensity.

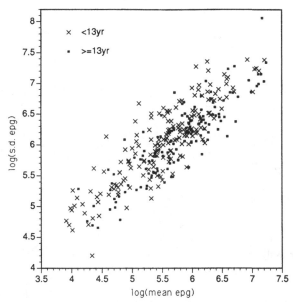

Figure 4. The relationship between estimates of standard deviation and mean of untransformed eggs per gram. The children in each school are grouped into one-year age bands and each point corresponds to one such group. Only groups of size greater than 15 are plotted. Data from 39 schools in the Kangundo and Kambu areas – reproduced from Fulford *et al.* (1992).

Both approaches sidestep some of the problems of confounding between exposure and development of immunity and of quantifying age-related changes in λ and μ, but introduce other drawbacks. Firstly, the dependence of λ and/or μ upon $M(a)$ (density dependence), while it does not cause the profile to peak, is similar to immunity in its effects on both the decline in dispersion and peak shift. Secondly, the single-parameter model usually considered for heterogeneity between individuals, while analytically convenient, is rather simplistic: it is assumed that individuals differ only by an age-independent factor in $\lambda(a)$ – the 'proportional force of infection' model of heterogeneity. Our Kenyan water contact data do not support this assumption (figure 5). Other simple models of heterogeneity do, under the null hypothesis, give rise to both age-dependence in variance-mean relationship and peak shift with intensity. For instance, any pattern in which heterogeneity of exposure itself was age-dependent would usually result in age-dependence of the variance-mean relationship. Evidence from our observations in Kenya indicates that the variation of water contact relative to its mean may indeed decrease with age (figure 6), i.e. that adults tend to be more uniform in their patterns of behaviour. Any pattern of heterogeneity, such as variation in the age of first

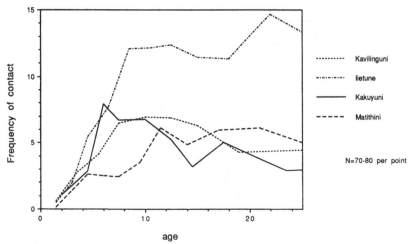

Figure 5. Mean frequency of water contact vs age focusing on ages 0 to 25 years. Same observations as in figure 3.

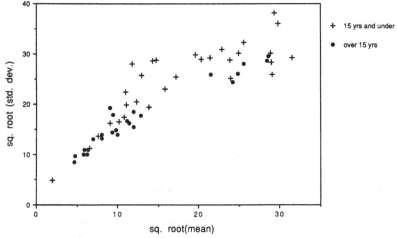

Figure 6. The relationship between standard deviation and mean weighted water contact score by age. The square roots of both s.d. and mean are plotted to assist visual interpretation. Data from the four Kangundo communities have been combined: the relationship appears to be continuous between the communities and the data are well balanced with respect to age and community.

contact, which tends to cause a peak shift to the *left* with increasing intensity, will usually also tend to cause a *decline* in dispersion with age.

The two approaches also have their own specific problems. In the case of the decline in dispersion, there is a problem with the clustering of events. In the usual models considered (for instance, Pacala and Dobson 1988) the

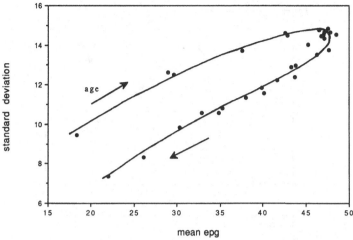

Figure 7. Variance-mean relationship for a simulated model with aggregated infection events but no density dependence. Reproduced from Fulford *et al.* (1992).

stochastic events are not clustered, although in reality both infection and parasite death are likely to be so. When clustering of infection events is introduced the variance-mean relationship can again become age-dependent under the null hypothesis (figure 7). It appears that dispersion decreases with age in this model because, while clustered infection events predominate before the peak intensity is achieved, unclustered death events assume greater importance in older individuals: thus the differential clustering between infection and death and the peaking of the profile are significant features of the model.

A problem specific to the peak shift approach arises from long term temporal fluctuations. From snail data (Sturrock *et al.* 1994) and reinfection rates (Roberts *et al.* 1993) it is clear that transmission within a community fluctuates from year to year. These fluctuations will of course affect both the age and the height of the peak intensity. It is not obvious how such fluctuations should be modelled since, because of the ethical requirement to intervene, transmission data for communities at equilibrium are difficult to collect. Preliminary simulation studies indicate that, when transmission is strongly autocorrelated over several years, there is a tendency for later peaks to be lower in amplitude than earlier ones (unpublished observations). However, the situation is rather complicated and it is even possible to reverse this correlation for certain combinations of parameters. More modelling work, in which observed patterns of fluctuation in transmission are accurately reflected, would be needed to confirm the importance of this effect.

An 'intuitive', non-mathematical explanation is as follows: Consider a typical asymmetrical age-intensity profile: rising steeply and falling more gently.

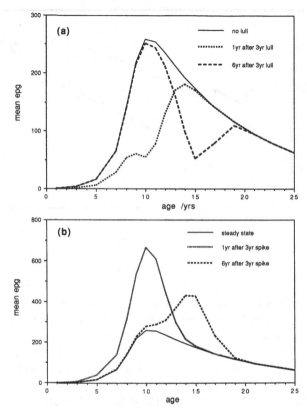

Figure 8. The effect of (a) a lull in transmission and (b) a transmission spike on a simulated age-intensity profile. $\lambda(a)$ peaks at 8 years and μ is constant.

Imagine a 'chunk' taken out of this by a few years' lull in transmission (figure 8a); the chunk will be deepest in the younger age groups where transmission is greatest. If the progress of this hypothetical community is followed for a few years, it will be seen that as the chunk moves through the age groups, it causes the peak to shift. When it lies under the usual peak the observed peak is both smaller and shifted to the right. Because the curve is asymmetrical, similar shifts to the left are less pronounced and are not accompanied by as large a reduction in the peak height. A similar effect is seen if a transmission spike is introduced (figure 8b).

It is true that some of the phenomena that potentially interfere with these tests might be detected and quantified. For instance, patterns of exposure that might give rise to the peak shift or decline in dispersion should themselves correlate with intensity of infection. The cost of checking this, however, would be dear in terms of the ease and elegance of the methods. To correlate patterns of exposure with intensity of infection, for instance, would require detailed water contact data on far more communities than our group, or anyone else, has available.

Finally, looking beyond the goal of simply detecting acquired immunity, neither method seems well suited to the quantization of immune protection. Not only are peak location and dispersion awkward to estimate, but their relationship with immunity would probably be rather complex.

5 Reinfection studies

The main advantages that treatment-reinfection studies have over simpler cross-sectional studies is that they effectively remove the blurring caused by worm longevity and the complication of differential worm death rates. Age-specific reinfection levels, at least over the short term, ought to be approximately proportional to $\lambda(a)$: if $\lambda(a) = \Lambda(a).L(t)$, $d\Lambda(a)/dt \approx 0$ and $\mu(a)$ =constant, then

$$M(a,t) \approx \Lambda(a).[\int_t^0 L(x).e^{\mu(x-t)}dx].$$

However, they are not without their disadvantages: reinfection levels can be too low to be estimated accurately and they are uninformative about worm death. Lack of compliance (with both treatment and stool samples) and treatment failure cause additional complications for these studies.

The converse experiment, in which transmission is broken and rates of natural worm death are observed among untreated individuals has been performed in the past (Wilkins *et al.* 1984). With the advent of better chemotherapy, in particular the drug praziquantel, these studies would no longer be considered to be ethically acceptable.

It is perhaps surprising that the two 'ecological' tests have not been applied to reinfection data. Provided that immunity operates on parasite invasion rather than death, both ought still to be valid and yet many of the objections listed above would be removed. We have relevant data from Kenya and intend to run these tests in due course. However, the direct link between intensity of reinfection and $\lambda(a)$ leads most naturally to regression analysis. It is the complications that arise from this type of analysis with which we intend to deal in the rest of the paper.

Transformations and distributional matters

In this section we concentrate specifically upon the schistosome that we study, *S. mansoni*; only the broader priciples will apply to other species.

There are at least three levels of variation to consider when analysing egg

	Number of stools									
	1	**2**	**3**	**4**	**5**	**6**	**7**	**8**	**9**	**10**
1	69.9	49.4	40.3	34.9	31.2	28.5	26.4	24.7	23.3	22.1
2	59.3	42.0	34.3	29.7	26.5	24.2	22.4	21.0	19.8	18.8
3	55.4	39.2	32.0	27.7	24.8	22.6	20.9	19.6	18.5	17.5
4	53.3	37.7	30.8	26.6	23.8	21.8	20.1	18.8	17.8	16.9
5	52.0	36.8	30.0	26.0	23.3	21.2	19.7	18.4	17.3	16.4
6	51.1	36.2	29.5	25.6	22.9	20.9	19.3	18.1	17.0	16.2
7	50.5	35.7	29.2	25.2	22.6	20.6	19.1	17.9	16.8	16.0
8	50.0	35.4	28.9	25.0	22.4	20.4	18.9	17.7	16.7	15.8
9	49.6	35.1	28.7	24.8	22.2	20.3	18.8	17.5	16.5	15.7
10	49.3	34.9	28.5	24.7	22.1	20.1	18.6	17.4	16.4	15.6

(Row labels at left: **Number of slides**)

Table 1. % Coefficient of variation for egg output estimates tabulated by numbers of stools and slides for an individual whose true output is 100epg.

output (usually measured as eggs per gram of faeces, epg):

(i) between slides, within stool,

(ii) between stools, within individual and

(iii) between individuals, within group.

Empirically, the variance is approximately proportional to the mean for (i), while the standard deviation is approximately proportional to the mean for (ii) and (iii). Between-stool variation is greater than is often appreciated so that, especially for smaller, detailed investigations in which individuals are the unit of study, the necessity to take many stool specimens to obtain sufficient precision cannot be over emphasised. In our own reinfection studies (Dunne *et al.* 1992), correlations between intensity of reinfection and immunological variables only became clear when we pooled stool results from six surveys, each of three stools, giving a total of 18 stools per individual, taken over a three year period. Multiple slides from a single stool cannot improve the accuracy beyond a certain point, as is demonstrated in Table 1. Slides are prepared from a single small sample from each stool. In a recent small study in Kenya we estimated that the variability between samples from a single stool only accounts for 30% of the variance between stools: the cumbersome process of taking multiple samples from each stool would give only marginal benefit.

It is often assumed that egg counts (raw counts per slide, rather than epg) follow a negative binomial distribution. The error structure resulting from the various components of variance approximately yield the following variance-mean relationship:

$$\text{var(mean)} = \phi.\text{mean} + \psi.\text{mean}^2 \tag{2}$$

where $\phi > 1$. For the negative binomial $\phi = 1$, but this distribution might serve as a starting point for analysis: both the index $k(= 1/\psi)$ and ϕ would need to be estimated and ought strictly to be functions of host age. The multiplicative nature of the model (see below) suggests that the link function should be the logarithm, although this is not the canonical link and hence not 'statistically optimal' (McCullagh and Nelder 1983).

But this analysis is rather more complicated than most researchers would want, and not necessarily very much more informative than simpler regression models. It is conventional to take logarithms of egg counts – usually log(epg + 1) – before performing the regression and there are theoretical justifications for this. Firstly, from the deterministic point of view, most factors should be multiplicative. Thus:

$$\text{epg} \quad = \quad e^{\alpha} \cdot \text{'exposure'}^{\beta} / \text{'immunity'}^{\gamma} \tag{3a}$$

$$\log(\text{epg}) \quad = \quad \alpha + \beta . \log(\text{'exposure'}) - \gamma . \log(\text{'immunity'}). \tag{3b}$$

Usually we think in terms of H^0: $\beta = 1$, $\gamma = 0$ vs. H^1: $\beta = 1$, $\gamma = 1$ but allowing β and γ more flexibility makes the model more robust. Since immunological variables, such as antibody levels, are measured on an arbitrary scale not necessarily proportional to their impact on intensity, initially there is no need to take their logarithms in equation (3b).

Egg counts present two distributional problems: skewness and heteroscedasticity (variance instability). Taking logarithms will stabilise the variance when the standard deviation is proportional to the mean (e.g. for the gamma distribution) and helps in the case of egg counts, since the second term in equation (2) is the dominant one, but does not completely cure the problem. The variance and mean of log(epg+1) typically plot as a partial inverted parabola. A variance-stabilising transformation for the relationship in equation (2) does exist but is rather complicated and involves an unknown constant, ψ/ϕ, which would need to be estimated, probably iteratively. Taking logarithms will also remove some of the skewness from the distribution but rarely does a completely symmetrical distribution result: the cluster at zero, which dominates the distribution when the prevalence is low, is not diffused by any (deterministic) transformation while the logarithm can reverse the skewness in intensely infected populations.

Frequently these distributional problems are ameliorated because the data are analysed as means. If each individual's egg output is the average of a number of stool results then the distribution becomes more continuous, with standard deviation proportional to the mean, i.e more like the gamma distribution. Means of egg counts of large enough groups of individuals should, according to the central limit theorem, become almost normally distributed. Bootstrap simulations indicate that Normal-theory based inference for logged egg counts is quite reliable when the sample size is above 25 and the prevalence is greater than 16% (Table 2).

While the logarithm has some beneficial effects on variance stability and

1000 samples from 'typical' *S. mansoni* egg count data: Matithini
Community pre- and posttreatment (1984 and 1989).

Details of source data.

	pretreatment	posttreatment
N	1223.	1228.
prevalence (%)	62.	16.
arithmetic mean (epg)	219.	22.6
geometric mean (epg)	20.2	0.88

**Reliablility of Normal-assumption inference: frequency
(%) with which 95% confidence intervals estimated from
bootstrap samples enclosed "true" mean.**

Bootstrap sampe size	--Pretreatment--		--Posttreatment--	
	untransf.	log.	untransf.	log.
25	84.5	94.2	64.6	88.8
50	90.2	95.6	72.8	93.4
100	90.1	94.5	82.3	93.0

**Distribution of sample means: 5th - 95th centiles
of bootstrap sample mean divided by "true" mean**

Bootstrap sample size	----Pretreatment-----		----Posttreatment----	
	arithmetic	geometric	arithmetic	geometric
25	0.42-1.78	0.38-2.40	0.04-3.26	0.18-2.53
50	0.57-1.58	0.52-1.87	0.15-2.55	0.41-1.92
100	0.66-1.36	0.62-1.59	0.34-2.05	0.51-1.63

Table 2. Bootstrap sampling comparison of arithmetic and geometric means

distributional symmetry it is not obvious that the overall performance of the
geometric mean is any better than that of the arithmetic mean. For instance,
in some preliminary simulation studies using sample of size 50 from the discretised gamma distribution we found that, while the arithmetic mean gives
an unbiased estimate of the true mean, the geometric mean underestimates it
considerably (by as much as 10 fold or more), and this bias increases rapidly
as the dispersion of the distribution increases. Also, at about the level of
dispersion that is actually observed between individuals, the proportionality
between the geometric mean and the true mean was lost. It can be demonstrated algebraically that the geometric mean (using the simple logarithm,
rather than $\log(\cdot + 1)$) of gamma distributed data (not discretised) ought
to be proportional to the true mean. The simulation results are borne out

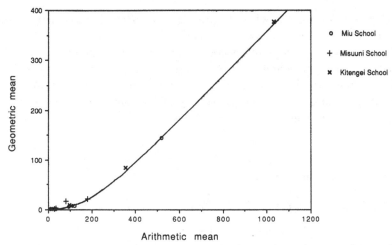

Figure 9. Geometric vs. arithmetic mean epg for five single-stool surveys from each of three schools. Sample sizes per survey ranged between 220 and 550.

by field data (figure 9). However, this bias of the geometric mean could be corrected and, on the whole, our bootstrap simulations indicate that the geometric mean is superior both with respect to reliability of Normal-theory based inference and the precision of its estimates, especially when the prevalence is low.

On the positive side, the proportionality between the geometric mean and the true number of worm pairs may be less affected by density dependent fecundity. In simulations of egg output data from a negative binomial distribution of worm pairs ($k = 0.5$) we found this to be so (unpublished observations). However, these results are questionable since Medley and Anderson's (1985) results, which we used to model the relationship between worm pairs and fecundity, do not fit well with our field data, predicting a far lower prevalence than we actually observe.

We, like many others in this field, have accumulated large quantities of egg count data over the years and are in a position to quantify quite accurately the dependence of the variance upon the mean, age and possibly other variables. In principle, therefore, it would be possible to apply this information to the analysis of further studies that would otherwise be too small to permit an accurate estimation of variance. An additional advantage would be that comparison of the observed and expected residual errors would provide a convenient test of goodness of fit. This sort of analysis would be most easily performed using programs such as GLIM, which, unlike simpler packages, can readily handle complex variance functions. In that case more attention to the error structure, perhaps returning to a model related to the negative binomial, would be appropriate.

Sometimes, for instance when the prevalence is so low that the distribution of egg counts is seriously distorted, it may be desirable to analyse prevalence, rather than intensity (epg), of infection. Prevalence is obviously not linearly related to worm burden and at high levels it is rather an insensitive variable. Its distribution can also be difficult to determine. In reinfection studies, the probability of infection (or the probability of infection being detected), P, should increase with exposure, X, as follows:

$$\frac{dP}{dX} = c.X.(1 - P). \tag{4a}$$

Hence, for a given individual:

$$-\log(1 - P) = \frac{1}{2}c.X^2$$
$$\log(-\log(1 - P)) = \log(c) + 2\log(X) + \text{const.} \tag{4b}$$

This would lead most naturally to binomial error regression with the complementary log-log link function. The problem is the familiar one of overdispersion: an individual's exposure cannot be measured accurately and, while this inaccuracy may be averaged out for groups of individuals, there will be considerable variation in exposure between individuals. A common device applied when overdispersion affects binomial data is to fit the beta-binomial distribution (Williams 1982). This distribution results if the binomial probability itself follows a beta distribution (i.e. the beta-binomial is a beta mixture of binomial distributions in the same way that the negative binomial is a gamma mixture of Poissons). If exposure, and hence $-\log(1 - P)$, follows a gamma distribution (a reasonable assumption for both measurement error and between individual variation) then it can be numerically demonstrated that the beta-binomial is a poor model. The reason that the beta-binomial is popular is that it is algebraically tractable; the distribution generated by assuming a gamma distribution for exposure is not. In principle it would be possible to establish an approximate model empirically but currently we have no data base suitable for this. A solution to this problem is required not only to find the error structure of prevalence estimates but also to establish the relationship between prevalence and mean exposure. To the authors' knowledge the problem remains unresolved.

Covariable matters

When factors affecting the rate of reinfection are investigated, two familiar problems which dog epidemiology immediately arise: confounding and 'error-in-X'. Confounding almost seems to be built into immunological data: immunity, since it requires experience of infection, must correlate with age and hence will be confounded with the many other variables that also correlate with age. In our studies, reinfection correlates very strongly with age;

so much so in Study H that very few individuals over 16 years of age were reinfected. To allow (control) for confounding variables in an analysis, the significance of the variable of interest (immunological) is tested by looking at the improvement in the fit of the model when the variable of interest is added to the model already containing the confounding variable. However, if the confounding variable is inaccurately or imprecisely estimated its effects may not be fully removed and spurious associations may appear to be significant.

The safest analysis would be to control for age since not only is this variable estimated accurately but it would also remove most of the confounding effects. Significance after controlling for age has been achieved for some IgE responses (Hagan *et al.* 1991, Dunne *et al.* 1992). However, controlling for age could drastically reduce genuine immunological effects. It might be preferable, therefore, to control for those factors which underlie the changes with age, since these may be less strongly confounded with immunity. The problem would be to identify all of these factors, but it is generally assumed that exposure is the most important. Since it should have a profound effected on infection rates, an additional incentive for controlling for exposure, whether or not it is age-related, is that it ought to increase the power of statistical tests simply by reducing the residual variance.

The measurement of exposure, however, is fraught with difficulties of precision, accuracy and 'over-parameterisation'. Precision can be estimated by dividing the available observations into two equal, balanced sets. For instance, if each site were observed on two days each month then each set would contain one day's observations for each site each month. The variance of the precision of exposure scores may then be calculated from what amounts to duplicate observations for each individual and the expected effect upon correlations can be estimated from the correlation between the duplicates. Denoting the imprecise, 'duplicate' exposure scores as x_{1i} and x_{2i}, theoretical (precisely measured) exposure score as X_i and the intensity (epg) as Y_i, $\text{corr}(Y_i, X_i) = \rho$, $\text{corr}(Y_i, x_{1i} + x_{2i}) = R$ and $\text{corr}(x_{1i}, x_{2i}) = R^*$, the following relationship may be easily derived:

$$R^2 = \frac{2R^*}{(R^* + 1)}\rho^2. \tag{5}$$

Thus, an obvious adjustment for estimates of R^2 would be the factor $(r^* + 1)/2r^*$, where r^* is the (estimated) coefficient of correlation between the duplicates. Typically we obtain values for r^* of around 0.6 for our better water contact observations, implying that some 25% of this powerful variable's effect has not been removed.

Accuracy, on the other hand, is impossible to assess: we do not know how to weight correctly the various aspects of contact nor whether we are recording all the pertinent aspects. Most researchers, including ourselves, have usually

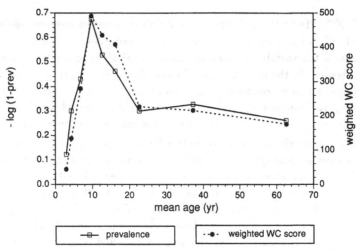

Figure 10. Iietune community weighted water contact and reinfection prevalence vs, age.
$N = 100$ for each point.

applied arbitrary weightings, based on what is known about cercarial activity
and body surface area, but our knowledge is scanty and there is a danger that
our choice may reflect our prejudices. It is possible to adjust the weightings
in order to improve their explanatory power but there are many parameters
and it is difficult to know when to stop. In an attempt to systematize this
approach, we have fitted these data to egg output using a non-linear model
of the form:

$$Y_i = c + \sum_{j}^{n_i} w_{1ij}.w_{2ij}.w_{3ij}. \ldots (\text{‘duration of contact’}_{ij}),$$

where w_{1ij}, w_{2ij},... are the weights given to the various aspects of the ith
individual's jth observed contact. In theory the parameter values estimated
by the fitting process ought to have maximised the explanatory power of
exposure. In practice the large number of parameters made the model unstable: it would not converge to a solution unless the parameter values were
constrained. It is also inevitable that some of the many parameters will be
age-related and, when these are emphasised, the age-exposure profile can be
moulded to mirror that of the age-reinfection curve (figure 10).

The problem of age confounding is so marked that we believe that new
approaches must lie in study design rather than analysis. An early study
in which experience of infection was uncoupled from age was undertaken in
Brazil by Kloetzel and Da Silva (1967). This study, in which the intensity
of infection among adult immigrants was shown to be related to years spent
in the endemic area rather than age, is still among the best evidence for acquired immunity to schistosomiasis. There are two further promising studies

of this sort currently under way in Africa. In northern Senegal an epidemic of *schistosomiasis mansoni* has occurred in the town of Richard Toll since the construction of a large dam over the Senegal River, exposing many adults to infection for the first time. This is the focus of intensive study by several groups as part of the ESPOIR project under the coordination of Prof. A. Capron of the Institut Pasteur, Lille, France. In Kenya, a tract of previously uninhabited bush at Masongaleni, adjacent to the Kambu area that we have been studying, has recently been cleared and settled by Wakamba immigrants from the Chyulu Hills, an area known to be devoid of schistosomiasis. A neighbouring community, who are infected with *S. mansoni* and who use the same water sources, should form a near perfect control group.

6   Concluding remarks

It is hoped that this review of the statistical problems associated with assessing the evidence for human immunity to schistosomiasis has drawn attention to the limitations of existing cross-sectional and reinfection studies. We hope also to have illustrated the fact that, beyond a certain degree of complexity, systems fail to yield to yet more complicated analysis: they must be simplified. Some of the problems outlined may be overcome by appropriate analysis and more detailed observation, while others, inherent in the study design, will not. The development of micro-simulation packages, for instance, may assist in determining the distribution of variables and with study design. However, in our opinion, mathematical modelling is a tool better applied to synthesis than to analysis: it has a greater role in the design of control programmes and in generating ideas than in providing scientific proof of biological phenomena. Major advances, we believe, will come from studies such as those in Senegal and Masongaleni, which overcome the enormous practical, though trivial theoretical, problem of age confounding.

References

Anderson, R.M. and Gordon, D.M. (1982) 'Processes influencing the distribution of parasite numbers within populations with special emphasis on parasite-induced host mortality', *Parasitology* 85, 373–398.

Anderson, R.M. and May, R.M. (1985) 'Herd immunity to helminth infection and implications for parasite control', *Nature* 315, 493–496.

Bradley, D.J. and McCullough, F.S. (1973) 'Egg output stability and the epidemiology of *Schistosoma haematobium*. Part II: An analysis of the epidemiology of endemic *S. haematobium*', *Trans. Roy. Soc. Trop. Med. Hyg.* 67, 491–500.

Bundy, D.A.P., Cooper, E.S., Thompson, D.E., Anderson, R.M. and Didier, J.M. (1987) 'Age-related prevalence and intensity of *Trichuris trichuris* infection in a St. Lucian community', *Trans. Roy. Soc. Trop. Med. Hyg.* 81, 85–94.

Butterworth, A.E., Dunne, D.W., Fulford, A.J.C., Capron, M., Khalife, J., Capron, A., Koech, D., Ouma, J.H. and Sturrock, R.S. (1988) 'Immunity in human schistosomiasis mansoni: cross-reactive IgM and IgG2 anti-carbohydrate antibodies block the expression of immunity', *Biochimie* **70**, 1053–1063.

Butterworth, A.E., Sturrock, R.F., Ouma, J.H., Mbugua, G.G., Fulford, A.J.C., Kariuki, H.C. and Koech, D. (1991) 'Comparison of different chemotherapy strategies against *Schistosoma mansoni* in Machakos District, Kenya. 1: Effects on human infection and morbidity', *Parasitology* **103**, 339–355.

Chandiwana, S.K., and Woolhouse, M.E.J. (1991) 'Heterogeneities in water contact patterns and the epidemiology of *Schistosoma haematobium*', *Parasitology* **103**, 363–370.

Dalton, P.R. and Poole, D. (1978) 'Water contact patterns in relation to *Schistosoma haematobium* infection', *Bull. WHO* **56**, 417–428.

Dessein, A.J., Begley, M., Demeure, C., Caillol, D., Galvao dos Reis, M., Andrade, Z.A., Prata, A. and Bina, J.C. (1988) 'Human resistance to *Schistosoma mansoni* is associated with IgG reactivity to a 37kDa larval surface antigen', *J. Immunol.* **140**, 2727–2736.

Dunne, D.W., Butterworth, A.E., Fulford, A.J.C., Kariuki, H.C., Langley, J.G., Ouma, J.H., Capron, A., Pierce, R.J. and Sturrock, R.S. (1992) 'Immunity after treatment of human schistosomiasis: asociation between IgE antibodies to adult worm antigens and resistance to reinfection', *Euro. J. Immunol.* **22**, 1483–1494.

Fulford, A.J.C., Mbugua, G.G., Ouma, J.H., Kariuki, H.C., Sturrock, R.F. and Butterworth, A.E. (1991) 'Differences in the rate of hepatosplenomegaly due to *Schistosoma mansoni* infection between two areas in Machakos District, Kenya', *Trans. Roy. Soc. Trop. Med. Hyg.* **85**, 481–488.

Fulford, A.J.C., Butterworth, A.E., Sturrock, R.F. and Ouma, J.H. (1992) 'On the use of age-intensity data to detect immunity to parasitic infections, with special reference to *Schistosoma mansoni* in Kenya', *Parasitology* **105**, 219–227.

Fulford, A.J.C., Butterworth, A.E., Ouma, J.H. and Sturrock, R.F. (1995) 'A statistical approach to schistosome population dynamics and estimation of the lifespan of *Schistosoma mansoni* in man', *Parasitology*, in press.

Hagan, P., Blumenthal, U.J., Dunn, D., Simpson, A.J.G. and Wilkins, H.A. (1991) 'Human IgE, IgG4 and resistance to infection with *Schistosoma haematobium*', *Nature* **349**, 243–245.

de Jonge, N., Gryseels, B., Hilberath, G.W., Ponderman, A.M., Deelder, A.M. (1988) 'Detection of circulating anodic antigens by ELISA for seroepidemiology of *Schistosomiasis mansoni*', *Trans. Roy. Soc. Trop. Med. Hyg.* **82**, 591–594.

Kloetzel. K., Da Silva, J.R. (1967) '*Schistosomasis mansoni* acquired in adulthood: behaviour of egg counts and the intradermal test', *Am. J. Trop. Med. Hyg.* **16**, 167–169.

Medley, G.F. and Anderson, R.M. (1985) 'Density-dependent fecundity in *Schistosoma mansoni* infections in man', *Trans. Roy. Soc. Trop. Med. Hyg.* **79**, 532–534.

McCullagh, P. and Nelder, J.A. (1983) *General Linear Models*, Chapman and Hall, London.

Ouma, J.H., (1987) *Transmission of* Schistosoma mansoni *in an Endemic Area of Kenya with Special Reference to the Role of Human Defaecation Behaviour and Sanitary Practices*, PhD thesis.

Pacala, S.W. and Dobson, A.P. (1988) 'The relationship between the number of parasites/host and the host age: population dynamic causes and maximum likelihood estimation', *Parasitology* **96**, 197–210.

Roberts, M., Gachuhi, K., Kamau, T., Fulford, A.J.C., Dunne, D.W., Ouma, J.H., Sturrock, R.S. and Butterworth, A.E. (1993) 'Immunity after treatment of human schistosomiasis: association between cellular responser and resistance to reinfection', *Inf. Immun.* **61**, 4984–4993.

Sturrock, R.S., Klumpp, R.K., Ouma, J.H., Butterworth, A.E., Fulford, A.J.C., Kariuki, H.C., Thiongo, F.W. and Koech, D. (1994) 'Observations on the effects of different chemotherapy strategies on the transmission of *Schistosoma mansoni* in Machakos District, Kenya, measured by long term snail sampling and cercariometry', *Parasitology* **109**, 443–453.

Warren, K.S. (1973) 'Regulation of the prevalence and intensity of schistosomiasis in man: immunity or ecology?', *J. Inf. Dis.* **127**, 595–609.

Warren, K.S., Mahmoud, A.A.F., Cummings, P., Murphy D.J. and Houser, H.B. (1974) 'Schistosomiasis mansoni in Yemeni in California: duration of infection, presence of disease, therapeutic management', *Am. J. Trop. Med. Hyg.* **23**, 902–909.

Webbe, G., James, C., Nelson, G.S., Smithers, S.R. and Terry, R.J. (1976) 'Acquired resistance to *Schistosoma haematobium* in the baboon (*Papio anubis*) after cercarial exposure and adult worm transplantation', *Ann. Trop. Med. Parasitol.* **70**, 411–424.

Wilkins, H.A., Goll, P.H., Marshall, T.F.de C. and Moore, P.J. (1984) 'Dynamics of *Schistosoma haematobium* infection in a Gambian community. III. Acquisition and loss of infection', *Trans. Roy. Soc. Trop. Med. Hyg.* **78**, 227–232.

Wilkins, H.A., Blumenthal, U.J., Hagan, P., Hayes, R.J. and Tullock, S. (1987) 'Resistance to reinfection after treatment of urinary schistosomiasis', *Trans. Roy. Soc. Trop. Med. Hyg.* **81**, 29–35.

Williams, D.A. (1982) 'Extra-binomial variation in logistic linear models', *Appl. Stat.* **31**, 144–148.

Woolhouse, M.E.J., Taylor, P., Matanhire, D. and Chandiwana, S.K. (1991) 'Acquired immunity and epidemiology of *Schistosoma haematobium*', *Nature* **351**, 757–759.

Woolhouse, M.E.J. (1992) 'A theoretical framework for the immunoepidemiology of helminth infection', *Paras. Immunol.* **14**, 563–578.

Virulence and Transmissibility in *P. falciparum* Malaria

Sunetra Gupta and Karen Day

1 Introduction

The relationship between virulence and transmissibility is an important theme in analysis of host-parasite interactions in natural populations (Anderson and May 1991). However, there are few studies of the effects of parasite virulence on the population dynamics of major infectious diseases of humans. Data from the era of malaria therapy (James 1932, Covell 1951) and recent molecular studies (reviewed by Marsh 1992) indicate that there may be considerable variation in virulence within the *Plasmodium falciparum* parasite, which causes over 1 million malaria deaths each year. In this paper we explore the population dynamic and genetic implications of such proposed parasite diversity to ask whether they may explain some of the now well-defined epidemiological features of malarial disease.

In African children, amongst whom the great majority of malaria deaths occur, *Plasmodium falciparum* malaria can be clinically resolved into 'mild' and 'severe' types. This distinction describes a clear, and readily recognisable, clinical differentiation of malaria into a majority (about 99%) of uncomplicated cases with a very low mortality ($\ll 1\%$), and a small number of severe cases with a mortality of 10-20% under treatment (Brewster 1990). Furthermore, severe malarial disease manifests as either severe malarial anaemia or cerebral malaria, both pathologically distinct from mild malaria. Hence, this classification is not just an arbitrary division of a continuum of disease severity, but reflects a clear bimodality in the severity of malarial disease.

There is strong evidence that host genetic susceptibility influences the clinical outcome of malarial infection; the immunological, nutritional and sociological status of the host may also be of varying degrees of importance (reviewed by Greenwood *et al..* (1991)). Disease severity may also depend on the size of initial parasite inoculum (McGregor 1965). The variability in the clinical outcome of *P. falciparum* infection may also be a consequence of heterogeneity in parasite phenotypes associated with the pathology of severe disease. It is apparent that whether an individual develops mild or severe malaria must depend on a complex combination of host and parasite factors. However, the epidemiological patterns of mild and severe disease observed within the population at large may be predominantly influenced by a few key variables. In this paper, we propose that certain characteristic epidemiological features of mild and severe disease may be best explained by heterogeneity in parasite virulence.

The paper is organised into five sections. We begin with a brief discussion of putative virulence factors in *P. falciparum* malaria, and their relationship to severe disease. Many of the parasite phenotypes designated as putative 'virulence factors' are likely to have some effect on the production and maintenance of transmissible sexual stages or gametocytes. In the second section, we explore the possible influence of the virulence factors on parasite transmissibility, and discuss the implications for the maintenance of heterogeneity in parasite virulence. In the third section, we interpret age-structured patterns of malarial disease as the epidemiological consequence of an association between parasite virulence and transmissibility. We use observed age-structured patterns of mild and severe disease, and recent molecular observations, to define a population structure of *P. falciparum* in terms of parasite virulence and transmissibility. The fourth section demonstrates how heterogeneity in host resistance may facilitate the maintenance of diversity in parasite virulence. In the final section, we discuss how the results of bednet trials can be explained by heterogeneity in parasite virulence. We thereby provide a coherent theoretical framework for the design and analysis of field and laboratory studies regarding parasite virulence.

2 Virulence factors

Although data from animal models (Cox 1988) and induced malaria experiments (James 1932, Covell 1951) indicate that isolates can vary in the severity of disease that they cause, differences in *P. falciparum* virulence have yet to be conclusively demonstrated in the field. Recently, however, a number of parasite phenotypes have been identified as possible virulence factors; these include cytoadherence (adherence of infected cells to epithelial surfaces), rosetting (of uninfected erythrocytes by infected erythrocytes), cytokine production, and less specifically, immune evasion mechanisms and variation in the intrinsic growth rate of the parasite. We provide below a brief summary of the importance of these parasite functions in the pathogenesis of severe malarial anaemia and cerebral malaria, to illustrate how polymorphism in any of these phenotypes could result in heterogeneity of parasite virulence.

The proximate cause of severe malarial anaemia is the destruction of parasitised erythrocytes, which may be associated with chronicity or high density of infection. High density and/or chronicity may generally be related to superior mechanisms of immune evasion and high growth rate. More specifically, parasite survival (and hence, parasite density) may be enhanced by cytoadherence, as the sequestration of infected cells in the vasculature may benefit the parasite by permitting infected erythrocytes to avoid circulation through the spleen, where they would be recognised as abnormal and destroyed (Miller 1969). Furthermore, the metabolic (hypoxic) environment of post-capillary venules where cytoadherence occurs, may be favourable for parasite development. Sequestration and rosetting may also confer a steric advantage for reinvasion of uninfected cells, and thus elevate parasite densities (Berendt *et al.* 1990). Bone marrow depression and rapid clearance of unparasitised erythrocytes may also contribute to severe malarial anaemia; data from animal models indicate that TNF (Tumour Necrosis Factor: a cytokine) may influence these processes (Kwiatkowski 1993).

The main pathological feature of cerebral malaria is the obstruction of cerebral vessels with parasite infected erythrocytes. High density asexual parasitaemia may precipitate cerebral malaria, as saturation of other sites may be responsible for the accumulation of infected erythrocytes in the cerebral vasculature. Alternatively, cerebral malaria may be caused by the enhanced adherence of infected erythrocytes to brain tissue, or by the blockage of brain capillaries from rosetting of uninfected erythrocytes by infected erythrocytes. Higher degrees of rosetting have been found among parasites from children with cerebral malaria in the Gambia, in comparison with non-cerebral cases (Carlson *et al.* 1990). Circulating TNF levels have also been observed to be higher in patients with cerebral malaria; TNF may act as a co-factor in the pathogenesis of cerebral malaria by upregulating parasite cytoadherence (Kwiatkowski 1991).

The effect of virulence factors on transmissibility

Parasite transmissibility may be expressed as a combination of parameters, known as the basic reproductive ratio (R_0), which is a measure of the average number of secondary infections generated by one primary infection in a totally susceptible population. The basic reproductive rate of malaria may be given as:

$$R_0 = ma^2bLDc \qquad (1)$$

where m is the number of mosquitos per human host, a is the mosquito biting rate (which is raised to the second power as two biting events must take place to complete the cycle), b denotes the probability that an infective mosquito bite will produce an infection in the host, L is the average lifespan of the mosquito, D is the average duration of infectiousness in the human host, and c is the probability an infectious 'feed' will lead to sporozoite production in the vector (Aron and May 1982). The relationships of these terms to the parasite functions associated with virulence may be complex.

The parameters in (1) that may be influenced by virulence factors are essentially those associated with infectiousness, namely the duration, D, and the intensity, c, of infectiousness. Certain of these parasite functions may also affect the initial establishment of infection, b, such as the ability to invade hepatocytes. Alternatively, these parasite functions may be genetically linked to factors affecting transmission, in which case it could modify almost any or all of the parameters in the equation, with the exception of the vector-host density ratio, m. We choose to illustrate the complexities of the relationship betwen virulence factors and transmissibility by limiting the discussion to effects of virulence factors on the infectiousness of the parasite within the human host.

The transmission of the parasite from the human host to the mosquito vector can only be achieved by the production of gametocytes (sexual stages). The factors that stimulate the production of gametocytes have yet to be clearly identified. High parasitaemia may enhance gametocyte production, if the latter is dependent on the density of asexual stages in the blood. There is *in vitro* evidence to suggest that gametocyte production is positively correlated with the density of asexual parasitaemia (Carter and Miller 1979). Furthermore, the consistent lag of 8–10 days between high parasitaemia/fever and the occurence of gametocytes in the peripheral circulation for *P. falciparum* infections (Carter and Graves 1988) suggests that the former may act as a specific trigger for the production of sexual stages. Thus virulence factors leading to high density of parasitaemia, such as cytoadherence, may increase the duration and intensity of infectiousness. Splenic evasion through cytoadherence may play a more direct role in increasing infectiousness as developing gametocytes of *P. falciparum* also sequester until mature and infectious (Garnham 1966).

A negative effect on transmission of all virulence factors occurs as a consequence of host mortality (reducing the population average of the duration of infectiousness, D). However, the adverse effects may be more subtle. For instance, high parasitaemia could induce a severe non-specific immune response, that could act to reduce the infectiousness of gametocytes. Fever/paroxysms are associated with high plasma levels of the pyrogenic cytokine TNF (Kwiatkowski 1989, Mendis *et al.* 1990) which, along with other cytokines such as IFN, appear to affect circulating gametocytes, as demonstrated by membrane feeding experiments on *P. vivax* infections in Sri Lanka (Gamagemendis *et al.* 1992).

As a result of these tensions between the different effects of parasite phenotypes associated with virulence, the relationship between virulence and transmissibility (R_0) is non linear, with the latter likely to peak at some intermediate value of virulence. Though in contrast to the classical coevolutionary paradigm where host and parasite are expected to attain some state of mutual harmlessness, selection for intermediate levels of virulence has been widely demonstrated, both experimentally and through theoretical exercises

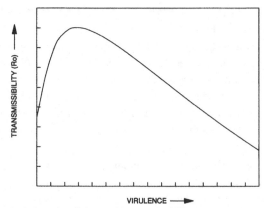

Figure 1. A typical functional form of transmissibility vs. virulence. Transmissibility may be measured as the basic reproductive ratio, R_0, while virulence may be represented by a theoretical measure of morbidity and mortality.

(Anderson and May 1982, Levin and Pimental 1981, May and Anderson 1983, 1990). Figure 1 shows a typical functional form of transmissibility vs. virulence, where R_0 is measure of the former, and the latter axis is a composite measure of morbidity and mortality. Parasite types with the intermediate degree of virulence that maximises transmission (R_0) will have an evolutionary advantage over other types, provided there is competition between the different parasite types. Under these circumstances, the system may be expected to evolve towards the intermediate degree of virulence that maximises transmissibility.

The question then arises of how polymorphisms are maintained at genetic loci governing the expression of virulence factors, given that selection will occur for alleles that maximise transmissibility. In a situation where there is strong competition between different parasite types (as a result of shared immune responses, for instance), coexistence is only possible if the strains have similar, if not identical, basic reproductive ratios (Gupta *et al.* 1994). Thus a more virulent strain must compensate for higher host mortality (which reduces the population average of duration of infectiousness, D) through higher infectiousness (c) and/or higher probabilities of establishment (b). The resulting relationship between virulence and transmissibility is shown in Figure 2a, where the first peak in transmissibility (R_0) represents mild malaria, and the second peak, of similar height, permits the existence of a more virulent strain of similar transmissibility.

However, selection for optimum virulence (i.e. maximum transmissibility) will only occur if the different strains are in competition. If there is no competition between the strains, the constraint that the basic reproductive ratios must be similar can be relaxed (Gupta *et al.* 1994). Thus R_0 will peak

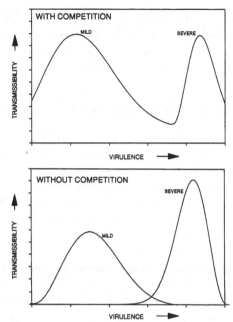

Figure 2. The relationships between parasites of differing virulence (a) with competition and (b) without competition. If the parasites are in competition, then they may coexist only under circumstances where the basic reproductive ratios of mild and severe types are identical, as shown in Figure 2a. If the parasite types are not in competition (i.e. constitute independently transmitted strains) then they may be represented by separate functional forms that independently dictate the optimum virulence of each strain, as shown in Figure 2b.

at some higher value of virulence for the 'severe' strain than for the 'mild' strain, but does not necessarily have to be of similar value, as demonstrated in Figure 2b. This scenario is favoured by the observed persistence of high prevalence of parasitaemia in older children, which suggests that infection-blocking immunity is either mainly strain specific, or develops only after a long history of exposure to shared determinants (Day and Marsh 1990). The typically abrupt decline in parasite rates between the ages of 10-15 years in endemic areas suggests the existence of a dynamically determined threshold in the immune response to shared determinants that is effective in blocking further infection (Gupta and Day 1994). This delayed development of 'cross-immunity' may serve as a weak source of competition, and limit the range of variation in R_0 between the parasite types (Gupta, Swinton and Anderson 1994).

We thus conclude that the maintenance of heterogeneity in parasite virulence is made possible by the virtual lack of effective 'cross-immunity' between strains of differing virulence, given that they are unlikely to be of similar transmissibility. These variously virulent strains thus essentially constitute separate transmission systems. In the following section, we show that this argument can offer a satisfactory basis for the hitherto unexplained age-structured patterns of severe and mild disease.

3   Age-structured patterns of disease

Figure 3 documents age-structured patterns of mild and severe malaria in The Gambia, West Africa. Figure 3a (adapted from Marsh 1992) records the age distribution of cases of mild malaria, in terms of average number of clinical episodes per year. Similar patterns have been recorded in other malaria endemic areas (Cattani *et al.* 1986, Rooth and Bjorkman 1992, Cox *et al.* 19943). Figure 3b shows the age distribution of cases of cerebral malaria (henceforth, CM) and severe malarial anaemia (henceforth, SMA) observed in a large case-control hospital-based study in the Gambia (see Hill *et al.* 1991); a similar study in coastal Kenya reports the same disjunction between the two age profiles (Marsh 1992). The average age of children with SMA has been reported as 27 months, and that of CM as 45 months, in The Gambia (Brewster *et al.* 1990). The corresponding ages in Coastal Kenya are 22 months and 40 months (Marsh 1992).

The steep rise and slow decline with age in the incidence of mild malaria (Figure 3a) can be explained by the existence of a number of independently transmitted antigenic types or 'strains', that each induce some degree of 'anti-disease' or protective immunity upon exposure (i.e. first infection).

The average age of exposure to mild malaria, defined as the experience of any one of n different strains is given by:

$$A_n = \frac{H}{\sum R_{0i}} \qquad (2)$$

where R_{0i} is the basic reproductive rate of strain i and H is the average duration of immunity against reinfection by the same strain (Gupta *et al.* 1993). The latter is determined by the relative proportions of the population who are immune (mostly adults) and non-immune (mostly children) to a given strain, rather than by the rate of decay of immunity, which does not appear to occur in endemic situations (either as a consequence of repeated boosting or as a natural characteristic of the immune response (Deloran and Chougnet 1992). In the limit where each strain induces lifelong strain-specific immunity against reinfection, H is equal to the average lifespan of the human host (Gupta *et al.* 1994).

Equation (2) implies that a large bulk of children will have experienced mild malaria at a very young age (< 1 year), as a consequence of the large number of strains circulating within a given region, even if the basic reproductive ratio of each strain (and hence of mild malaria as a whole) is very low.

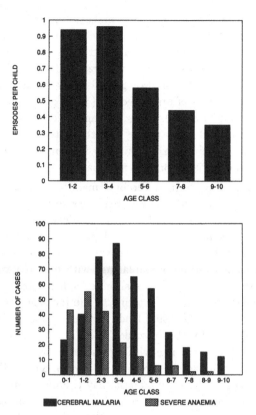

Figure 3. Age-structured patterns of mild and severe malaria in The Gambia, West Africa. Figure 3a (adapted from Marsh (1992)) records the age distribution of cases of mild malaria, in terms of average number of clinical episodes per year. Figure 3b shows the age distribution of cases of cerebral malaria and severe malarial anaemia observed in a large case-control hospital-based study in the Gambia (for details, see Hill *et al.* (1991))

The circulation of a large number of strains that each induce strain-specific 'anti-disease' (protective) immunity upon exposure can explain the slow, uniform decline in the incidence of mild disease. As the experience of different strains accumulates, the probability of infection with a new strain diminishes. Thus, the incidence of disease will decline slowly with age, as shown in Figure 3a. The broken lines in Figure 4a record the output of a mathematical model based on the above assumptions, where the number of strains of mild malaria is 50 (see Appendix A for mathematical details). Exposure to mild malaria, defined as the experience of any one of these strains, rises rapidly, as does the incidence of mild disease. The incidence of mild disease subsequently declines, as the number of 'new' strains encountered diminishes.

Both severe malaria syndromes appear to decline more rapidly with age than mild malaria. In the case of severe malarial anaemia (SMA), this may be an effect of protection from past exposure to mild malaria, as the sharp decline with age in the incidence of SMA correlates with the steep rise with age in the proportion exposed to mild malaria. The dotted line in Figure 4a shows the pattern of incidence of SMA generated by the assumption that the latter is a rare consequence of first infection (= exposure) with mild malaria parasites (any of the 50 strains). Thus, the age-specific pattern of incidence of SMA may be explained by assuming that the latter is a rare complication of infection with any mild malaria strain, occuring mainly among those who have little previous experience of mild malaria.

The age-structured pattern of cerebral malaria cannot however be explained by an association with lack of exposure to mild malaria. Furthermore, a recent study in The Gambia clearly indicates that lack of previous exposure is not a risk factor for the development of CM (Erunkulu 1992). Children with CM, in this study, were shown to recognise as wide a diversity of parasite isolates as children of similar age with mild malaria. This result suggests that CM may be caused by a an independently transmitted parasite type. The observed time-space clustering of the incidence of severe malaria in coastal Kenya (Snow et al. 1993) lends further support to this hypothesis. The higher average age of CM as recorded in Figure 3b can be thus explained as a consequence of a slower rise with age in exposure to parasites causing CM, in comparison with parasites causing mild malaria (and SMA). Equation 2 indicates that exposure to mild malaria may rise more rapidly than to CM because the former may be caused by a larger number of strains. Within this framework, the more rapid decline in the incidence of CM with age, in comparison with mild malaria, can be explained as characteristic of a disease caused by a single or a few strains.

The rise in exposure to mild malaria, defined as the experience of any one of a large number strains, will occur on a more rapid scale than for the few strains capable of causing CM, even if the transmissibility of mild malaria (a weighted average of the R_0 values of the constituent strains) is lower than the R_0 of CM (Gupta et al. 1994). As the proportion unexposed to each type diminishes, the incidence of the associated severe disease will decline. Figure 4a contrasts the respective patterns of CM and SMA, generated by a mathematical model in which CM is caused by a single parasite strain, while mild malaria may be caused by any of 50 strains. The solid lines record the slow rise in exposure to the CM strain, and the corresponding pattern of decline in incidence of CM. The incidence of both CM and SMA have been magnified by a factor of 10 for purposes of comparison with mild malaria. Figure 4b shows more clearly the relative patterns of decline for SMA and CM and mild malaria, where each has been rescaled to a maximum value of unity.

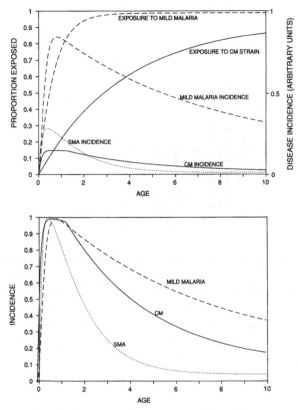

Figure 4. The simulations of a mathematical model with 50 strains of mild malaria and a single strain of cerebral malaria, as described in Appendix A. Figure 4a records the patterns of exposure to mild malaria and cerebral malaria parasites, and the associated patterns of mild and severe disease. The incidence of severe malarial anaemia and cerebral malaria is magnified 10 times to bring their respective patterns into view. Figure 4b compares patterns of decline in mild malaria, cerebral malaria and severe malarial anaemia, by normalising incidence to a maximum of unity for each disease.

In order to recover the precise patterns recorded in Figure 3, it is necessary to incorporate the effects of 'maternal immunity' on disease incidence. In the absence of 'maternal immunity', the highest incidence of disease is likely to occur in the youngest age class, as it contains the highest concentration of susceptibles. Clearly, this is not the case for either mild or severe malaria. Thus, a significant degree of protection against disease at birth, decaying rapidly with age, must be invoked to account for the low numbers in the first few years of life. The incidence of disease will thus, in all cases, appear to peak at a given age, rather than exhibiting a monotonic decline. The age at which incidence peaks will be determined by the rate of decline of

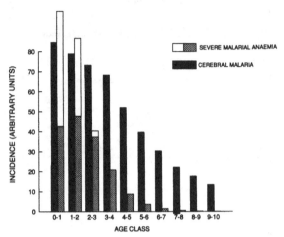

Figure 5. The effects of maternal immunity on the patterns of incidence of severe malarial anaemia and cerbral malaria. Without maternal immunity, disease incidence would decay uniformly, and at a faster rate for severe malarial anaemia. However, in the early age classes a certain proportion of these potential disease events are prevented, shown in white for SMA and grey for CM (not drawn to scale). SMA will nonetheless peak in the 1-2 age class, as a result of its rapid rate of decline. Because of its slow rate of decline, CM will however peak in a later age-class. We assume that maternal immunity is 70% in the 0-1 age class, and declines exponentially thereafter at a rate of 80%.

disease incidence in the absence of maternal immunity. The later peak in the case of CM thus essentially reflects a slower decline in disease incidence in comparison with SMA. This is shown in Figure 5, where the same degree of reduction in incidence in the early age classes, as a result of maternal protection, causes SMA to peak in an earlier age class than CM. We assume that maternal immunity decays exponentially at a rate of 80%, such that a significant proportion of children in the 0–1 and 1–2 age classes and a small fraction of the 2–3 year olds are protected against disease. With the incidences in the first three age classes accordingly scaled down, the age distributions of SMA and CM peak respectively in the 1–2 and 3–4 age classes.

Certain molecular observations support the stratification of the parasite population into strains of differing virulence and transmissibility, where those causing CM constitute a distinct subset. Although a multiplicity of parasite factors is associated with the diverse pathological consequences of malaria, we assume that the main cause of CM is the blockage of brain vessels by cytoadherence of infected erythrocytes. A high molecular weight antigen designated Pf EMP1 has been associated with the expression of the cytoadherence phenotype (Howard 1988). Polymorphisms in this molecule, leading to variability in cytoadherence, have been suggested as a possible explanation for heterogeneity in parasite virulence (Berendt *et al.* 1990, Ockenhouse *et al.* 1991, Marsh *et al.* 1988). The putative parasite cytoadherence ligand Pf EMP1 is believed to be the target of agglutinating antibodies which are isolate- and variant-specific (Newbold *et al.* 1992). These antibodies have been shown to correlate with protection against mild disease (Marsh *et al.* 1989). Epidemiological patterns of seroconversion to these antigenic types (as defined by the agglutinating antibodies) recorded in the Madang region of Papua New Guinea suggest that they are independently transmitted (Gupta *et al.* 1994). The stratification of the parasite population into independently transmitted strains of varying degrees of virulence may thus possibly be achieved with respect to this phenotype.

Differences in site-specificity of cytoadherence of gametocytes and asexual stages has led to the belief that cytoadherence mechanisms associated with the two developmental pathways are distinct (Howard 1988). Recent molecular experiments suggest that this may not be the case. Karyotype analysis of *P. falciparum* has shown that a 0.3 mb subtelomeric deletion on the right end of chromososme 9 results in the simultaneous loss of expression of asexual cytoadherence and gametocytogenesis (Day *et al.* 1993). This deletion also results in loss of expression of Pf EMP1, and the agglutination phenotype. The localisation of the expression of these phenotypes to a small region of chromosome 9 suggests that gametocytes and asexual stages may share the same cytoadherence mechanism, possibly mediated through Pf EMP1. This hypothesis is supported by the observation that early gametocytes utilise the same cytoadherence receptor (CD36) on host target cells (Day, unpublished data). The Pf EMP1 genotype may thus directly define the transmissibility of a strain, and thus consolidate the stratification of the parasite population into strains of differing virulence and transmissibility.

4   Host heterogeneity and parasite virulence

We have shown how a large diversity in virulence and transmissibility can exist within a *P. falciparum* transmission system, as a result of the long delay in the development of 'cross-immune' infection-blocking responses, which serve only as a very weak source of inter-strain competition. Host genetic factors that protect against severe disease will serve to further weaken the intensity of competition by providing an alternative transmission system. In the limit where a strain is lethal in all but a certain host genotype, the strain may linger at low levels within the latter (causing a small fraction of deaths when it is transmitted to non-immune host genotypes) instead of vanishing from the system. Mathematical models (Appendix B) predict that, under these circumstances, rapid selection for the 'resistant' host genotype will eventu-

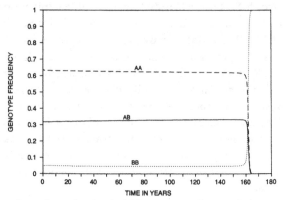

Figure 6. The effect of a reduction in biting rate on the population prevalence of two different parasite 'strains' where the basic reproductive rate of strain A is 5 times that of strain B, in the absence of bednets ($a = 0.4/$day). The effect of bednet use is shown as a shift in biting rate from 0.4/day to 0.3/day; the impact of this change on prevalence of infection is minimal for strain A, and significant for strain B. Thus if strain B is the more virulent strain, there will be a reduction in disease, that is not accompanied by a reduction in prevalence of parasitaemia in the population.

ally occur, as a sudden massive epidemic wipes out most of the susceptible population, as shown in Figure 6. However, for a certain narrow range of initial gene frequencies, the time to fixation will be very large and in theory could approach infinity. While it is not unlikely that initial frequencies of the resistance gene will be concentrated in this low range, the distribution of severe malaria among host genotypes indicate that it is far from the limit where the associated parasite is tolerated exclusively within a single genotype. Fixation of a resistant allele/trait/etc. is thus unlikely to occur on a sudden short timescale as shown in Figure 6. Nonetheless, the abstraction serves to illustrate the important point that strains that are extremely virulent within the population in general, can exist within their own sub-system involving a resistant host genotype. Hence, the observed variation in genetically determined host susceptibility to malaria may facilitate the maintenance of rare virulent parasite strains within the population.

5   Effects of heterogeneity in parasite virulence on vector control

The stratification of the parasite population into strains of differing virulence and transmissibility, where most such strains induce mild disease, can be used to explain the observation that the use of bednets can reduce the incidence of mild disease without inducing any significant change in prevalence of infection

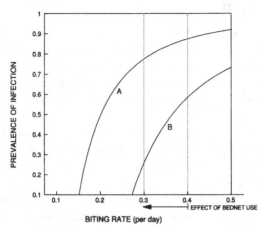

Figure 7. The lack of change in genotype frequency over 150 years in the host population, where BB represents a homozygous type resistant to a highly virulent parasite strain, that kills AA and AB types upon infection. The highly virulent strain may be contained at low levels within the resistant population, BB, as a result of this association (see Appendix B for details).

(Snow *et al.* 1988, Alonso *et al.* 1991). The latter has previously been explained by assuming that the development of malarial disease is a function of the size and frequency of innoculation. Within the strain framework, the effect of bednets may be very simply explained as a reduction in the number of new strains encountered (i.e. those capable of causing disease). Although a similar proportionate reduction will have occured in the total number of strains (i.e. those capable of causing infection) encountered, the effects of this will be lost due to saturation in the prevalence of parasitaemia. Disease incidence, however, will not have saturated, since not every infection leads to disease, and because the duration of disease is short in comparison with duration of parasitaemia. Therefore, a reduction in the number of new strains encountered may manifest itself in a reduction in disease.

Alternatively, the effect of bednet use may be interpreted as the consequence of the differential impact of reduction in transmission (by bednet use) upon parasite types associated with disease. Figure 7 demonstrates the effect of a reduction in biting rate (a) on the population prevalence of two different parasite 'strains' where the basic reproductive rate of strain A is 5 times that of strain B, in the absence of bednets ($a = 0.4/$day). It is clear that the differential impact of reducing access to hosts will be much greater in the case of strain B. The reduction in mild disease may thus be explained by a sub-spectrum of virulence among mild strains, where the more virulent strains are less transmissible than those that lead to asymptomatic infections.

6   Discussion

The spectrum of disease severity in *P. falciparum* malaria may be explained
by differences in virulence of parasite types. A number of parasite phenotypes
have been suggested as factors of virulence. As these factors are likely to have
both negative and positive effects on parasite transmission, it can be argued
that the relationship between virulence and transmissibility is generally non-
linear, with the latter peaking at some intermediate value of virulence, to
which the system may be expected to evolve if there is competition between
the variously virulent parasite types. However, in the absence of strong competition, a large degree of variation in virulence and transmissibility will be
tolerated within the system.

We may thus construct a coherent system to explain the spectrum of malarial disease by postulating the existence of several different antigenic types,
that each induce some degree of strain-specific anti-disease immunity upon
infection, but may or may not not elicit adequate infection blocking responses.
The development of immunity against a conserved or shared determinant can
serve as a source of weak competition between the strains, since there is effectively a long delay in the establishment of such a 'cross-immune' response,
as evidenced by age-profiles of parasite prevalence. As a result, a wide degree
of variation in the basic reproductive ratios of the different strains may be
maintained.

Age-specific patterns of incidence of severe and mild disease may be explained by assuming that majority of these antigenic types are associated
with mild disease. Epidemiological and molecular studies, viewed within this
framework, strongly suggest that while severe malarial anaemia may be a
complication occuring in a certain proportion of early infections with 'mild'
parasites, cerebral malaria is almost certainly caused by a few distinct antigenic types. Thus, exposure to mild malaria rises more rapidly than to cerebral malaria (as manifest in the higher average age of cerebral malaria cases),
simply because the former can be caused by any of a large number of strains.
Conversely, the incidence of mild malaria declines at a much slower (and
more uniform) manner than the sharp non-linear decline observed in cerebral malaria cases that is more typical of a disease associated with a single
strain. The extremely rapid decline in incidence of severe malarial anaemia
with age can be explained by assuming that the probability of developing
the syndrome drops rapidly with number of past infections with mild malaria
parasites. Any mild malaria strain is assumed to be capable of precipitating
severe malarial anaemia, provided the host has not been infected with malaria
more than a few times.

The definition of a *P. falciparum* 'strain' is not strict, as we have used it, in
this paper, to distinguish independently transmitted antigenic types, rather
than to represent a stable multilocus genotype. The definition of a strain

will depend on the number of polymorphic loci involved in distinguishing an independent antigenic type, and the relative contribution of recombination to the pool of genotypes. Rates of recombination will depend on the intensity of transmission, and may be a relatively rare event in areas of low transmission, given the short duration of infectiousness. Evidence is gradually emerging that a large degree of clonality may prevail in endemic situations (Day, unpublished data), which agrees with observed sex ratios in male and female gametes (Read *et al.* 1991). Any departure from panmixia will have a disproportionate effect on rarer strains (such as those associated with severe disease) in reducing the opportunity for recombination. The structure of the transmission system may thus, itself, suffice, to isolate 'strains' differing in virulence and transmissibility.

We have focussed on cytoadherence as a major determinant of parasite virulence, that may also be used to stratify the parasite population into independently transmitted antigenic types or 'strains'. The putative cytoadherence ligand PfEMP-1 and the associated the agglutination phenotype have both been shown to undergo clonal antigenic variation (Biggs *et al.* 1991, Roberts *et al.* 1992). This does not however complicate the definition of a malaria 'strain', since *in vitro* studies (Roberts *et al.* 1992) reveal very rapid rates of emergence of new antigenic variants that are inconsistent with the slow accumulation of experience of agglutination phenotypes of field isolates (Gupta *et al.* 1994). It seems likely that antigenic variation through switching of agglutination phenotypes during clonal expansion within the host is of significance in extending the duration of a single infection, but not in protecting against a range of 'strains', possibly because there is little overlap between the variants associated with each 'strain'. Thus, a cytoadherence genotype, comprising a series of variants, may function in the same manner as Trypanosome serodemes (distinct repertoires of variable antigen types), which have been shown to co-circulate within a transmission system (Masake *et al.* 1987).

The large variation in parasite virulence, as a factor of malarial disease, can essentially be attributed to the absence of competition between the various parasite strains, arising from weak shared immune responses, small overlap in antigenic variants of the different strains, and the low probabilities of recombination occuring as a result of short infectious periods. Heterogeneity in host resistance is a further factor in the maintenance of parasite polymorphisms associated with virulence. The theoretical framework presented in this paper serves to explain several epidemiological observations, and should stimulate further research on the population genetics and dynamics of parasite virulence.

Appendix A

Let $y_i(a, t)$ denote the proportion of the population of age a, at time t, with experience of i strains of mild malaria. The dynamics of the system may be represented by the following set of equations:

$$\frac{\delta y_1}{\delta t} + \frac{\delta y_1}{\delta a} = n\lambda(1 - \sum y_i) - ((n-1)\lambda + \mu)y_i$$

$$\frac{\delta y_i}{\delta t} + \frac{\delta y_i}{\delta a} = (n - i + 1)\lambda y_{i-1} - ((n-i)\lambda + \mu)y_i$$

where the total number of strains circulating within the system is n, and λ is the per capita force of infection ($= R_0/H$). We seek solutions to these equations at equilibrium, and thus set the time derivates to zero.

The proportion unexposed to mild malaria (defined as the experience of any one of the n strains) at age a is given by:

$$X(a) = 1 - \sum y_i(a)$$

The incidence of mild disease between the ages a_1 and a_2 is given by $Z(a_2) - Z(a_1)$, where:

$$\frac{dZ(a)}{da} = \lambda(\sum(n - i)y_i(a) + nX(a))$$

where mild disease is assumed to be a consequence of infection with a new strain.

The incidence of severe malarial anaemia between the ages a_1 and a_2 is given by $Z'(a_2) - Z'(a_1)$, where

$$\frac{dZ'(a)}{da} = n\lambda X(a)$$

in the extreme where SMA can be precipitated by any malaria strain among those without past experience of mild malaria.

The same set of equations can be adapted to calculate exposure to and incidence of cerebral malaria, by reducing the number of strains, n.

Appendix B

We examine the effects of host heterogeneity at one locus with two alleles, r and s, associated respectively with resistance and susceptibility to disease. The genotypes rr, ss and rs develop a fatal disease upon infection with probabilities α_{rr}, α_{ss} and α_{rs} respectively. The dynamics of the host population may thus be expressed as:

$$\frac{dx_{ij}}{dt} = p_i p_j(1 + \delta_{ij}) - \alpha_{ij}\lambda(x_{ij} - z_{ij}) - \mu x_{ij}$$

$$\frac{dz_{ij}}{dt} = (1 - \alpha_{ij})\lambda(x_{ij} - z_{ij}) - (\gamma + \mu)z_{ij}$$

where x_{ij} is the density of the subgroup of genotype ij, z_{ij} is the density of immunes in subgroup ij, p_i is the frequency of allele i, λ is the force of infection, $1/\gamma$ ($= H$, in the text) is the average duration of immunity, and δ_{ij} is defined as zero when $i = j$, and 1 otherwise.

The proportion infectious, w_{ij}, may thus be expressed as:

$$w_{ij} = \frac{\lambda(x_{ij} - z_{ij})}{\sigma}$$

where $1/\sigma$ ($= D$, in the text) is the average duration of infectiousness. The latter is assumed to be very short in comparison to the average duration of immunity; hence the proportion infectious is assumed to instantaneously adjust to the proportion non-immune, and can be expressed in the above form.

The force of infection may be defined (after Aron and May 1982) as $\lambda = maby$, where y is the proportion of infected mosquitoes, and the other parameters have the same interpretation as in equation (1) in the text. The dynamics of the infected mosquito population may be given as:

$$\frac{dy}{dt} = a \sum \frac{w_{ij}}{N}(1 - y) - \mu_m y$$

Together, these equations define a system where host heterogeneity influences the transmission dynamics of a virulent parasite strain, which in turn modifies the structure of the host population. Figure 7 presents numerical solutions to these equations in the limit where $\alpha_{rr} = 0$, $\alpha_{ss} = \alpha_{rs} = 1$

References

Alonso, P.L., Lindsay, S.W., Armstrong, J.R.M., Conteh, M., Hill, A.G., David, P.H., Fegan, G., de Francisco, A., Hall, A.J., Shenton, F.C., Cham, K. and Greenwood, B.M. (1991) 'The effect of insecticide-treated bed nets on mortality of Gambian children', *Lancet* **337**, 1499–1502.

Anderson, R.M. and May, R.M. (1991) *Infectious Diseases of Humans: Dynamics and Control*, Oxford University Press, Oxford.

Anderson, R.M. and May, R.M. (1982) 'Coevolution of hosts and parasites', *Parasitology* **85**, 411–426.

Aron, J.L. and May, R.M. (1982) 'The population dynamics of malaria'. In *Population Dynamics of Infectious Diseases*, R.M. Anderson (ed.), Chapman and Hall, London, 139–179.

Berendt A.R., Ferguson, D.J.P. and Newbold, C.I. (1990) 'Sequestration in *Plasmodium falciparum* malaria: sticky cells and sticky problems', *Parasitol. Today* **6**, 247–254.

Biggs, B.A., Gooze, L., Wycherly, K., Wollish, W., Southwell, B., Leech, J.H. and Brown, G.V. (1991) 'Antigenic variation in *Plasmodium falciparum*', *Proc. Nat. Acad. Sci.* **88**, 9171–9174.

Brewster, D.R., Kwiatkowski, D. and White, N.J. (1990) 'Neurological sequelae of cerebral malaria in children', *Lancet* **336**, 1039–1043.

Carlson, J., Helmby, H., Hill, A.V.S., Brewster, D. Greenwood, B.M. and Wahlgren, M. (1990) 'Human cerebral malaria: association with erythrocyte rosetting and lack of anti-rosetting antibodies', *Lancet* **336**, 1457–1460.

Carter, R. and Graves, P. 'Gametocytes'. In *Malaria: Principles and Practice of Malariology*, W.H. Wernsdorfer and I. McGregor (eds.), Churchill Livingstone, 253–305.

Carter, R. and Miller, L.H. (1979) 'Evidence for environmental modulation of gametocytogenesis in *Plasmodium* in continuous culture', *Bull. WHO (suppl. 1)* 37–52.

Cattani, J.A., Tulloch, J.L., Vrbova, H., Jolley, D., Gibson, F.D., Moir, J.S., Heywood, P.F., Alpers, M.P., Stevenson, A. and Clancy, R. (1986) 'The epidemiology of malaria in a population surrounding Madang, Papua New Guinea', *Am. J. Trop. Med. Hyg.* **35**, 3–15.

Covell, G. (1951) 'Clinical, chemotherapeutic, and immunological studies on induced malaria', *Brit. Med. Bull.* **8**, 51–55.

Cox, F.E.G. (1988) 'Major animal models in malaria research: rodent'. In *Malaria: Principles and Practice of Malariology*, W.H. Wernsdorfer and I. McGregor (eds.), Churchill Livingstone, 1503–1543.

Cox, M.J., Kum, D., Tavul, L., Narara, A. Raiko, A., Baisor, M., Alpers, M., Medley, G. and Day, K.P. (1994) 'Dynamics of malaria parasitaemia associated with febrile illness in children from a rural area of Madang, Papua New Guinea', *Trans. Roy. Soc. Trop. Med. Hyg.* **88**, 191–197.

Day, K.P. and Marsh, K. (1990) 'Naturally acquired immunity to *Plasmodium falciparum*', *Parasitol. Today* **6**, 68–71.

Day, K.P., Karamalis, F., Thompson, J., Barnes, D. Brown, H., Brown, G.V. and Kemp, D. (1993) 'Virulence and transmissibility of *Plasmodium falciparum* map to chromosome 9', *Proc. Nat. Acad. Sci.* **90**, 8292–8296.

Deloran, P. and Chougnet, C. (1992) 'Is immunity to malaria short-lived?', *Parasitol. Today* **8**, 375–378.

Erunkulu, O.A., Hill, A.V.S, Kwiatkowski, D., Todd, J.E., Iqbal, J., Berzins, K., Riley, E.M. and Greenwood, B.M. (1992) 'Severe malaria in Gambian children is not due to lack of previous exposure to malaria', *Cli. Exp. Immunol.* **89**, 296–300.

Gamagemendis, A.C., Rajakaruna, J., Carter, R. and Mendis, K.N. (1992) 'Transmission blocking immunity to human *Plasmodium vivax* malaria in an endemic population in Kataragama, Sri Lanka', *Para. Immunol.* **14**, 385–396.

Garnham, P.C.C. (1966) *Malaria Parasites and other Haemosporidia*, Blackwell Scientific Publications, Oxford.

Greenwood, B.M., Marsh, K. and Snow R. (1991) 'Why do some African children develop severe malaria?', *Parasitol. Today* **8**, 239–242.

Gupta, S., Trenholme, K., Anderson, R.M. and Day, K.P. (1994) 'Antigenic diversity and the transmission dynamics of *P. falciparum*', *Science* 263, 961–963.

Gupta, S., Swinton, J. and Anderson, R.M. (1994) 'Theoretical studies of the effects of heterogeneity in the parasite population on the transmission dynamics of malaria', *Proc. R. Soc. Lond. B* 256, 231–238.

Gupta, S. and Day, K.P. (1994) 'A theoretical framework for the immunoepidemiology of *Plasmodium falciparum* malaria', *Para. Immunol.* 16, 361–370.

Hill, A.V.S., Allsopp, C.E.M., Kwiatkowski, D., Anstey, N.M., Twumasi, P., Rowe, P.A., Bennet, S., Brewster, D. McMichael, A.J. and Greenwood, B.M. (1991) 'Common West African HLA antigens are associated with protection from severe malaria', *Nature* 352, 595–600.

Howard, R.J. (1988) 'Malarial proteins at the membrane of *Plasmodium falciparum* infected erythrocytes and their involvement in cytoadherence to endothelial cells', *Prog. Allergy* 41, 98–147.

James, S.P., Nicol, W.D. and Shute, P.G. (1932) 'A study of induced malignant tertian malaria', *Proc. Roy. Soc. Med.* 25, 1153–1186.

Kwiatkowski, D. (1989) 'Febrile temeperatures can sychronise the growth of *Palsmodium falciparum in vitro*', *J. Exp. Med.* 169, 357–361.

Kwiatkowski, D. (1991) 'Cytokine and anti-disease immunity to malaria', *Res. Immunol.* 142, 707–712.

Kwiatkowski, D. (1993) 'Prospects of an anti-disease vaccine'. In *Molecular Considerations in Malaria Vaccine Development*.

Levin, S. and Pimental, D. (1981) 'Selection and the evolution of virulence in bacteria: An ecumenical excursion', *Am. Nat.* 117, 300–315.

Marsh, K., Marsh, V.M., Brown, J., Whittle, H.C. and Greenwood, B.M. (1988) '*Plasmodium falciparum*: The behaviour of clinical isolates in an *in vitro* model of infected red blood cell sequestration', *Exp. Parasitol.* 65, 202–208.

Marsh, K. (1992) 'Malaria – a neglected disease?', *Parasitology* 104, S53–S69.

Marsh, K., Hayes, R.H., Otoo, L., Carson, D.C. and Greenwood, B.M. (1989) 'Antibodies to blood stage antigens of *Plasmodium falciparum* in rural Gambians and their relationship to protection against infection', *Trans. Roy. Soc. Trop. Med. Hyg.* 83, 293–303.

Masake, R.A., Nantulya, V.M., Musoke, A.J., Moloo, S.K. and Nguli, K. (1987) 'Characterisation of Trypanosoma congolese serodemes in stocks isolated from cattle introduced onto a ranch in Kilifi, Kenya', *Parasitology* 94, 349–357.

May, R.M. and Anderson, R.M. (1983) 'Epidemiology and genetics in the coevolution of parasites and hosts', *Proc. R. Soc. Lond. B* 219, 281–313.

May, R.M. and Anderson, R.M. (1990) 'Parasite-host coevolution', *Parasitology* 100, S89–S101.

McGregor, I.A. (1965) 'Consideration of some aspects of malaria', *Trans. Roy. Soc. Trop. Med. Hyg.* 59, 145–152.

Mendis K., Naotunne, T. de S., Karunaweera, N.D., *et al.* (1990) 'Anti-parasite effects of cytokines in malaria', *Immunol. Lett.* **25**, 217–220.

Miller, L.H. (1969) 'Distribution of mature trophozoites and schizonts of *Plasmodium falciparum* in the organs of *Aotus trivigatus*, the night monkey', *Am. J. Trop. Med. Hyg.* **18**, 860–865.

Newbold, C.I, Pinches, D.J, Roberts, D.J. and Marsh, K. (1992) '*Plasmodium falciparum*: The human agglutinating antibody response to the infected red cell surface is predominantly variant specific', *Exp. Parasitol.* **75**, 281–292.

Ockenhouse, C.F., Ho, M., Tandon, N.N., van Seventer, A., Shaw, S., White, N.J., Jamieson, G.A., Chulay, J.D. and Webster, H.K. (1991) 'Molecular basis of sequestration in severe and uncomplicated *Plasmodium falciparum* malaria: Differential adhesion of infected erythrocytes', *J. Inf. Dis.* **164**, 163–169.

Read, A.F., Narara, A., Nee, S., Keymer, A.E. and Day, K.P. (1991) 'Gametocyte sex ratios as indirect measures of outcrossing rates in malaria', *Parasitology* **104**, 387–395.

Roberts, D.J., Craig, A.G., Berendt, A.R., Pinches, R., Nash, G., Marsh, K. and Newbold, C.I. (1992) 'Rapid switching to multiple antigenic and adhesive phenotypes in malaria', *Nature* **357**, 689–692.

Rooth, I. and Bjorkman, A (1992) 'Fever episodes in a holoendemic malaria area of Tanzania: parasitological and clinical findings and diagnostic aspects related to malaria', *Trans. Roy. Soc. Trop. Med. Hyg.* **86**, 479–482.

Snow, R.W., Rowan, K.M. and Greenwood, B.M. (1988) 'A trial of permethrin-treated bed-nets in the prevention of malaria in Gambian children', *Trans. Roy. Soc. Trop. Med. Hyg.* **82**, 838–842.

Invited Discussion

Angela R. McLean

What's so special about within-host dynamics?

When an epidemiology conference hosts a session on 'within-host dynamics', three questions immediately come to a discussant's mind: 'Why are we doing this?', 'What are we doing here?' and 'What difference does being within a host make?' The first of these three questions is answered by the quality of the papers presented in this session. There are many fascinating questions about the pathogenesis of infectious diseases, and about the dynamics of host responses to infectious organisms. These questions often involve highly non-linear interactions between host and pathogen within the host organism. The rigour and clarity of thought required by mathematical description of such interactions is a great aid in developing an intuitive understanding of which processes are important, and of what patterns those processes might generate.

The subject matter of the four talks: two on HIV, one on malaria and one on schistosomiasis is probably a fair representation of the field. The enigma of HIV's pathogenesis has prompted many theoretical (and empirical) investigations. Nowak's theory is one elegant example of the numerous theories proposed to explain the long period between infection with HIV and illness with AIDS (reviewed in McLean 1993). In contrast to the care and rigour with which Nowak's theory has been expounded, some of the 'verbal theories' of HIV's pathogenesis are classic examples of why biologists ought to make mathematical models; so that they can see when the predictions made by their verbal models simply cannot be matched up with the patterns they aim to explain. A cogent argument for the use of mathematical models in an exploratory fashion by biologists is given by Hillis (1993). AIDS does not just generate problems of explaining the observed patterns: the great variability in the course of disease between individuals has generated fascinating statistical questions concerning how to characterise the observed patterns. Taylor addresses the question of whether it is possible to find consistent linear trends in the decline of an individual's CD4+ cell count. A question that relates to both HIV papers presented here concerns the relation between measured variables that are useful predictors of an individual's prognosis (e.g. CD4+ cell count and degree of immune activation) and mechanisms of HIV pathogenesis. Phillips (1992) gives a lucid account of some of the important issues. Fulford describes the problems associated with epidemiological studies which try to detect the effects of an acquired immune response to schistosomiasis infection. Since the time-scale over which an immune response is acquired is the same as the time-scale over which individuals mature and change their behaviour, age appears as a confounding effect in all such studies. Gupta shows how a clearer understanding of events within an individual can lead to a better understanding of the between-host dynamics of malaria.

Thus the first question is answered, we do this because there are many extremely interesting questions which can be elucidated with the help of models of within-host dynamics of infectious diseases. The second two questions are answered in tandem. A session on within-host dynamics is appropriate at an epidemiology conference for at least two reasons. As Gupta has shown, a clearer understanding at the within-host level sheds light on events at the between-host level. There are also issues of methodology. Many of the models employed in the consideration of within-host population dynamics of infectious disease are very similar to models that have been used for almost a century to describe the spread of infectious organisms between individuals. Perhaps more importantly the lesson that has been learned in epidemiology, that modelling becomes most powerful when tightly tied in with experimental data, does not have to be relearned. All the papers presented this morning were exemplary in their efforts to compare models with data. So is the study of within-host population dynamics simply the application of the same old set of models to a different set of biological variables? I think not. Infections within individuals have many different properties from infections within communities. The first of these is that the place of 'host' is usually taken by cells within the individual. These turnover on time sclaes similar to those of the parasite. This is a quite different scenario from that usually observed in epidemiology, where it is almost invariably the case that the parasitising organism turns over on time-scales that are much faster than those of the parasitised organism. Thus whether it be turnover of infected cells or the generation of specific immune responses, pathogens within hosts inhabit a rapidly changing environment. It is therefore no longer sensible to make the simplifying assumption that host dynamics occur on time-scale that are so slow that they can be ignored. A second important difference is that in some sense each man (or mouse) is an island. Thus every time a pathogen newly infects an individual, events begin afresh. Transient effects then become of much more interest. Another vitally important implication of this second difference is that experiments become possible. Both planned experiments in animal models and natural experiments in the form of treatment intervention in humans become possible, and repeatable. Thus there is scope for testing predictions made by models of within-host dynamics to a far greater extent than has been possible in 'mainstream' theoretical epidemiology. Such experiments are bound to encounter the issue of redundancy in the immune system—already widely apparent in studies of gene knockout mice. Models of the competition for antigen between different arms of the immune system will be needed.

The dynamics of infectious organsims within their hosts are fascinatingly interesting, important and tractable. The subject is a vigorous and exciting one where new techniques of observation are generating patterns that need explaining at an ever greater rate. Theoretical epidemiologists, whether from a mathematical or a statistical background, should consider joining the fun!

References

Hillis, W.D. (1993) 'Why physicists like models and why biologists should', *Curr. Biol.* **3** 79–81.

McLean, A.R. (1993) 'The balance of power between HIV and the immune system', *Trends Microbiol.* **1** 9–13.

Phillips, A.N. (1992) 'Studies of prognostic markers in HIV infections: implications for pathogenesis', *AIDS* **8** 63–64.

Invited Discussion

Andy Dobson

Parasite Diversity and Parasite Coexistence

These papers deal with different aspects of understanding how hosts cope with the diversity of antigenic challenges that pathogens provide. These comments examine common threads underlying three of the presentations and describe some recent work on the more general problem of the diversity of pathogens that any host population can sustain.

The work of Martin Nowak and his colleagues at Oxford, Imperial College and Amsterdam University epitomizes the challenges that mathematical models present to empirical epidemiologists. As with other recent work on the mathematics of the immune system and infection with HIV (McLean 1993), the work suggests alternative interpretations of epidemiological data and has stimulated the collection (and analysis) of data not normally collected by immunologists and clinicians. At the heart of the Nowak model is the interaction between the diversity of HIV quasi-species in individual patients and the ability of the host to produce a sufficient diversity of antigens to cope with this. At a crucial level of quasi-species diversity, the diversity threshold, the immune system is overwhelmed, CD4 counts decline precipitously and the patient succumbs to full-blown AIDS. The length of time until this occurs is dependent upon a variety of factors, but most importantly upon the replication and mutation rate of the virus, and upon the host's ability to mount an efficient and diverse immune response. My main questions are about this diversity threshold; the diversity levels presented in the model seem much higher than the diversity levels observed in individually infected HIV/AIDS patients. Is this because the antigen tests used to measure the diversity of antibody in HIV patients are only developed for a subset of antigens, or does the V3 loop which produces the majority of this antigenic diversity mutate at a very high rate? If information is available on the genetic structure of the V3 loop for different quasi-species variants, would it be possible to use some of the techniques that Marty Kreitman and his colleagues (McDonald and Kreitman 1991) have developed to look for selection at specific sites in this loop?

These questions are not meant as 'persnickety' concerns about parameterization. More specifically, I want to direct the discussion towards the more general question: how important is mutation in generating the large levels of parasite diversity and what determines the limit on the diversity of pathogens and parasites that any host population can support?

In the conference held in 1993 on wildlife diseases (Grenfell and Dobson 1995), a number of evolutionary biologists argued that it is wrong to consider evolutionary processes to operate on different time scales from ecological processes and then went on to suggest that selection was more important than mutation, in determining observed levels of diversity in host parasite systems. Yet, parasitic organisms reproduce at rates 3–4 orders of magnitude faster than their free-living relatives (Dobson *et al.* 1992). Similarly, the dynamics of viruses and bacteria may operate on time scales 5–6 orders of magnitude faster than those of the vertebrate hosts they parasitize. This suggests that mutation may be highly important as a mechanism by which many pathogens produce new challenges for vertebrate populations. In contrast, the age-structure of vertebrate populations may produce significant viscosity that acts to reduce considerably the rate at which hosts will respond to any individual strain of the pathogen.

The work by Gupta and Day on the diversity of different strains of malaria infecting humans eloquently illustrates that an individual host population can support a diversity of strains of the same pathogen species. Their analysis suggests that this diversity would not be maintained if the transmission dynamics of each strain were identical. Under these circumstances, the strain that optimizes R_0 through the physiological play-off between pathogenicity and transmission will ultimately dominate. Nevertheless, differences in the use of vectors by different malaria strains seem to either allow persistence or at least slows the transient dynamics by which one strain drives the others to extinction.

If we look at parasites of white tailed deer, 90% of allozyme diversity in the eastern United States is seen at the level of the individual (Mulvey, Aho *et al.* 1991). In the case of malaria, how much of the total genetic variability in the population is seen at the level of infections in individual hosts? Is there geographical variation in the distribution of the different strains and is there any evidence for reciprocal changes in the genetic structure of the human or vector populations?

I would like to mention some work on parasitic helminths that addresses two of the points raised in the talks mentioned above and also some of the questions raised in the talk on schistosomiasis. If we wish to calculate R_0 for a direct life cycle macroparasite we have to consider possible pay-offs between parasite fecundity and parasite induced host mortality (Dobson and Merenlender 1990). These would occur if fecundity involves converting host resources and supportive tissue into parasite eggs, or if the production of eggs or other transmission stages led to an increasingly diverse immune response from the host. Inclusion of such an effect into the standard expression for R_0 in a macroparasite produces essentially the same relationship between virulence and R_0 as we see for microparasites in the classic studies of myxomatosis

(Anderson and May 1982, Dwyer *et al.* 1990, Fenner 1983). However, there is empirical support for the relationships in macroparasites and we could select parameter values that produce much less dramatic peaks.

The obverse side of the debate about selection for parasite strains that maximize R_0, considers whether hosts can support a variety of pathogens and how similar species can coexist. Models for simple two macroparasite, one host communities suggest that persistence is enhanced by aggregation in the distribution of each parasite species, and that the host's ability to sustain the pathogen is dependent on the parasite's birth and transmission rates (Dobson 1985, Roberts and Dobson 1995). Interactions between parasite species (or different strains of the same parasite species) enter the model as covariance terms – these can be positive (if the parasites utilize the same intermediate host species or jointly reduce the efficiency of the host immune response), or negative if direct competition or cross-immunity occurs between species (or strains). The main effect of these covariance terms in the simple two species model is to bend the isoclines, this alters the position of their intersection, but not their points of origin on each axis. This suggests that covariance terms, such as cross-immunity, may alter the size of the population of each parasite species, but will not have any effect on their persistence. A similar result is implied in the paper by Gupta and Day who suggest that the absence of direct competition and weak cross-immunity between different malaria strains permits the coexistence of a number of malaria strains in some human populations.

Mick Roberts and I have been extending this model to consider the dynamics of a more general community of n species of macroparasite in one host species (Roberts and Dobson 1995, Dobson and Roberts 1994). These models again emphasize that aggregation of parasites is crucial in allowing persistence – but strains with different R_0 can persist in the same population. One key feature of the expression for host population size in these models is a function that contains a diversity threshold, D_T, (similar in form to that described in Nowak and May 1991) – once parasite diversity exceeds this level, the host population is no longer able to support the parasite community and either some parasite species, or the host and all the parasite species collapse to extinction:

$$D_T = \frac{H_0}{\dfrac{\sum k_i \lambda_i}{r + \sum k_i(a + \mu_i + \alpha_i)} - 1}.$$

Here H_0 is an index of transmission that varies inversely with the efficiency with which the parasites locate the host, r is the growth rate of the host population, a is the birth rate of the host population, k is the degree of aggregation of each parasite species, and λ, μ, and α are the instantaneous birth, death and parasite induced host death rates for each parasite species. The expression for the diversity threshold suggests that the life history variables that determine fecundity, virulence and transmission and observed degree of aggregation are crucial in determining the number of parasite species (or strains) that can persist in a host population. If I subscribed to the fundamentalist Popperian school of community ecology I might believe that the sets of parameter values observed for each species in the community were random and independent sets from those of other species. More likely they are not, but instead reflect the life history constraints that characterize different parasite species. Thus the observed degree of aggregation and rates of parasite induced host mortality are ineluctably linked to the transmission and mortality rates of the parasite and host. Teasing out the relationships between these variables will require careful field studies such as those described by Fulford *et al.* and laboratory studies similar to those of Taylor *et al.* In this area the recent work by (Woolhouse 1992) and the work of Grenfell *et al.* (1995) will be important in understanding how changes in exposure rates, cross immunity and loss of immunological memory will lead to systematic changes in the mean and higher order moments of levels of infection.

I would like to conclude by suggesting that we constantly underestimated the level of diversity that parasites have generated through mutation and large reproductive rates. In humans infected by HIV this mutational diversity may lead to the collapse of the immune system. In contrast, at the population level, mechanisms exist which reduce diversity by selecting for strains with optimal life histories. Nevertheless, the persistence of a diverse community of parasites and a variety of different genetic strains may be achieved through spatial heterogeneities and differences in the life history strategies of the parasite species involved.

References

Anderson, R.M. and May, R.M. (1982) 'Coevolution of hosts and parasites', *Parasitology* **85**, 411–426.

Dobson, A.P. (1985). 'The population dynamics of competition between parasites', *Parasitology* **91**, 317–347.

Dobson, A.P., Hudson, P.J. and Lyles, A.M. (1992) 'Macroparasites: worms and others'. In *Natural Enemies. The Population Biology of Predators, Parasites and Diseases*, M.J. Crawley (ed.), Blackwell Scientific Publications, Oxford, 329–348.

Dobson, A.P. and Merenlender, A. (1990). 'Coevolution of macroparasites and their hosts. In *Parasite-Host Association. Coexistence or Conflict?*, C.A. Toft, A. Aeschlimann and L. Bolis (eds.), Oxford Scientific Publications, Oxford, 83–101.

Dobson, A.P. and Roberts, M. (1994) 'The population dynamics of parasitic helminth communities', *Parasitology* **109**, S97–S108.

Dwyer, G., Levin, S.A., and Buttel, L. (1990) 'A simulation model of the population dynamics and evolution of myxomatosis', *Ecol. Monogr.* **60**, 423–447.

Fenner, F. (1983) 'Biological control as exemplified by small pox eradication and myxomatosis', *Proc. Roy. Soc. Lond. B* **218**, 489–511.

Grenfell, B.T., Dietz, K., and Roberts, M.G. (1995) 'Modelling the immuno-epidemiology of macroparasites in naturally-fluctuating host populations'. In *Ecology of Infectious Diseases in Natural Populations*, B.T. Grenfell and A.P. Dobson (eds.), Cambridge University Press, Cambridge, 362–383.

Grenfell, B.T. and Dobson, A.P. (eds.) (1995) *Ecology of Infectious Diseases in Natural Populations*, Cambridge University Press, Cambridge.

McDonald, J.H. and Kreitman, M. (1991) 'Adaptive protein evolution at the Adh locus in *Drosophila*', *Nature* **351**, 652–654.

McLean, A.R. (1993) 'The balance of power between HIV and the immune system', *Trends in Microbiol.* **1**, 1–7.

Mulvey, M., Aho, J.M., Lydeard, C., Leberg, P.L., and Smith, M.H. (1991) 'Comparative population genetics structure of a parasite (*Fascioloides magna*) and its definitive host', *Evolution* **45**, 1628–1640.

Roberts, M.G. and Dobson, A.P. (1995) 'The population dynamics of communities of parasitic helminths', *Math. Biosci.* **126**, 191–214.

Woolhouse, M.E.J. (1992) 'A theoretical framework for the immunoepidemiology of helminth infection', *Paras. Immunol.* **14**, 563–578.

Invited Discussion

Graham Medley

There was fascinating dichotomy presented this morning by the papers of Nowak and Taylor. This dichotomy has been given several names during this meeting, and my favourite is the distinction between thought experiments to understand the processes that generate observed patterns, and the analysis of real experimental data. These two papers are essentially addressing the same subject: the pattern of CD4 counts over time, and it appears to me that both approaches would benefit from consideration of the other. On one hand, Taylor explains much of the variability in the observed counts as being derived from an underlying stochastic process, whereas it may well be due to a highly non-linear process changing on a time-scale faster than the sampling interval. On the other hand, Nowak does not use his model to produce predictions of CD4 numbers which may actually be testable by comparison with such data.

There is general problem here with the use of deterministic models, i.e. those that produce a single value or set of single value results for each time point without any measure of variability. Differential equations are an invaluable tool for mathematical descriptions of disease processes, but suffer from the fact that data-derived estimates are required for the processes embedded in the equation system, for example density dependent transmission. There are methods available for fitting equations directly to observations of the system over time, but these tend to regard the variability in data as some form of random error, and the fitting involves simple reduction of the average difference between observation and model. However, the variability itself is developed by the dynamic processes and contains much information about the dynamic processes. A simple death process results in loss of variability over time, whereas a birth-death process results in increasing heterogeneity over time, and the changes in variability over time in data can give as much information about the parameter values and structure of the process as can the mean value.

Generally, population biological processes can be described by the following equation:

$$\dot{x}(t) = B(x) - D(x)$$

where the functions $B(\cdot)$ and $D(\cdot)$ represent the input and output rates respectively for the quantity, x, under consideration. For most biological populations, x is an integer valued quantity, and this equation can be rewritten as an infinite set of differential equations describing the probabilities of observing x individuals, $p_x(t)$:

$$\dot{p}_x(t) = p_{x-1}B(x-1) + p_{x+1}D(x+1) - p_x[B(x) + D(x)]$$

189

with appropriate modifications and additional definitions for the boundary equations. Note that the functions, $B(\cdot)$ and $D(\cdot)$, in this set of equations are functionally equivalent and have the same units and same parameterisation as the functions in the equivalent deterministic equation. Preliminary attempts to test the validity of estimating parameters of differential equation systems directly from observational data using this formulation appear to give enough encouraging results to warrant further consideration of the method (Medley and Blythe, unpublished observations). This method is at present restricted by the computational problems in dealing with large numbers of differential equations.

Lifespan of Human T Lymphocytes

Angela R. McLean and Colin A. Michie

The lifespan of T lymphocytes is of particular interest because of their central role in immunological memory. Is the recall of a vaccination or early infection, which may be demonstrated clinically up to 50 years after antigen exposure, retained by a long-lived cell, or its progeny? Using the observation that T lymphocyte expression of isoforms of CD45 corresponds with their ability to respond to recall antigens, we have investigated the lifespan of both CD45RO (the subset containing responders, or 'memory' cells) and CD45RA (the unresponsive, or 'naive' subset) lymphocytes in a group of patients after radiotherapy (Michie *et al.* 1992). We have found a rapid loss of unstable chromosomes (which result in cell death in mitosis) from the CD45RO but not the CD45RA pool. Immunological memory therefore apparently resides in a population with a more rapid rate of division. The survival curves for the two populations are best described by a model in which there is also reversion *in vivo* from the CD45RO to the CD45RA phenotype. Expression of CD45RO in T cells may therefore be reversible. Further data showing survival curves of T lymphocytes with stable radiation damage (passed to one daughter cell during mitosis) is also considered. These curves show very little loss of such cells. The difference between the two populations (stable and unstable damage) allows an estimate of their proliferation rates and death rates. These parameter estimates may be of interest to people modelling the dynamics of the immune response as they give some rough indicators of the timescales on which T lymphocytes turn over (McLean and Michie 1993).

References

Michie, C.A., McLean, A.R., Alcock, C. and Beverley, P.C.L. (1992) 'The lifespan of human T lymphocyte subsets defined by CD45 isoforms', *Nature* **360**, 264–5.

McLean, A.R. and Michie, C.A. (1993) 'Vival burden in AIDS', *Nature* **365**, 365, 301.

Discussion

HADELER** McLean has pointed out that the human immune system is highly redundant and that different 'arms' compete in fighting an infective agent. I propose to consider the analogy with the saccadic motion of the eye. If our eyes follow a moving object then the head and eyeballs 'compete'. The head and eyeballs perform rather irregular rotations which may be different in each run of the experiment, but the total rotation follows the object smoothly.

DE BOER If one takes the usual assumption that 10% of immune cells are activated, is there any information in McLean and Michie's data on the differential mortality of activated and in-activated cells?

REPLY There are numerous definitions of activated lymphocytes. If one were to use a definition such as, 'activated T lymphocytes are those which are expressing high affinity interleukin-2 receptors', then this study can not help answer de Boer's question. However, the finding that CD45RO is only transiently expressed (albeit for quite a long time) has lead some authors to call CD45RO+ cells 'primed' or 'more activated' rather than 'memory' cells, and to view CD45RO simply as a marker of recent activation. Our data gives a direct measure of the differential mortality of CD45RA+ and CD45RO+ T lymphocytes.

DOBSON** The results that McLean presents raise some intriguing questions about the population dynamics of the immune system and its organisation. Is it possible that T-cells or other components of the immune system change their role as they age? In models that have been made for social insects (Oster and Wilson 1978, Seeley 1985), it was found that the most efficient way to organise a colony of individuals who perform a variety of tasks was to have each individual perform each task sequentially. The extreme alternative to this is to have each individual specialise on a particular task. Is it possible that the immune system is organised to that some individual cell types are specialists, while others sequentially perform a range of tasks? Obviously, if a range of tasks is being undertaken, the most vital ones should be performed early in the cell's life, while the more dangerous (to the cell) tasks should be performed later. Do you think the differences you see in CD4 cell survival may reflect this?

REPLY Dobson's comment is most interesting. At the moment any such interpretation of our data would be rather speculative. However I think that this type of argument, source of so much rich insight in animal ecology, would be equally well applied to the immune system.

References

Oster, G.F. and Wilson, E.O. (1978) *Caste and Ecology in the Social Insects*, Princeton University Press, Princeton, NJ.

Seeley, R. (1985) *The Honey Bee*, Princeton Monographs in Behavioral Ecology, Princeton University Press, Princeton, NJ.

Diversity and Virulence Thresholds in AIDS

Rob J. de Boer and Maarten C. Boerlijst

We propose a novel model for the interaction between HIV and the immune system. Two differential equations describe the interactions between one strain of virus and one clone of T-lymphocytes. We employ the model to generalize earlier results on the AIDS diversity threshold (Nowak *et al.* 1990, Nowak *et al.* 1991). Virus diversity is implemented in the model by assuming that all virus strains and all T-cell clones are identical. Given this assumption, diversity is represented as a parameter.

First we confirm the earlier results by showing that our model has a diversity threshold corresponding to a saddle-node bifurcation. We derive an analytical expression for the local bifurcation point in terms of the parameters. This shows that the diversity threshold corresponds to a linear combination of the diversity, infectivity, and antigenicity of the virus quasi-species. The mechanism by which an increase in diversity causes AIDS is by increasing the total virus concentration.

Secondly we derive a 'virulence' threshold corresponding to a global bifurcation involving the basins of attraction. Here 'virulence' is defined as the infectivity and antigenicity of a virus strain. We derive an analytical expression for the global bifurcation point in terms of the parameters. A numerical study of the relation between the diversity and virulence thresholds suggests that the condition for the development of AIDS is a linear combination of diversity and virulence.

References

Nowak, M.A., May, R.M. and Anderson, R.M. (1990) *AIDS* **4**, 1095–1103.

Nowak, M.A., Anderson, R.M., McLean, A.R., Wolfs, T.F.W., Goudsmit, J. and May, R.M. (1991) *Science* **254**, 963–969.

De Boer, R.J. and Boerlijst, M.C. (1994) 'Virulence and diversity thresholds in AIDS', *Proc. Nat. Acad. Sci. USA* **94**, 544–548.

Statistical Analysis of AZT Effect on CD4 Cell Counts in HIV Disease

A.J. McNeil, S.M. Gore, R.P. Brettle, and A.G. Bird

We explore the fitting of a class of hierarchical regression models to longitudinal CD4 lymphocyte count data from the Edinburgh City Hospital cohort. This mainly drug-using (IDU) cohort provides an excellent resource for the study of HIV disease progression for several reasons: seroconversions have been estimated for a large proportion of the cohort on the basis of stored sera retrospectively tested for HIV antibodies and knowledge of needle-sharing behaviour; immunological monitoring has been thorough since 1985 with blood taken at most clinic visits and regular attendance behaviour encouraged; immunological measurements are considered accurate from quality control comparisons between UK laboratories.

Thus we are able to consider a set of 164 seropositives who have well-estimated seroconversions and at least 10 CD4 counts each to the end of 1991; 102 of these subjects have at least 15 counts and 51 have at least 20 giving good longitudinal marker series. We also have checking data from 1992 which are not used in the initial modelling but which are used later to compare the models we fit.

Our basic model is a hierarchical regression model for the square root of CD4 count which we find to decay in a plausibly linear fashion. We fit the model using Markov chain Monte Carlo techniques, specifically the Gibbs sampler. This approach is easily implemented and takes in its stride the highly unbalanced time 'design' of the data which would cause great problems in conventional modelling. Our model could also be described as a random effects growth curve and bears similarities to recent work by Lange *et al.* (1992).

We are able to entertain various adjustments to our basic model, including heterogeneous errors and robustification to outlying individuals, and we make comparisons by using a predictive methodology and the 1992 checking data. We suggest uses of our best model, including prediction of subsequent CD4 paths and estimation of the time of the landmark immunological event CD4^{200} (soon to be included in the AIDS definition in the USA and used as a surrogate endpoint for clinical trials). Moreover, we are able to use our model as a framework for the study of treatment (zidovudine) effects on CD4 trajectories.

We consider a variety of ways in which treatment effects can be modelled. Our best models postulate a change of level and change of slope at initiation of treatment and find both effects to be significant. According to these

models, zidovudine causes an elevation of CD4 counts but a slight accelera-
tion of the slope of CD4 decay, although it nonetheless represents a beneficial
intervention for a long period into the future. We describe the strategy for
intervention which is the logical implication of our modelling and discuss interpretations of our results. Using the 1992 checking data we find that our
best treatment effect models fit better than the basic models which do not
take the effect into account; see McNeil (1993) for further details.

References

Lange, N., Carlin, B.P. and Gelfand, A.E. (1992) 'Hierarchical Bayes models for
the progression of HIV infection using CD4 T-cell numbers', *J. Amer. Statist.
Assoc.* **87**, 615–626 (see also 631–632).

McNeil, A. (1993) *Statistical Methods in AIDS Progression Studies with an Analysis
of the Edinburgh City Hospital Cohort*. PhD thesis, University of Cambridge.

Discussion

AGUR It has been shown that one of the toxic side effects of AZT is temporarily to increase the density of immature white blood cells. Does McNeil's
analysis take this into account or is it reflected in the results of the analysis?

REPLY The model we propose looks simply for temporary increases in serial
CD4 measurements; it does not possess the subtlety to take into account
suggested increases in the density of immature white cells. It is conceivable
that changes of this kind could explain in part (or whole) the apparent
recovery in CD4 levels; it is not clear, on the basis of the fitted model,
whether a genuine recovery in immune function is being found.

JACQUEZ It would be unusual if the decrease in CD4 cells was purely linear.
Is the observed linear decrease in McNeil's data due to the short period of
observation?

REPLY Linear decay of root CD4 is a good working description of longitudinal
CD4 behaviour in the period where data is usually available; it may be that
it does not adequately model the initial fast decline of CD4 cells which
is reported to take place in the immediate aftermath of seroconversion,
but few patients have data covering this phase. Moreover, the period
of observation represented by our data is not that short: most patients
have three or four years of CD4 measurements and some have five due
to the requirement that included patients should have at least 10 CD4
determinations; this length of follow-up seems sufficient to characterize
individual rates of CD4 decay based on a linear model.

ISHAM Has McNeil tried a piece-wise linear model to test for or take into
account a possible non-linear decrease?

REPLY We have not tried a piece-wise linear model. Lange *et al.* (1992) experimented with such a model which had two linear pieces and a random change point. However their data did not support this level of model sophistication and they too found linear decline in root of CD4 to be an adequate description of their data.

BLOWER Has McNeil investigated the possibility of gender effects in the rate of loss of CD4 counts? How do his results relate to those derived from the cohorts of homosexual men?

REPLY There was an indication of a gender effect on CD4 whereby women started from higher levels and decayed more slowly. This was not a statistically significant effect but it is certainly something which merits further investigation.

Modelling Progression of HIV Infection: Staging and the Chicago MACS Cohort

John A. Jacquez, James S. Koopman, Carl P. Simon and Ira M. Longini, Jr.

The long incubation period of AIDS, with variation in infectiousness over its course, has emphasized the need to model progression of the disease process. The models used for progression of HIV infection to AIDS have generally been staged Markov models that imply a one-way progression from infection to AIDS to death and so do not allow for temporary remissions in the progression of the disease. Such models have negative exponential distributions for the transit times in a stage and independence of transit times in successive stages (Longini *et al.* 1992, Longini *et al.* 1991). In our studies to estimate transmission probabilities from data on the Chicago MACS cohort, by stage of infection, we found it necessary to examine progression in the cohort.

The Multicenter AIDS Cohort Study (MACS) involves 4 cohorts of male homosexuals recruited in 1984 in 4 cities: Baltimore, Chicago, Los Angeles and Pittsburgh (Kaslow *et al.* 1987). Approximately every 6 months, the participants had physical examinations, had blood drawn and filled out a questionnaire on sexual practices. We examine progression in the Chicago MACS cohort which consisted of 1020 individuals at the start of the study. We present data on the first to twelfth waves of examinations, covering the period 1984–90.

Cumulative plots of seropositivity for HIV-1 show that approximately 40% of the Chicago cohort was HIV(+) by the first wave and that about 70 more seroconversions occurred from wave 1 to wave 12. The experience of the other cohorts was similar. Thus roughly 85% of the infections occurred before the first wave of examinations.

MACS questionnaires obtained data on total number of partners, number of anonymous partners, and number of anal and oral partners, both insertive and receptive. They show a small decrease in all such activities in the 18 months up to wave 1. Much more change occurred after the first wave. By wave 4 the number of partners per month had fallen to approximately 1/4th the level reported for the period 18 months before wave 1.

For HIV seropositives at wave 1, the distributions of CD4+ T-cell counts show a steady drift downwards from wave 1 to wave 12. Those who were seronegative at wave 1 and remained seronegative showed only small changes in the T4 cell counts. However, the temporal changes in histograms of distributions and the plots of the means hide an extensive variation in the time courses of counts in the individuals. There was extensive short term and long term variation in the time plots. The short term variability can be ascribed to laboratory error and to biological processes unrelated to the HIV infection; it is well known that many forms of stress and intercurrent infections affect CD4 cell counts. However there can also be longer term variations in the time course of the disease process which may include temporary improvements in the cell counts.

For the stages, we used the same CD4 counts for boundaries as were used by Longini *et al.* (1991). However the numbering was different; the first antibody positive stage was stage 3 (CD4 count ≥ 900). The raw counts were smoothed with a 3-point linear smoother. For each individual, we then interpolated the smoothed data points to obtain a stage-by-month file for each individual. From that we calculated histograms of transit times in stages, for those who exit a stage by going down to the next stage, and for those who go back up to the next lower numbered stage. The histograms of transit times exhibited evidence of non-exponential distributions for the later stages; there were fewer short transit times than would be expected for an exponential distribution. The histograms for the later stages were all unimodal with modes at 5-10 months and long tails to the distributions. However, the histograms for the first two stages were closer to exponential. Regarding the direction of flow, for the first antibody stage all exits were to the next stage. For all other stages but the last, about four times as many individuals exited a stage in the forward direction as compared to the backwards direction. Finally, pairwise correlations between the transit times of successive stages gave no evidence of correlation between the early stages, stages 3 and 4, and stages 4 and 5, but did suggest increasing correlations between the later stages, 5 and 6, 6 and 7, and 7 and 8. However, the largest correlation coefficient, that between the transit times in stages 7 and 8, was 0.5, and considering that the smoothing technique introduces some short range correlations, it seems unlikely that the correlations are important even if they were to turn out to be statistically significant.

The results suggest that we should look at staged semi-Markov models with backflow. For the individual stages, a model consisting of a few compartments to give a gamma density for transit times may suffice. The ideal would be to find a good model of the basic pathological processes at work.

References

Longini, I.M., Byers, R.H., Hessol, N.A. and Tan, W.Y. (1992) 'Estimating the stage-specific numbers of HIV infection using a Markov model and back-calculation', *Stat. Med.* 11, 831–843.

Longini, I.M., Clark, W.S., Gardner, L.I. and Brundage, J.F. (1991) 'The dynamics of CD4+ T-lymphocyte decline in HIV-infected individuals: a Markov modeling approach', *J. AIDS* **4**, 1141–1147.

Kaslow, R.A., Ostrow, D.G., Detels, R., *et al.* (1987) 'The multicenter AIDS Cohort Study: rationale, organization, and selected characteristics of the participants', *Am. J. Epidemiol.* **126**, 310–318.

The Interpretation of Immunoepidemiological Data for Helminth Infections

M.E.J. Woolhouse

Introduction

Acquired immunity is a particular type of density-dependent process that may affect the establishment, mortality or fecundity of parasitic helminths, as functions both of current infection and of past infection; that is, a density-dependent process with 'memory'. This type of process is likely to have complicated impacts on parasite population dynamics because of this memory component (Woolhouse 1992a). The epidemiological impact of acquired immunity will also depend on which parasite life-cycle stage provides the antigen stimulating a protective response and on which stage is the target of the response. For human schistosomes (the main example used here), the relevant life cycle stages are larvae (cercariae and schistosomulae) (L), adult worms (A), and eggs (E). The evidence for different forms of immunity to schistosomes has been elegantly reviewed in Hagan and Wilkins (1993); possible combinations of target and response are: larval antigen/anti-larval response (an LL process); adult antigen/anti-larval response (an AL process); and adult antigen/antiadult response (an AA process).

Mathematical models

The models used here are described in detail elsewhere (Woolhouse 1992b, 1993, 1994) and are based on earlier elaborations of a simple immigration-death process (Anderson and May 1985, Roberts and Grenfell 1991). The models describe the dynamics of the worm burden, experience of infection, and level of resistance for a set of individuals in a population. Worm burden is self explanatory. Experience of infection corresponds to the (discounted) cumulative exposure to parasite antigens and can be interpreted as related to the numbers of specific memory cells. Level of resistance corresponds to the impact of acquired immunity on parasite establishment or mortality and is a function of the experience of infection, and, for current purposes, can be interpreted as related to levels of protective antibodies or eosinophilia. The dynamics of these variables are determined by parameters representing the rate of infection, parasite mortality rate, the rate of loss of immunological memory, and an index of the strength of the immune response. The rate of infection and parasite mortality rate are self explanatory. The rate of loss of immunological memory corresponds to the decay through time in the ability to mount a protective response, and can be interpreted as related to the turnover of the memory cell population. The strength of the immune response can be interpreted as related to the proliferation and activity of effector cells and specific antibodies. The models can incorporate heterogeneities between individuals as heterogeneities in parameter values. Heterogeneities in the rate of infection, for example, can be interpreted as life-long differences between individuals in exposure to infection and/or innate susceptibility.

The behaviour of models corresponding to LL, AL and AA processes was evaluated with respect to host age (assuming an equilibrium with respect to time), using a fourth order Runge-Kutta approximation, for a range of parameter values (see Woolhouse 1992, 1994). Model predictions were compared with observed immunoepidemiological patterns as described below. This procedure was repeated for a variety of models which invoke age dependent patterns of exposure to infection, but not acquired immunity or other density-dependent processes.

Age-intensity patterns

The age-intensity curve for human schistosomes is typically convex, with peak intensities in either older children or young adults (Fisher 1934, Clarke 1966). This pattern is reproduced by the LL, AL and AA models, provided there is significant immunological memory. The pattern must also, at least partly, reflect age-dependent exposure, although there are doubts that this alone can explain the high degrees of convexity observed (Butterworth *et al.* 1988).

The age-intensity curves for populations subject to different rates of transmission show a 'peak shift', higher peak levels of infection are associated with those peaks occuring in younger age classes for *S. haematobium* (Woolhouse *et al.* 1991) and *S. mansoni* (Fulford *et al.* 1992). This pattern is also reproduced by models of acquired immunity, but not by models with age-dependent exposure alone unless there are systematic variations in the shape of the age-exposure curve.

Age-intensity curves show that significant levels of infection are found in the oldest age classes (e.g. Clarke 1966), although exceptions have been reported (Fisher 1934). Populations with higher levels of infection in younger age classes tend to have higher levels of infection in older age classes (Fulford *et al.* 1992). These patterns are reproduced by the AL and AA models but not by the LL models. The differences arise because, in LL processes, acquired immunity does not (directly) influence subsequent exposure to antigen, whereas in AL and AA processes acquired immunity reduces subsequent exposure to antigen.

Predisposition

Predisposition may be operationally defined as a positive correlation between worm burdens before and after chemotherapy. It has been reported for *S. mansoni* infection and appears to be age dependent, statistically significant correlations occuring only in younger age classes (Tingley *et al.* 1988). Models of acquired immunity predict age dependent predisposition, with highest values in the youngest and oldest age classes.

Reinfection and specific antibody levels

Negative correlations between reinfection rates and specific IgE levels have been reported for *S. haematobium* (Hagan *et al.* 1991) and *S. mansoni* (Dunne *et al.* 1992), and interpreted as indicating a protective role for IgE. There are indications that, for *S. mansoni*, these correlations may be age dependent. The LL and AL models predict age dependent correlations, though the shape of the relationship may differ between the models – for the LL model the correlation declines monotonically with age, for the AL model the correlation may increase again in older age classes. Importantly, the correlation may be positive at all ages despite significant acquired immunity. The AA model predicts a positive correlation throughout. These results require at least some consistency in relative rates of exposure before and after chemotherapy.

Implications and predictions

The epidemiological evidence for human schistosome infection appears most consistent with the predictions of a model incorporating an AL process. This model can reproduce the shape of the age-intensity curve, the 'peak shift', age dependent predisposition and a negative correlation between levels of protective antibodies and reinfection rates. Given the models used, these results require significant immunological memory, but not necessarily that this memory is lifelong.

Neither the LL nor AA models are consistent with all these epidemiological patterns, and must be rejected as complete descriptions of schistosome immunoepidemiology. Many of the observed epidemiological patterns can also be explained by models invoking age related patterns of exposure to infection, though the patterns required might be considered somewhat arbitrary with respect to field observations. Conversely, the results presented here may be somewhat dependent on the details of the assumptions regarding patterns of exposure and infection, such as the long term stability of relative rates of exposure, the form of the differences between age dependent exposure rates between communities, and the use of continuous infection as opposed to discrete infection events.

References

Anderson, R.M. and May, R.M. (1985) 'Herd immunity to helminth infection and implications for parasite control', *Nature* **315**, 493–496.

Butterworth, A.E.*et al.* (1988) 'Longitudinal studies on schistosomiasis', *Philos. Trans. R. Soc. Lon. B.* **321**, 495–511.

Clarke, V. de V. (1966) 'The influence of acquired resistance in the epidemiology of bilharzia', *C. Afr. J. Med.* **12** (Suppl), 1–30.

Dunne, D.W.*et al.* (1992) 'Immunity after treatment of human schistosomiasis – association between IgE antibodies to adult worm antigens and resistance to reinfection', *Eur. J. Immunol.* **22**, 1483–1494.

Fisher, A.C. (1934) 'A study of schistosomiasis in the Stanleyville district of the Belgian Congo', *Trans. R. Soc. Trop. Med. Hyg.* **28**, 277–306.

Fulford, A.J.C.*et al.* (1992) 'On the use of age-intensity data to detect immunity to parasite infections, with special reference to *schistosoma mansoni* in Kenya', *Parasitology* **105**, 219–228.

Hagan, P.*et al.* (1991) *Nature* **349**, 243–245.

Hagan, P. and Wilkins, H.A. (1993) 'Parasitology yesterday – concomitant immunity in schistosomiasis', *Parasitol. Today* **9**, 3–6.

Roberts, M.G. and Grenfell, B.T. (1991) 'The population dynamics of nematode infections of ruminants: periodic perturbations as a model for management', *IMA J. Math. Appl. Med. Biol.* **8**, 83–93.

Tingley, G.A.*et al.* (1988) 'Water contact as a measure of exposure to infection in human schistosomiasis: the relationship to faecal egg counts', *Trans. R. Soc. Trop. Med. Hyg.* **82**, 448–452.

Woolhouse, M.E.J. (1992a) 'Immunoepidemiology of intestinal helminths – pattern and process', *Parasitol. Today* **8**, 111.

Woolhouse, M.E.J. (1992b) 'A theoretical framework for the immunoepidemiology of helminth infection', *Parasite Immunol.* **14**, 563–578.

Woolhouse, M.E.J. (1993) 'A theoretical framework for immune-responses and predisposition to helminth infection', *Parasite Immunol.* **15**, 583–594.

Woolhouse, M.E.J. (1994) 'Immunoepidemiology of human schistosomes – taking the theory into the field', *Parasitol. Today* **10**, 196–202.

Woolhouse, M.E.J.*et al.* (1991) 'Acquired-immunity and epidemiology of schistosoma-haematobium', *Nature* **351**, 757–759.

The Distribution of Malaria Parasites in the Mosquito Vector: Consequences for Assessing Infection Intensity in the Field

G.F. Medley, P. Billingsley and R.E. Sinden

The most common measures of mosquito infection with *Plasmodium* estimated in the field are the prevalence and intensity of malarial parasites. Of these quantities, the prevalence is the simplest to measure. We are interested in the effect of sample size (numbers of mosquitoes examined) on the accuracy of estimation of these quantities, and the relationship between the distribution of infectious stages within the mosquitoes and the population dynamics and genetics of malaria.

Previous work has shown that the distribution of malaria oocysts within their vector hosts is empirically well described by a negative binomial distribution with varying mean and overdispersion (Medley *et al.* 1993). Although this research was carried out on laboratory derived infections, the relationship appears consistent over a variety of malaria and vector species combinations. The implication is that the relationship is an intrinsic feature of the population biology of malaria parasites within their vectors.

In this presentation, we use data from wild caught mosquitoes (*Anopheles gambiae s.l.* and *A. funestus*) infected with *Plasmodium falciparum*. There were a total of 1112 mosquitoes within 64 samples (mean 17.4 mosquitoes, range 2–60): each sample being the total number of mosquitoes caught in a household. The total number of oocysts found in the mosquitos was 960 (mean intensity within samples 1.34, range 0.023–24). For further details see Billingsley *et al.* (1994). The distribution of oocysts was found to be consistent with the laboratory derived infections, and no difference was detected between the distributions in the different vector species, further suggesting that the distribution is a conserved feature of the population biology of different parasite and host species. The analysis of laboratory infections showed decreasing heterogeneity with increasing intensity of infection, but there was no such effect in the wild caught mosquitoes. This is probably due to the much reduced infection intensity in natural infections.

The distribution of oocysts was estimated from the relationship between prevalence and mean intensity. Our conjecture is that the mean intensity is determined by the level of infection in the human host to which the group of mosquitoes was exposed, but that the distribution is generated by the mosquito/malaria relationship. Using the estimated relationship between prevalence and mean intensity of infection, the comparison between observed and expected distributions and the bivariate confidence regions indicate that this conjecture is not in conflict with the data. In particular, the observed frequency distribution of oocysts is well reproduced as a mixture of negative binomial distributions with a constant degree of heterogeneity (as measured by the parameter k) and means determined by the distribution of infection within households.

The results of the simulations also give the conditional distributions of prevalences and mean intensities. These show that there is considerable variability in mean intensity given a particular prevalence, but that some inference can be drawn from the prevalence. For example, it is possible to say that for two samples of 25 mosquitos with prevalences of infection of 10% and 30%, they will have a different mean intensity. Any inference of mean intensity from prevalence has not been quantified previously. The ability to draw inferences of means from prevalence depends dramatically on sample size—it improves greatly up to samples of 500 mosquitoes but no great improvement is gained beyond that number. This result has direct relevance to the number of mosquitoes that should be sampled to detect reduction in transmission.

The distribution of oocysts in mosquito vectors has several important consequences in terms of the transmission of malaria. First, sexual reproduction occurs in the vector, and the resulting oocyst population is a skewed sample of the genetic recombinants that occurred in the blood meal. Second, the genetic composition of the sporozoite inoculum given to humans may well have an overdispersed distribution. At present, the number of sporozoites received at biting is thought not to be important in determining the resultant infection in humans, but the number and genetic diversity within an inoculum of sporozoites must have some effect on the overall population dynamics and genetics of malaria. Third, prevalence is the most common measurement of mosquito infection; our results suggest that this can be used to derive confidence intervals for mean intensities.

References

Billingsley, P., Medley, G.F., Charlwood, J.D. and Sinden, R.E. (1994) 'Relationship between prevalence and intensity of *Plasmodium falciparum* infection in wild caught *Anopheles* mosquitoes', *Am. J. Trop. Med. Hyg.* **51**, 260–270.

Medley, G.F., Sinden, R.E., Fleck, S., Billingsley, P.F., Tirawanchai, N. and Rodriguez, M.H. (1993) 'Heterogeneity in patterns of malarial oocyst infections in the mosquito vector', *Parasitology* **106**, 441–449.

When Susceptible and Infective Human Hosts are not Equally Attractive to Mosquitoes: a Generalization of the Ross Malaria Model

Günther Hasibeder

1 Introduction

Models for vector-transmitted infections are always based on several homogeneity assumptions, even when some aspects of heterogeneity are incorporated in the model. Usually most of these assumptions are not stated explicitly, and among these is the implicit assumption that susceptible and infective hosts are bitten homogeneously by insect vectors. Some experiments and a field study documented in the literature (Baylis and Nambiro (1993) and references therein) seem to indicate the possibility that vectors have a feeding preference for infected hosts. On the other hand, if infective human hosts are especially protected against mosquito bites, for example through the use of bed nets, susceptible hosts could on average be bitten more frequently.

2 The model

In order to investigate effects when biting of insect vectors is non-homogeneous between susceptible and infective hosts, we consider a generalization of the Ross malaria model (which is a type of model applicable not only to malaria transmission), allowing both for increased or decreased attractiveness of infective hosts, but disregarding other kinds of heterogeneity which have e.g. been dealt with by Hasibeder and Dye (1988). We characterize the degree of heterogeneity between susceptible and infective hosts by one single parameter and, unlike the analysis in Kingsolver (1987), we start at the level of individuals:

Let $\pi_1(X)$ denote the proportion of adequate contacts (bites or blood meals facilitating transmission) of infective vectors which they have with susceptible hosts, and $\pi_2(X)$ the proportion of adequate contacts of uninfected vectors which they have with infective hosts. Then

$$\frac{dX}{dt} = \alpha \pi_1(X)Y - \rho X$$

$$\frac{dY}{dt} = \beta \pi_2(X)(V - Y) - \delta Y,$$

where X and Y are the numbers of infective hosts and vectors, respectively, V denotes the constant total number of vectors, α and β are the transmission rates, ρ is the recovery rate of hosts, δ the death rate of infective vectors, and t is chronological time (see Hasibeder and Dye (1988) for a more detailed interpretation of symbols and discussion of the underlying assumptions).

We assume

$$\pi_1(X) + \pi_2(X) = 1$$

and, with H denoting the total number of hosts,

$$\frac{\pi_2(X)}{X} = p\frac{\pi_1(X)}{H - X},$$

i.e. that each infective host is adequately contacted by vectors p times as frequently as each susceptible host, and this positive constant p can be called the relative vector preference for infective hosts (which is now independent of the infection status of the vector). Consequently

$$\pi_1(X) = \frac{H - X}{H - X + pX}$$

$$\pi_2(X) = \frac{pX}{H - X + pX}.$$

Higher vector preference for infective hosts is characterized by $p > 1$, whereas $p < 1$ symbolizes that susceptible hosts are contacted more frequently. $p = 1$ recovers the basic Ross model.

Denoting with $b_s(p, X)$ the proportion of bites taken from each susceptible host, and with $b_i(p, X)$ the proportion of bites taken from each infective host, it can nicely be demonstrated that they remain within realistic limits for this modelling approach: In the standard Ross model both proportions are $\frac{1}{H}$; in case $p > 1$

$$\frac{1}{H} \geq b_s(p, X) \geq \frac{p^{-1}}{H}$$

$$\frac{p}{H} \geq b_i(p, X) \geq \frac{1}{H},$$

and similarly for $p < 1$.

3   Basic reproduction number, equilibria, stability

According to this model, the basic reproduction number (basic reproduction ratio) of the infection, which we denote with $R_0(p)$ since it depends on p, is

$$R_0(p) = p\frac{\alpha\beta V}{\rho\delta H}.$$

With respect to the existence of stationary states and their stability properties, four different patterns — with one, two, or even three equilibrium points in the state space — are possible:

[A] There is one globally stable endemic equilibrium, and the infection-free equilibrium is unstable.

[B] The infection-free equilibrium is globally stable.

[C] The infection-free equilibrium is locally stable, and in addition there are one unstable and one locally stable endemic equilibrium; host prevalence is greater at the stable equilibrium than at the unstable equilibrium.

[D] The infection-free equilibrium is locally stable, and in addition there is one endemic equilibrium which is unstable.

We define

$$r = \frac{\alpha V}{\rho H}, \quad s = \frac{\beta}{\delta}.$$

Then

$$R_0(p) = prs,$$

and the above four possible equilibrium patterns occur according to the following parameter conditions:

1. $R_0(p) > 1 \implies$ [A]

2. $R_0(p) = 1$

    2.1. $r > 1 + \frac{2}{s} \implies$ [A]

    2.2. $r \leq 1 + \frac{2}{s} \longrightarrow$ [B]

3. $R_0(p) < 1$

    3.1. $r \geq 1 + \frac{2}{s} + \frac{2\sqrt{s+1}}{s} \wedge 0 < p < \frac{1}{rs} \implies$ [C]

    3.2. $1 + \frac{2}{s} < r < 1 + \frac{2}{s} + \frac{2\sqrt{s+1}}{s}$

        3.2.1. $\frac{4-s(r+r^{-1}-2)}{4(s+1)} < p < \frac{1}{rs} \implies$ [C]

        3.2.2. $p = \frac{4-s(r+r^{-1}-2)}{4(s+1)} \implies$ [D]

        3.2.3. $0 < p < \frac{4-s(r+r^{-1}-2)}{4(s+1)} \implies$ [B]

    3.3. $r \leq 1 + \frac{2}{s} \wedge 0 < p < \frac{1}{rs} \implies$ [B]

4 Interpretation

In case $R_0 > 1$ even only very few initial infection cases always lead to an endemic equilibrium (pattern **A**), as in the basic Ross model. However, if $R_0 \leq 1$ the equilibrium pattern of this epidemic model does not only depend on R_0, but also on additional parameter conditions: while it is possible, as in the Ross model, that the infection becomes extinct independent of the initial state (pattern **B**), it is also possible that extinction occurs if there are only few initial infection cases, but that prevalence moves towards a positive equilibrium if it is sufficiently high at the beginning (pattern **C**). If $R_0 = 1$ even the same pattern **A** as for $R_0 > 1$ is possible.

Also, the fact that the basic reproduction ratio R_0 is proportional to p, and thus increases with increasing p, is somewhat surprising and not immediately plausible: A higher relative vector preference for infective hosts leads to a higher proportion of bites taken from infective hosts, and thus on the one side to higher transmission from infective hosts to susceptible vectors, but on the other side also to reduced transmission from infective vectors to susceptible hosts.

References

Baylis, M. and Nambiro, C.O. (1993) 'The effect of cattle infection by *Trypanosoma congolense* on the attraction, and feeding success, of the tsetse fly *Glossina pallidipes*', *Parasitology* **106**, 357–361.

Hasibeder, G. and Dye, C. (1988) 'Population dynamics of mosquito-borne disease: persistence in a completely heterogeneous environment', *Theor. Pop. Biol.* **33**, 31–53.

Kingsolver, J.G. (1987) 'Mosquito host choice and the epidemiology of malaria', *Am. Nat.* **130**, 811–827.

The Dynamics of Blood Stage Malaria: Modelling Strain Specific and Strain Transcending Immunity

Jonathan Swinton

There is a great deal of interest among malariologists about the effect of antigenic diversity on the transmission dynamics of malaria (Day and Marsh 1991). Complementing other modelling studies on this effect at a population level (Gupta *et al.* 1994), we explore the within-host dynamics of blood stage malaria in a single individual infected with a basket of different parasite strains. By generalising a previous model (Anderson *et al.* 1989) to account for this situation and calibrating it against the observed data on the time course of malaria infection, we are able to include the effects of the host immune response despite the difficulty of obtaining quantitative data on this component.

We intend to use our model to investigate the effects of different types of immune response: for example the relative success of a fast, quickly decaying strain-specific response combined with a slowly generated but persistent strain-transcending response.

We will discuss whether combinations of strain specific and strain transcending responses to a basket of infections at the blood stage of malaria account for the observed patterns of parasitaemia in malaria endemic areas.

Following Anderson *et al.* (1989), and similarly to Hellriegel (1992), we define $x(t)$ as the number of uninfected erythrocytes, $m(t)$ as the number of free merozoites and $y(t)$ as the number of infected red blood cells. We assume that red blood cells are produced at a constant rate Λ and die at a per-capita rate μ with a mean life-span of $1/\mu$. Free merozoites infect unparasitised cells at a rate $\beta x m$; these cells rupture after a mean time of $1/\alpha$ to produce r more free merozoites.

The conclusion (Anderson *et al.* 1989) that immunity directed against the relatively shortlived merozoites was less important dynamically than immunity against the longer lived parasitised erythrocytes leads us initially to consider only immunity directed against the latter.

We assume that there may be up to N strains of parasite, and we use a subscript i to denote the density of free merozoites of each strain and of the red cells they infect by y_i and m_i respectively for each of the strains $i = 1, \ldots, N$.

We assume that each strain can elicit a strain-specific immune response, and we aggregate the effect of this response on the density of the strain into a single variable u_i.

We assume that there is also a cross-strain immune response which we denote by u_0. In the absence of convincing data on the dynamics of the response u, we assume, unlike Anderson, May and Gupta, that this response is stimulated at a rate proportional by a factor k to the density of parasite alone. We set the killing effect of this immune response u to occur at a rate guy, and allow the response to decay at a rate b.

Both in this model and *in vivo*, both acute and chronic infections are capable of producing substantially depressed red blood cell levels. There is controversy about the role of anaemia in malaria (Phillips and Pasvol 1992), and in order to accommodate different assumptions about the erythropoietic response to infection we include a further dynamic variable into the model: the rate of erythropoiesis Λ.

This leads to the following set of equations:

$$\frac{dx}{dt} = \Lambda - \mu x - x \sum_{i=1}^{N} \beta_i m_i$$

$$\frac{dy_i}{dt} = \beta_i x m_i - \alpha_i y_i - g_i u_i y_i - g_0 u_0 y_i$$

$$\frac{dm_i}{dt} = r_i \alpha_i y_i - d_i m_i - \beta_i x m_i$$

$$\frac{du_i}{dt} = k_i y_i - b_i u_i \qquad i = 0 \ldots n$$

$$\frac{d\Lambda}{dt} = \epsilon \left(1 - \frac{(x + \sum y_i)}{\Lambda_0/\mu} \right)$$

for $i = 1, \ldots, N$.

Further extensions to this model, to account for the possibility of reinfection of parasitised erythrocytes and of the known preference of *P. falciparum* for reticulocytes are possible and have been explored by Hetzel (1993).

References

Anderson, R.M., May, R.M. and Gupta, S. (1989) 'Non-linear phenomena in host-parasite interactions', *Parasitology* 99, S59–S79.

Day, K.P. and Marsh, K. (1991) 'Naturally acquired immunity to *Plasmodium falciparum*'. In *Immunoparasitology Today*, C. Ash and R.B. Gallagher (eds.), Elsevier Trends Journals, Cambridge, A68–A71.

Gupta, S., Anderson, R.M., Trenholme, K. and Day, K.P. (1994) 'Antigenic diversity and the transmission dynamics of *P. falciparum*', *Science* **263**, 961–963.

Hellriegel, B. (1992) 'Modelling the immune response to malaria with ecological concepts: short-term behaviour against long-term equilibrium', *Proc. Roy. Soc. Lond. B* **250**, 249–256.

Hetzel, C. (1993) *The dynamics of the immune response to infection: mathematical models and experimental investigation*. PhD thesis, Imperial College, University of London.

Phillips, R.E. and Pasvol, G. (1992) 'Anaemia of *Plasmodium falciparum* malaria', *Ballière's Clin. Haematol.* **5**, 315–330.

Part 3
Population heterogeneity (mixing)

Modeling Heterogeneous Mixing in Infectious Disease Dynamics

H. W. Hethcote

1 Introduction

The spread of many infectious diseases occurs in a diverse population, so that it is desirable to include heterogeneity in the formulation of the epidemiological model in order to improve its predictive and explanatory power and its applicability. Often the heterogeneous population is divided into subpopulations or groups, each of which is homogeneous in the sense that the group members have similar characteristics. This division into groups can be based not only on disease-related factors such as mode of transmission, latent period, infectious period, genetic susceptibility or resistance, and amount of vaccination or chemotherapy, but also on social, cultural, economic, demographic or geographic factors. For example, the mixing behavior may depend on the age of the individuals. If any of the epidemiological characteristics are gender dependent, then groups of men and women may be necessary.

The transmission of sexually transmitted diseases (STDs) often occurs in a very heterogeneous population. People with many different sexual partners have many more opportunities to be infected and to infect others than people who have fewer partners. Thus for STDs it is often necessary to divide the population on the basis of the amount of sexual activity. Frequently, the epidemiological characteristics of STDs are different for men and women. For example, the probability of transmission per partner of gonorrhea from male to female is greater than that from female to male. Moreover, the fraction of women with gonorrhea who are asymptomatic is larger than the fraction for men (Hethcote and Yorke 1984).

In recent years the human immunodeficiency virus (HIV), which leads to acquired immunodeficiency syndrome (AIDS), has emerged as an important new infectious disease. There is a tremendous amount of heterogeneity associated with HIV/AIDS. Some common modes of transmission are heterosexual intercourse, homosexual intercourse and sharing of needles by injecting drug users (IDUs). Thus a general model for HIV/AIDS could include groups of people based on their sexual behavior, e.g. homosexual men, bisexual men, heterosexual women, and heterosexual men. Moreover, the IDUs can be divided into those who are homosexual men, bisexual men, heterosexual women, and heterosexual men. It may be necessary to further subdivide all of the previous groups into subgroups based on their numbers of sexual or needle-sharing partners. Since perinatal transmission can occur from an infected mother to her child, groups of children of female IDUs and of heterosexual women can be included. Moreover, there are many differences based on social, demographic and geographic factors. Because of the great diversity and heterogeneity among those at risk to HIV/AIDS, modeling this disease is a challenging task (Castillo-Chavez 1989, Anderson and May 1991, Anderson *et. al.* 1986, May and Anderson 1987, Anderson 1988, Blythe and Castillo-Chavez (1989), Hethcote *et. al.* 1991a,b, Hethcote and Van Ark 1992a, Hethcote 1994, Hyman and Stanley 1988, Jacquez *et al.* 1988, Lin *et al.* 1993). See Isham (1988) and Schwager *et. al.* (1989) for reviews of mathematical and statistical approaches in HIV/AIDS modeling. See Hethcote and Van Ark (1992b) for modeling of HIV/AIDS in the major risk groups in fifteen regions of the United States.

In this paper we focus on heterogeneity based on differences in the mixing done by individuals in the population. For STDs this is related to the numbers and types of sexual partners. Models can be formulated with either a continuous distribution of social/sexual behaviors or the population can be stratified into subpopulations or groups using specific social/sexual criteria. Models for HIV/AIDS with a continuous distribution of sexual activity levels have been considered by Hyman and Stanley (1988). Becker and Marschner (1990), Castillo-Chavez and Blythe (1989) and Busenberg and Castillo-Chavez (1991) have studied these types of models with various preference mixing functions, have shown that proportionate mixing is the only separable solution, have found the general solution for a homosexual population, and have found expressions for the basic reproduction number in the proportionate mixing case. Models with a continuous distribution of sexual behavior are not considered here; we focus on the formulation and estimation of the contact or mixing matrix between members of the groups in multigroup models.

In Section 2 the incidence term for a multigroup model is formulated in terms of a contact or mixing matrix. A major problem in models with many groups is the estimation of the n^2 entries in the matrix for the contacts among the n groups. Both proportionate and preferred mixing formulations of the mixing matrix are reviewed. Estimation methods using these formulations are discussed.

In Section 3 the effects of heterogeneity on estimates of the basic reproduction number and on estimates of the amount of vaccination needed to obtain herd immunity are considered. Several authors have concluded that the estimate of R_0, under the false assumption that a heterogeneously mixing population is homogeneously mixing, is not greater than the actual R_0 for the heterogeneous population. The 'homogeneous mixing fallacy' estimates can cause epidemiologists to underestimate how much uniform vaccination is necessary in order to eradicate diseases.

Often the mixing behavior depends on the age of the individuals so the age must be considered as a variable in an epidemiological model. For example, school children may have many more opportunities to contract and spread diseases such as measles, mumps, rubella and chickenpox than most adults have. Age-structured models are considered in Section 4. The proportionate and preferred mixing approaches to the formulation of the contact rate between people of different ages are presented for models with a continuous dependence on age. Multigroup models with groups based on age intervals are special cases. Estimates of the force of infection as a function of age have been obtained from epidemiological data. Here methods are presented for estimating proportionate and preferred mixing matrices from age-specific force of infection data. Estimates of mixing activities and mixing matrices are given for measles in two locations.

2   Mixing heterogeneity in socially-defined groups

Often the heterogeneity in disease transmission is based on differences in the social behavior of the population at risk for the disease. Thus the division of the population into groups is based on 'who mixes with whom'. Members of some groups may have lots of contacts with people in certain groups and fewer contacts with people in other groups. The mixing pattern between social groups is particularly important for STDs. Numerous authors have formulated epidemiological models with multiple groups and have defined contact matrices for the interactions between members of the groups (Watson 1972, Lajmanovich and Yorke 1976, Hethcote 1978, Nold 1980, Hethcote and Yorke 1984, Dietz 1981, Anderson and May 1985c, Anderson *et. al.* 1986, Hethcote and Van Ark 1987, Sattenspiel 1987, Jacquez *et. al.* 1988, Becker and Marschner 1990, Castillo-Chavez 1989, Castillo-Chavez *et. al.* 1989, Diekmann *et. al.* 1990, Hethcote and Van Ark 1992a, 1992b, Anderson and May 1991, Lin *et. al.* 1993). The mixing pattern between people with different sexual activity levels influences the speed and asymptotic behavior of the epidemic (Hyman and Stanley 1988, Jacquez *et. al.* 1988). An infectious disease spreads faster in a multigroup population when the groups are closely connected by mixing which is nearly random (proportionate mixing) and spreads more slowly when the groups are weakly connected (Kaplan and Lee 1990).

Perhaps the simplest form of the transmission matrix is the diagonal matrix corresponding to the situation in which there is only internal mixing within each group. Of course, the groups are really not interacting at all in this case, so the internal mixing matrix is not of much interest. The simplest form of the transmission matrix when the groups are connected seems to be the proportionate mixing contact matrix (Hethcote and Yorke 1984, Nold 1980, Hethcote and Van Ark 1987, Anderson *et. al.* 1986). In the proportionate mixing approach there is a mixing activity associated with each group and the contacts between groups are proportional to the product of their activities. When members of the groups are interacting, but there is a tendency for people to mix more within their own group, then modelers often use a preferred mixing matrix, which is a convex combination of a proportionate mixing matrix and an internal mixing matrix. This type of matrix was used by Hethcote *et. al.* (1992) and by Hethcote and Yorke (1984) in modeling gonorrhea in eight risk groups. For modeling HIV/AIDS preferred mixing matrices have been used by Jacquez *et. al.* (1988), Blythe and Castillo-Chavez (1989), Hethcote and Van Ark (1992b), and Kaplan *et al.* (1989). Here we consider both proportionate and preferred mixing matrices.

Since we are interested in providing a review of the basic results and in illustrating estimation procedures, we consider only proportionate and preferred mixing; however, other more complex approaches to mixing matrices in socially-defined groups have been used. In modeling the spread of hepatitis A among children in daycare centers in Albuquerque, Sattenspiel (1987) considered the mixing within each center and the movement of people between the centers. This structured mixing approach was extended by Jacquez *et. al.* (1988) into a two step process where the first step involves the choice of an activity group in which to make contacts and the second step involves selection of contacts within the activity group. Another extension by Koopman *et. al.* (1989) considered a three step process where sexual pairing results from 1) social contact, 2) acceptance as a potential sexual partner, and 3) initiation of sex in response to the needs and standards of each partner. Morris (1995) uses a general loglinear approach for the contact matrix of partnerships between people in groups. Thus a variety of approaches to the formulation and estimation of mixing matrices are available.

2.1   A mixing matrix for socially-defined groups

Before presenting special forms of mixing matrices, we formulate a general mixing matrix for a multigroup model of SI, SIS, SIRS or SEIRS type. Let N_i be the size of group i for $i = 1$ to n. Let X_i and Y_i be the numbers of people in group i who are susceptible and infectious. Let the contact rate η_{ij} be the average number of adequate contacts per unit time of a susceptible person in group i with people in group j. Here an adequate contact is an encounter which is sufficient for transmission of infection if the group i person is susceptible and the group j person is infectious. The total number of contacts per unit time of all susceptibles in group i with people in group j

is $\eta_{ij}X_i$. Since the fraction of the contacts in group j which are with an infective is Y_j/N_j, the incidence (new infections) per unit time in group i due to contacts with group j is $\eta_{ij}X_iY_j/N_j$. The total incidence in group i is

$$INC_i = \sum_{j=1}^{n} \eta_{ij}X_iY_j/N_j. \tag{2.1}$$

Thus the contact or mixing matrix $\mathbf{C}$ for the multigroup model formulated in terms of the differential equations for X_i and Y_i has entries given by

$$c_{ij} = \eta_{ij}/N_j. \tag{2.2}$$

2.2 The threshold result for SIS or SIRS models with n groups

If γ_i and μ_i are the removal rate constant and death rate constant in group i, then the differential equation for the infectives in group i is

$$Y_i' = \Big[\sum_{j=1}^{n} \eta_{ij}Y_j/N_j\Big]X_i - (\gamma_i + \mu_i)Y_i. \tag{2.3}$$

In a model with constant population sizes N_i in each group, susceptible fractions of the population given by $S_i = X_i/N_i$, and infectious fractions given by $I_i = Y_i/N_i$, the differential equation (2.3) becomes

$$I_i' = \Big[\sum_{j=1}^{n} \eta_{ij}I_j\Big]S_i - (\gamma_i + \mu_i)I_i. \tag{2.4}$$

The definition of the contact rate η_{ij} here has the advantage that this differential equation is independent of the group sizes N_i. The n differential equations given by (2.4) are simpler than equations (2.2) in Hethcote and Van Ark (1987), who defined the contact rate λ_{ij} to be the average number of adequate contacts per unit time of a person in group j with people in group i. The two different contact rates are related by $\lambda_{ij}N_j = \eta_{ij}N_i$. The adequate contact rate η_{ij} could be factored into a contact rate between groups i and j times a probability of transmission per contact from an infective in group j to a susceptible in group i. This formulation is sometimes useful, but it involves twice as many parameters and all of them cannot be estimated using the procedure in Section 2.5.

The stability of the disease-free equilibrium depends on the eigenvalues of the $n \times n$ irreducible matrix $\mathbf{A} = \mathbf{L} - \mathbf{D}$, where $\mathbf{L} = [\eta_{ij}]$ and $\mathbf{D}$ is the diagonal matrix with diagonal entries $(\gamma_i + \mu_i)$. The threshold condition for stability of the disease-free equilibrium is $s(\mathbf{A}) \leq 0$, where the stability modulus $s(\mathbf{A})$ is the maximum real part of the eigenvalues of $\mathbf{A}$ (Lajmanovich and Yorke

1976, Hethcote 1978). Now $AD^{-1} = T - E$, where D^{-1} is the diagonal matrix of mean infectious periods $1/(\gamma_j + \mu_j)$, E is the identity matrix, and $T = LD^{-1} = [\eta_{ij}/(\gamma_j + \mu_j)]$ is the next generation matrix (Diekmann *et. al.* 1990). The basic reproduction number R_0 is the spectral radius $\rho(T)$, which is the maximum absolute value of the eigenvalues of T. For the one group model, the basic reproduction number is $R_0 = \eta/(\gamma + \mu)$, so the next generation matrix T and $R_0 = \rho(T)$ are natural generalizations. Note that $s(A)$ has the same sign as $\rho(T) - 1$, so that $s(A) \le 0$ iff $R_0 = \rho(T) \le 1$ (Hethcote and Van Ark 1987). For the formulation (2.3) in terms of numbers of infectives, the next generation matrix is

$$K = [\eta_{ij} N_i / \{N_j(\gamma_j + \mu_j)\}] = [\lambda_{ij}/(\gamma_j + \mu_j)]. \qquad (2.5)$$

If N is the diagonal matrix of population sizes, then $\rho(K) = \rho(NTN^{-1}) = \rho(T) = R_0$, so the basic reproduction number R_0 is independent of the formulation used.

The threshold result for n group models of SIS or SIRS type (Lajmanovich and Yorke 1976, Hethcote and Van Ark 1987) is that the disease persists in the population iff the basic reproduction number $R_0 = \rho(T)$ is greater than 1. More formally, it is:

The threshold result *If $R_0 = \rho(T) \le 1$, then all solutions approach the disease-free equilibrium. If $R_0 = \rho(T) > 1$, then all solutions (except the disease-free equilibrium solution) approach the unique endemic equilibrium.*

2.3 Proportionate mixing in socially-defined groups

There is rarely enough information directly to estimate the n^2 entries in the contact matrix C without making some assumptions about the structure of the matrix C. The simplest assumption is based on the idea of proportionate mixing. This proportionate mixing approach (Hethcote and Yorke 1984, Nold 1980) assumes that the number of contacts between members of two groups is proportional to the activity levels and sizes of the two groups. Thus individuals in more active groups have more contacts per unit time. One advantage of this approach is that it reduces the number of parameters to be estimated from n^2 contact rates to n activity levels.

Let a_i be the mixing activity in group i, which is the average number of contacts per unit time of a person in group i, so $1/a_i$ is the average time between contacts. The total number of contacts per unit time made by all people in the population is $D = \sum_{k=1}^{n} a_k N_k$. Since D is also the total number of contacts received by all people, the fraction of these contacts received by all members of group j is $b_j = a_j N_j / D$. The proportionate mixing assumption is that the a_i contacts per unit time made by a person in group i are distributed among the groups in proportion to the fractions b_j of the contacts received by the groups. Thus $\eta_{ij} = a_i b_j$ so that the incidence in group i given by (2.1) becomes

$$INC_i = \sum_{j=1}^{n} a_i b_j X_i Y_j / N_j = \frac{a_i X_i}{D} \sum_{j=1}^{n} a_j Y_j. \tag{2.6}$$

Note that the contact matrix for proportionate mixing can be written as $c_{ij} = (a_i/D^{\frac{1}{2}})(a_j/D^{\frac{1}{2}})$ so that there are only n quantities $\{a_i\}$ or $\{a_i/D^{\frac{1}{2}}\}$ to be determined instead of the n^2 entries η_{ij} in the original contact matrix. Although the definition of the contact rate η_{ij} here is not the same as that of the contact rate λ_{ij} in Hethcote and Van Ark (1987), the proportionate mixing incidence here is the same as they obtained in their equation (6.6).

For a sexually transmitted disease such as gonorrhea or HIV/AIDS with activity levels based on numbers of new sexual partners per month, the proportionate mixing model can be conceptualized as the 'big bar' model. The frequency with which people visit the 'big bar' to choose a new sexual partner depends on their sexual activity level. For gonorrhea in a heterosexual population, the very sexually active men and women visit the 'big singles bar' to choose a partner of the opposite sex more often than those in the less active groups. For HIV/AIDS in a homosexual population, the very sexually active gay men visit the 'big gay bar' to choose a partner more often than the less active gay men. Sometimes proportionate mixing is called random mixing, since people at the 'big bar' on a given night choose their new sexual partner randomly from those who are there. But it is important to remember that they are not choosing randomly from all sexually active people; they are choosing randomly from those at the 'big bar' on that night and very sexually active people visit the 'big bar' more often.

2.4   Preferred mixing in socially-defined groups

Although the proportionate mixing matrix is the simplest matrix with intergroup interactions, it is not applicable when people in the groups are more likely to contact others in their group than they are to have random (i.e. proportionate mixing) contacts. The simplest matrix which allows this possibility is the preferred mixing matrix, which is a linear combination of a proportionate mixing matrix and a diagonal, internal mixing matrix. The preferred mixing matrix has entries

$$c_{ij} = \epsilon a_i a_j / D + (1 - \epsilon) a_i \delta_{ij} / N_j$$

where ϵ in the interval $[0, 1]$ is the convex combination parameter and δ_{ij} is the Kronecker delta. If the parameter ϵ is 1, then the contact matrix is a proportionate mixing matrix, and if the parameter ϵ is 0, then the matrix is diagonal so that each member of a group mixes only with other members of the same group. The convex combination parameter ϵ is related to the correlation between the activity level of the susceptible person and the activity level of the person contacted. Jacquez *et. al.* (1988) use the term *preferred mixing* to describe a more general formulation, which has n convex combination parameters $\{\epsilon_i\}$ for the n groups.

Hethcote and Yorke (1984) used an eight group model for gonorrhea, where the population was divided by gender (female or male), by being sexually very active or active, and by being symptomatic or asymptomatic when infected. In order to satisfy the fit criterion that the overall prevalence in women was 3% of the women at risk, the ϵ in the preferred mixing matrix was 0.8, so that 80% was proportionate mixing and 20% was internal mixing. This corresponds to a correlation coefficient r of 0.08 between the sexual activity level of a person and the sexual activity level of their partners. Note that 100% proportionate mixing did not satisfy the fit criterion.

In a model of HIV/AIDS in homosexual men in San Francisco, the population was divided into sexually very active and active groups (Hethcote *et al.* 1991a,b). The best fit to the HIV and AIDS incidence data occurred with $\epsilon = 0.82$, so that 82% was proportionate mixing and 18% was internal to the activity levels. However, in this case the fit with 100% proportionate mixing was nearly as good. Thus the proportionate mixing explanation was completely adequate. For more details on modeling HIV/AIDS in San Francisco and 15 other regions of the United States, see the book by Hethcote and Van Ark (1992b).

2.5   Estimation of mixing matrices for socially-defined groups

Estimating the mixing patterns which characterize networks of sexual behavior can be done in several ways. One possibility is to use information from sexual behavior surveys, but this approach is always subject to the difficulties associated with nonresponse bias, not enough respondents and untruthful answers by respondents. It may be more reliable to use data about the epidemiological status of people in the mixing groups.

First consider the proportionate mixing approach. Let μ be the natural death rate constant so $1/\mu$ is the average lifetime, and let γ be the rate constant for removal from the infectious classes so $1/(\gamma + \mu)$ is the (death-adjusted) average period of infection for all groups. The group i contact number $k_i = a_i/(\gamma + \mu)$ is the average number of contacts of a person in group i during the infectious period. The fractional activity levels b_i, and the group i contact numbers k_i in the proportionate mixing approach can be estimated directly from epidemiological data. For an epidemic in a heterogeneous population, these quantities can be estimated from the initial and final susceptible fractions in each group obtained from serosurvey data (Hethcote and Van Ark 1987, Section 8). This approach has been used to estimate the basic reproduction number for disease epidemics in a homogeneously mixing population by using the equation $R_0 = \ln(S_0/S_\infty)/(S_0 - S_\infty)$. Based on seropositivities of Yale University students at the beginning and end of their freshman year, the estimates of R_0 were 6.2 for rubella, 2.2 for Epstein-Barr virus, and 1.44 for influenza (Hethcote and Van Ark 1987, Hethcote 1989).

For an endemic disease in a heterogeneous population, the quantities b_i and k_i can be estimated from either the susceptible fraction in each group obtained from serosurvey data or from the average age of attack in each group obtained from clinical data (Hethcote and Van Ark 1987, Section 7). Suppose that the susceptible fractions, S_i^e, at the endemic equilibrium have been estimated for all of the groups by a serosurvey of an unvaccinated population and that the sizes N_i of the groups are known. Then it has been found (Hethcote and Van Ark 1987) that

$$b_i = \left(\frac{1}{S_i^e} - 1\right)N_i \Big/ \left[\sum_{j=1}^{n}\left(\frac{1}{S_j^e} - 1\right)N_j\right] \tag{2.7}$$

$$k_i = \left(\frac{1}{S_i^e} - 1\right)\sum_{j=1}^{n}\left(\frac{1}{S_j^e} - 1\right)N_j \Big/ \left[\sum_{j=1}^{n}\left(\frac{1}{S_j^e} - 1\right)^2 S_j^e N_j\right] \tag{2.8}$$

These formulas apply for SI, SIS and SIRS models. The basic reproduction number R_0 (also called the contact number) is given by

$$R_0 = \sum_{i=1}^{n} b_i k_i,$$

so it can also be estimated. Finding expressions for the confidence limits on these estimates is an open problem.

It would be desirable to also estimate the activity levels a_i and the proportionate mixing contact matrix c_{ij} from the endemic equilibrium fractions, S_i^e, but this is not possible since the a_i are contacts per unit time and time rates cannot be estimated from time independent equilibrium values. Note that the proportionate-mixing, next-generation matrix $\mathbf{K}$ with entries $b_i k_j$, can be estimated from the equilibrium values (Hethcote and Van Ark 1987). If the average infectious period, $1/(\gamma + \mu)$, is known, then the activities can be estimated from $a_j = k_j(\gamma + \mu)$, so that the proportionate mixing matrix with entries $a_i a_j / D$ can then be estimated.

The ability to estimate information about the mixing matrix from seropositivity data is an advantage of the proportionate mixing approach. We do not know of examples in which this proportionate mixing approach has been applied to seropositivity data for infectious diseases in heterogeneously mixing populations, but this would certainly be a worthwhile project. Note that somewhat similar methods have been used for stochastic models. Longini *et. al.* (1982) have used serologic data from the cities of Seattle, Washington and Tecumseh, Michigan to estimate the community probabilities of infection (CPI) and the secondary attack rates (SAR) within households for influenza and rotaviruses. A similar approach has been used by Becker and Angulo (1981) for variola minor (chickenpox) in Brazil.

For the preferred mixing matrix in an n group model, there are $n + 1$ parameter values, $\{a_i\}$ and ϵ, but these cannot be found from epidemic or endemic data for the n groups since the number of unknowns is greater than the number of known quantities. Methods need to be developed for estimating preferred mixing parameters from seropositivity data.

The proportionate mixing formulas above apply for SIS models, so they might be useful for STDs such as gonorrhea. They also apply for SI diseases, so they could theoretically be used for estimating parameters in multigroup models of HIV/AIDS; however, for this disease with a ten year average incubation period for AIDS, it would take many years before it might settle down to an equilibrium, particularly since many changes in behavior can occur in a ten year period. Thus estimation of mixing parameter values for HIV/AIDS may have to be estimated from survey information or from the initial growth of HIV in the groups. The estimation of mixing matrices from serologic data as advocated here complements their estimation from sexual behavior survey data as described in the next paper by Morris (1995).

3   Consequences of the homogeneous mixing fallacy

When a population, which is actually mixing heterogeneously is falsely assumed to be mixing homogeneously, this can affect estimates obtained from data on the population. The rule of thumb obtained from a variety of studies on heterogeneous mixing is that the estimate of the basic reproduction number R_0 (i.e. the contact number) obtained under the 'homogeneous mixing fallacy' is not greater than the actual R_0 for the heterogeneously mixing population. This means that the 'homogeneous mixing fallacy' estimate of the fraction $(1 - 1/R_0)$ which must be successfully immunized by vaccination uniformly in all groups in order to achieve herd immunity is too low. This is intuitively reasonable since uniform vaccination at an 'average' level in the entire population would not be adequate for herd immunity in those groups in which the disease is more easily spread.

May and Anderson (1984) used an SIR model with n groups to examine a spatially heterogeneous population with one transmission rate in each group and a lower transmission rate between the groups. They defined the optimum vaccination program as the program with different fractions vaccinated in each group which achieves eradication using the least total amount of vaccination. Thus the vaccination rates would be higher in groups with higher transmission rates and lower in groups with lower transmission rates. The uniform vaccination program is the program which achieves eradication by vaccinating the same fraction in every group. The 'homogeneous mixing fallacy' program also vaccinates uniformly, but vaccinates at the level obtained by falsely assuming that the population is homogeneously mixing; note that this program does not achieve eradication, in general.

In a 'city and villages' calculation, May and Anderson (1984) found that the total amount of vaccination was lower for the optimum vaccination program than for the uniform vaccination program. Their 'homogeneous mixing fallacy' estimate of the fraction necessary for eradication was between those for the optimum and the uniform vaccination programs. Using a model with a different mixing matrix formulation, Hethcote and Van Ark (1987) found the same ordering of the three vaccination programs, but their differences between the estimated fractions were less than those found by May and Anderson (1984). The uniform vaccination program consistently required more total vaccination than the optimum vaccination program. This is clearly reasonable since the uniform vaccination program would have to vaccinate at the level needed to eradicate the disease in the most difficult group, while the optimum vaccination program could vaccinate lower fractions in the lower transmission rate groups. The 'homogeneous mixing fallacy' program does not achieve eradication, in general, but in their calculations (Hethcote and Van Ark 1987), the estimate of the total vaccination needed using the 'homogeneous mixing fallacy' assumption was close to the total vaccination needed for the optimum vaccination program. Of course, the 'homogeneous mixing fallacy' program assumed uniform vaccination while the optimum program used higher vaccination levels in some groups and lower vaccination levels in other groups.

Other authors have examined the epidemiological consequences of homogenizing a heterogeneously mixing population. Adler (1992) showed that averaging the mixing patterns of behaviorally different groups caused the basic reproduction number R_0 to decrease or remain unaltered in epidemic models with symmetric transmission between groups. The effects of heterogeneity in mixing have also been studied for stochastic models by Becker and Marschner (1990) and Marschner (1992). Stratification of their population was achieved using a multitype branching process approximation to the epidemic. Except for a few unusual cases with asymmetric transmission, they found that the basic reproduction number R_0 (here it determines whether an epidemic might occur) was larger for the heterogeneously mixing model than for the equivalent homogeneously mixing model (i.e. with the same total number of contacts per day). However, the probability of a minor outbreak of the epidemic when $R_0 > 1$ was higher for the heterogeneously mixing model than for the homogeneously mixing equivalent. In the Ross host-vector malaria model, Hasibeder and Dye (1988) also found that the basic reproduction number R_0 for models with heterogeneous mixing was not less than that for the corresponding model with homogeneous mixing.

Thus a general conclusion from modeling analyses is that the basic reproduction number R_0 for a heterogeneously mixing model is higher than for the 'equivalent' model with homogeneous mixing. This is equivalent to the conclusion that the estimates of the fraction which must be uniformly vaccinated successfully in a population using the 'homogeneous mixing fallacy' is lower than the actual uniform successful vaccination necessary to achieve herd immunity.

4   Mixing heterogeneity in age-structured models

The different daily schedules of people of different ages implies that the number of encounters and the ages of those encountered vary greatly. For example, children going to school mix more with other school children than they do with adults while adults with jobs mix more with other adults. Although simple models which do not consider age-related mixing can give some useful insights, it is often appropriate for many infectious diseases to consider an age-structured model for their spread. Age-structured models have been studied and applied by numerous authors (Hoppensteadt 1975, Dietz 1975, 1981, Hethcote 1983, 1987, Anderson and May 1985c, 1991).

The spread of many childhood diseases such as measles, mumps, rubella and chickenpox may be governed by the pattern of contact among children and the infectivities (probabilities of transmission per contact) of the diseases. The pattern of contact among preschool and school age children depends on their daily contacts with other children in playgroups and in school classrooms. Thus it might be possible to determine one age-specific pattern of contacts for a country, which could be used for all of these childhood diseases by changing to a different infectivity factor for each disease. Then this pattern of contacts could be used in predicting the spread of a variety of diseases by merely changing the probability of transmission per contact. In order to get accurate estimates of the mixing matrix, one would need data on disease seropositivity for many age groups averaged over enough years or locations so that the seropositivity is independent of when epidemics occurred. Since vaccination affects age specific transmission and seropositivity, prevaccination data must be used. Alternatively, since we do not vaccinate for chickenpox, it might be possible to use recent data on chickenpox to establish the current contact pattern for the childhood diseases.

Since we are interested in mixing heterogeneity related to age, we consider only the incidence term without choosing any specific age-structured epidemiological model. Let $x(a,t)$ and $y(a,t)$ be the age distributions as a function of age a and time t for the susceptibles and the infectives. Thus, for example, at time t the number of infectives between ages a_1 and a_2 is $\int_{a_1}^{a_2} y(a',t)da'$. The incidence term for the number of new infections per unit time in the partial differential equations for the age-structured model is often written as $\lambda(a,t)x(a,t)$ where

$$\lambda(a,t) = \int_0^\infty c(a,a')y(a',t)da' \qquad (4.1)$$

is called the force of infection. The contact rate $c(a,a')$ is the per capita number of people of age a contacted by an infective of age a' per unit time. Here a contact is assumed to be an encounter which results in transmission of the infection if the person contacted is susceptible. The units of $c(a,a')$ are (people of age a contacted)/[people of age $a \times$ unit time $\times$ one infective of age a'], so that the units of $\lambda(a,t)$ are the reciprocal of time.

4.1 Proportionate mixing in age-structured models

Here we give the proportionate mixing form of the contact function $c(a,a')$ and then we show how to estimate it from data. This proportionate mixing is based on the same idea as used for the multigroup models in Section 2. Assume that the age distribution for the population at a steady state is given by $n(a)$. Let $l(a')$ be the average number of people contacted by a person of age a' per unit time, so that $D = \int_0^\infty l(a')n(a')da'$ is the total number of contacts per unit time made by all people. Here we consider only adequate contacts which are sufficient for transmission of the particular disease, but this is easily modified to consider general contacts by including a parameter for the probability of transmission per contact of the particular disease (Rouderfer *et. al.* 1994). Since D is also the total number of contacts per unit time received by all people, $l(a)/D$ is the fraction of all contacts which are received by a person of age a. The proportionate mixing assumption is that the $l(a')$ people contacted per unit time by a person of age a' are distributed among people of age a in proportion to the fraction $l(a)/D$ of all contacts per unit time received by people of age a. Thus

$$c(a,a') = l(a')l(a)/D. \qquad (4.2)$$

Now $\int_0^\infty l(a')y(a',t)da'$ is the number of infectious contacts per unit time at time t and $l(a)/D$ is the fraction of contacts received by people of age a per unit time at time t, so the force of infection $\lambda(a,t)$ given by (4.1) is the number of infectious contacts received by people of age a per unit time at time t and the incidence $\lambda(a,t)x(a,t)$ is the number of people of age a infected per unit time at time t.

At a steady state endemic disease situation, the equilibrium force of infection $\lambda(a)$ and distributions $x(a)$ and $y(a)$ are independent of t. Next we find an expression for $l(a)$ as a function of $\lambda(a)$, $y(a)$ and $n(a)$. From (4.1) and (4.2) we have

$$l(a) = D\lambda(a) \Big/ \int_0^\infty l(a')y(a')da'. \tag{4.3}$$

Multiplying both sides of the equation above by $y(a)$ and integrating from 0 to ∞ yields an expression for $\int_0^\infty l(a')y(a')da'$. Substitution of this expression into the denominator of (4.3) yields

$$l(a) = D^{\frac{1}{2}}\lambda(a) \Big/ \Big[\int_0^\infty \lambda(a')y(a')da'\Big]^{\frac{1}{2}}. \tag{4.4}$$

Multiplication of both sides of the equation above by $n(a)$ and integrating yields the expression

$$D^{\frac{1}{2}} = \int_0^\infty \lambda(a')n(a')da' \Big/ \Big[\int_0^\infty \lambda(a')y(a')da'\Big]^{\frac{1}{2}}. \tag{4.5}$$

Substitution of this expression into (4.4) yields

$$l(a) = \lambda(a) \int_0^\infty \lambda(a')n(a')da' \Big/ \int_0^\infty \lambda(a')y(a')da'. \tag{4.6}$$

Thus the mixing activity function $l(a)$ can be estimated from the force of infection $\lambda(a)$, the distribution $y(a)$ for the number of infectives and the distribution $n(a)$ for the population size.

Often the population is grouped by age-intervals such as $[0,4]$, $[5,9]$, $[10,14]$, $[15,19]$ and $[20,75]$. Let N_k denote the size of the age group k and Y_k be the number of infectives in group k. In this case the force of infection λ_j for those with age a corresponding to group j is found from (4.1) to be

$$\lambda_j = \sum_{k=1}^m c_{jk}Y_k. \tag{4.7}$$

For proportionate mixing, the mixing matrix corresponding to (4.2) has elements given by

$$c_{jk} = l_k l_j / D = (l_j/D^{\frac{1}{2}})(l_k/D^{\frac{1}{2}}) \tag{4.8}$$

where l_j is the average number of people contacted by a person in age group j per unit time and $D = \sum_{k=1}^m l_k N_k$ is the total number of people contacted per unit time. Then in the endemic steady state situation, the expressions (4.4) and (4.5) become

$$l_j/D^{\frac{1}{2}} = \lambda_j \Big/ \Big[\sum_{k=1}^m \lambda_k Y_k\Big]^{\frac{1}{2}}. \tag{4.9}$$

$$D = \left[\sum_{k=1}^{m} \lambda_k N_k\right]^2 \bigg/ \sum_{k=1}^{m} \lambda_k Y_k. \tag{4.10}$$

The expression (4.6) for the mixing activity l_j becomes

$$l_j = \lambda_j \sum_{k=1}^{m} \lambda_k N_k \bigg/ \sum_{k=1}^{m} \lambda_k Y_k. \tag{4.11}$$

Thus the mixing activity levels for those in age group j can be estimated from the forces of infection, the group sizes and the number of infectives in each group (Rouderfer et. al. 1994). Note that the mixing matrix entries c_{jk} can be found from the values of $l_j/D^{\frac{1}{2}}$, which can be estimated using (4.9) from the forces of infection and the numbers of infectives.

4.2 Preferred mixing in age-structured models

Preferred mixing formulations analogous to those in Section 2.3 can be derived for age-structured models. A preferred mixing contact function can be written as

$$c(a, a') = \epsilon l(a')l(a)/D + (1 - \epsilon)l(a)\delta(a' - a)/n(a'), \tag{4.12}$$

where ϵ in $[0, 1]$ is the convex combination parameter and δ is the Dirac delta function. The formulation (4.12) is unrealistic since infectives would only contact people of exactly the same age and no two people would be exactly the same age down to the microsecond. If there is a tendency for people to mix with others of nearby ages, then a Gaussian kernal could be used for the nearby mixing so that

$$c(a, a') = \epsilon l(a')l(a)/D + \left[(1 - \epsilon)l(a)/\left[n(a')\sqrt{2\pi}\sigma\right]\right] \exp\left[-(a' - a)^2/2\sigma^2\right], \tag{4.13}$$

where the Gaussian variance σ^2 determines which ages are 'nearby'.

The preferred mixing definitions are analogous for models with age-interval groups. If people tend to mix more with those in their same age-interval group, then the preferred mixing contact matrix has entries

$$c_{jk} = \epsilon l_k l_j/D + (1 - \epsilon)l_j\delta_{jk}/N_k, \tag{4.14}$$

where a_j is the mixing activity of a person in group j and δ_{jk} is the Kronecker delta.

For preferred mixing it is not possible to get explicit formulas similar to (4.11) for the activities l_j, but some simplifications are possible. For example, multiply both sides of (4.7) by N_j and sum to get $\sum \lambda_j N_j = \sum l_j Y_j$. Substituting this back into (4.7) leads to

$$l_j = \lambda_j/[\epsilon \sum \lambda_k N_k/D + (1 - \epsilon)Y_j/N_j] \tag{4.15}$$

where $D = \sum l_k N_k$. If ϵ is fixed, then these n equations can be solved iteratively to estimate the n activities l_j. Examples of this approach are given in Section 4.4.

4.3   Methods for estimating age-structured mixing

Direct data on the force of infection as a function of age are not available, but it can sometimes be estimated from available data. Using serological data or records of case notifications, a maximum likelihood method has been developed for estimating the forces of infection (Grenfell and Anderson 1985, Anderson and May 1991). Usually, it is assumed that the endemic disease has reached a steady state so that the force of infection λ and the epidemiological age distributions x, y and z for the number of susceptibles, infectives and those removed with immunity, respectively, are independent of time t. Although some authors do not do it, it is important to emphasize the assumption that the disease is at a steady state. If $\lambda(a)$ and the age distribution $n(a)$ for the population were known, then the steady-state age distributions $x(a)$, $y(a)$ and $z(a)$ could be found (analytically or numerically) from the differential equations for the model.

Sometimes the information available from a serological study is the cumulative fraction $z(a)/n(a)$ of the population which has been infected and is removed with immunity at age a. Sometimes the information available is the incidence $\lambda(a)x(a)$ as a function of age. In either case we need to find the force of infection function $\lambda(a)$ so that the solution of the differential equations gives the best fit to the data (Anderson and May 1991, pp. 160–162). If $\lambda(a)$ is assumed to be a quadratic or a cubic function of a, then the coefficients can be found which give the best fit to the data. For hepatitis B in developing countries, estimates of the force of infection as a polynomial function of age a have been obtained from data in 15 countries by Edmunds et. al. (1995). If $\lambda(a)$ is assumed to be a piecewise constant function on five age intervals, then the λ_1, λ_2, λ_3, λ_4, λ_5 constants are found which give the best fit. Once $\lambda(a)$, $y(a)$ and $n(a)$ are known, the proportionate mixing equations (4.2), (4.5) and (4.6) can be used to find the activity function $l(a)$, the total number D of contacts per unit time and the contact function $c(a, a')$. If the age-interval values λ_j, Y_j and N_j are known, then the equations (4.8), (4.9) and (4.11) can be used to find the analogous age-interval quantities.

For the proportionate mixing approach when the population is grouped by age intervals, information on the activities l_j can be found from the force of infection information. From (4.11) we see that the activity levels l_j in age-interval groups are a fixed constant times the forces of infection λ_j. Thus the activity level ratios l_j/l_1 relative to that in the first age interval are equal to λ_j/λ_1. Hence the relative mixing activity levels can be estimated directly from the force of infection estimates without knowledge of the group population sizes N_k or the number of infectives Y_k in the groups. If the force of infection estimates $\{\lambda_j\}$ are used in the differential equations for a specific model, then the prevalences $\{Y_j\}$ can be found numerically. These estimates and the group sizes $\{N_j\}$ can then be used in (4.8) to (4.11) to find the activity levels and the proportionate mixing matrix. This is illustrated in the next section. An important point of the discussion above is that data and methods are available so that proportionate mixing matrices can be estimated. Finding expressions for the confidence limits on these estimates of the activity levels and the entries in the contact matrix is an open problem.

For the preferred mixing approach there may not be enough information available to estimate all of the unknown quantities. For the continuous form given by (4.13), it is not possible to estimate $l(a)$, σ and ϵ from the force of infection function $\lambda(a)$. For the age-interval formulation, the preferred mixing matrix given by (4.14) has $m+1$ unknowns, $\{l_j\}$ and ϵ, but they cannot be estimated from the m known values, $\{\lambda_j\}$. However, if the convex combination parameter ϵ is chosen in advance, then the m equations (4.15) can be solved iteratively for the activities l_j if the values of $\{\lambda_j\}$, $\{N_j\}$, and $\{Y_j\}$ have been estimated. Note that the prevalences $\{Y_j\}$ can be estimated by numerically solving the differential equations for the specific model.

Anderson and May (1991, pp. 176–77) use four different mixing matrices which they label WAIFW (who acquires infection from whom). These four *ad hoc* matrices each have 5 unknown parameters, which can be estimated from the forces of infection in their 5 age groups. A disadvantage of using one of their WAIFW matrices is that one or more of the estimates of their matrix elements may turn out to be negative. They state (Anderson and May 1991, p. 177) that 'this indicates that a matrix structure inappropriate to the observed age dependence in λ has been chosen'. This problem never occurs in the proportionate mixing approach since explicit expressions (4.11) and (4.8) are given for the activity levels l_j and the contact matrix elements c_{jk}. Although the four WAIFW matrices of Anderson and May have some intuitive basis, there is no clear justification for choosing one of them instead of other mixing matrices.

4.4 Estimating age-structured mixing matrices from data

When the population is divided into m age groups, there are m forces of infection λ_j to be estimated from the data. Anderson and May (1985a, 1985c, 1991) present estimates of age specific forces of infection for various diseases. Their age classes are usually $[0, 4]$, $[5, 9]$, $[10, 14]$, $[15, 19]$ and $[20, 75]$. For measles in England and Wales in 1966 (Anderson and May 1991 p. 164), their forces of infection for the first four age groups are 0.184, 0.579, 0.202, 0.100 and 0.100. Here it is assumed that the force of infection in the 20–75 year old age group is the same as in the 15–19 year old age group. Now we consider preferred mixing and calculate relative activities, which are normalized so $l_1 = 1$, and find mixing matrices C_ϵ, which are normalized so $c_{11} = 1$. These normalized activities and mixing matrices give a good picture of the mixing patterns.

Note that preferred mixing with $\epsilon = 1$ is proportionate mixing. For proportionate mixing the relative activities are equal to the ratios of the forces of infection. Using the forces of infection above for measles in England and Wales in 1966, the relative mixing activities are 1, 3.1, 1.1, 0.5 and 0.5. The normalized mixing matrix is

$$\mathbf{C_1} = \begin{bmatrix} 1 & 3.1 & 1.1 & 0.5 & 0.5 \\ 3.1 & 9.9 & 3.4 & 1.7 & 1.7 \\ 1.1 & 3.4 & 1.2 & 0.6 & 0.6 \\ 0.5 & 1.7 & 0.6 & 0.3 & 0.3 \\ 0.5 & 1.7 & 0.6 & 0.3 & 0.3 \end{bmatrix} \qquad (4.16)$$

If specific parameter values are used in a model, then the differential equations in the model can be solved numerically using the forces of infection λ_k to obtain the number Y_k of infectives in each group. These values can then be used in equations (4.11) and (4.15). We have used an age-structured SIR model with an infectious period of one week and l_j as the number of contacts per week of a person in group j. We have assumed that everyone survives until age 75 (Anderson and May 1991, p. 62, type I) and have normalized the population size to one.

Using the numerical solution of the differential equations for the prevalences, we have found from the equations (4.11) that that the activities l_j are 2.7, 8.5, 3.0, 1.5, and 1.5 in the five age groups, respectively. Note that $c_{jk} = l_j l_k / D = (l_1^2 / D)(l_j / l_1)(l_k / l_1)$, so that the proportionate mixing matrix $\mathbf{C}$ given by (4.8) for the five age-interval groups is l_1^2 / D times the normalized mixing matrix $\mathbf{C_1}$ given by (4.16) above. The total contacts per week are given by $D = 4.5$ so that $l_1^2 / D = 7.4$. In a population of size N, the value of l_1^2 / D would be $7.4/N$. Thus the estimation of the proportionate mixing contact matrix for this case is complete.

Careful scrutiny of the normalized proportionate mixing matrix $\mathbf{C_1}$ in (4.16) above reveals some unrealistic aspects. For example, the internal contacts in groups 1, 3, 4 and 5 of 1, 1.2, 0.3 and 0.3, respectively, are less than the 3.1, 3.4, 1.7 and 1.7 contacts of people in these age groups with age group 2. This seem implausible since we might expect each group to have more internal contacts than external contacts. Thus the proportionate mixing matrix does not appear to be a good choice for this age-structured population. Since there does not seem to be enough internal mixing, we now try preferred mixing matrices.

Again using the forces of infection for measles in England and Wales in 1966, the differential equations for the SIR model described above are solved numerically for the prevalences and then the equations (4.15) are solved iteratively for the activities. The normalized preferred mixing matrices with

$\epsilon = 0.8$ and $\epsilon = 0.7$ are

$$
\mathbf{C}_{0.8} = \begin{bmatrix}
1 & 0.5 & 0.4 & 0.2 & 0.2 \\
0.5 & 5.2 & 1.4 & 0.7 & 0.7 \\
0.4 & 1.4 & 3.3 & 0.5 & 0.5 \\
0.2 & 0.7 & 0.5 & 1.5 & 0.3 \\
0.2 & 0.7 & 0.5 & 0.3 & 0.4
\end{bmatrix}, \tag{4.17}
$$

$$
\mathbf{C}_{0.7} = \begin{bmatrix}
1 & 0.2 & 0.3 & 0.1 & 0.1 \\
0.2 & 4.5 & 1.0 & 0.6 & 0.6 \\
0.3 & 1.0 & 7.3 & 0.9 & 0.9 \\
0.1 & 0.6 & 0.9 & 3.6 & 0.5 \\
0.1 & 0.6 & 0.9 & 0.5 & 0.8
\end{bmatrix}. \tag{4.18}
$$

These matrices seem more plausible since the first four diagonal elements (corresponding to within group mixing) are larger than the other elements in the same row or column (corresponding to mixing with other groups). It is interesting to observe from the matrices in (4.17) that the second age group of 5–9 year olds becomes less dominant as we move away from proportionate mixing by decreasing ϵ. For $\epsilon = 0.8$ the relative mixing activities are 1, 3.7, 2.7, 1.4 and 1.4. For $\epsilon = 0.7$ the relative mixing activities are 1, 4.0, 6.0, 3.3 and 3.4, so that the relative activity in the third group of 10–14 year olds is greater than that of the second group of 5–9 year olds.

For measles in Baltimore, Maryland, USA in 1963, the forces of infection are 0.2, 0.582, 0.379, 0.2 and 0.1 (Anderson and May 1991, p. 164). The differential equations in the SIR model above are solved to obtain the prevalences $\{Y_k\}$ and the equations (4.15) are then solved iteratively to find the activities. With the convex combination parameter $\epsilon = 0.8$, the relative mixing activities are 1, 3.8, 5.4, 3.0 and 1.5, and the normalized preferred mixing matrix is

$$
\mathbf{C}_{0.8} = \begin{bmatrix}
1 & 0.5 & 0.6 & 0.4 & 0.2 \\
0.5 & 5.0 & 2.4 & 1.3 & 0.7 \\
0.6 & 2.4 & 8.2 & 1.9 & 1.0 \\
0.4 & 1.3 & 1.9 & 3.7 & 0.5 \\
0.2 & 0.7 & 1.0 & 0.5 & 0.4
\end{bmatrix} \tag{4.19}
$$

This matrix seems plausible as a mixing matrix, since the diagonal elements in the first four age groups are larger than the other elements in the same row or column.

An important lesson from this section is that it is possible to estimate information about mixing activity levels and preferred mixing matrices in age groups from available data. We have demonstrated the feasibility of the methods, but have not undertaken a careful comparison of mixing matrices. Such a study of mixing matrices would be a worthwhile project. It is interesting to observe that the situation with about 80% proportionate mixing and

20% internal mixing seems to have been suitable in several instances, e.g. in the gonorrhea and HIV examples in Section 2.4 and in the two measles data sets here.

The matrices $C_{0.8}$ in (4.17) and (4.19) above are plausible and are appealing since they have a theoretical basis as a mixture of proportionate and internal mixing. However, their intuitive appeal does not indicate that they are any better than the *ad hoc* WAIFW matrices in Anderson and May (1991, p. 176–177). The proportionate mixing matrices do have the advantage that they are easily generalized to a situation with more groups corresponding to smaller age intervals. For example, one could use the preferred mixing approach with 32 groups consisting of one year age-interval groups from age 0 to age 19 and five year age-interval groups up to age 80. Deciding on a WAIFW matrix with 32 groups might be difficult. Of course, the possible mixing matrices should be compared methodically with age specific data on many diseases to decide which forms are most appropriate. For hepatitis A in Bulgaria, Greenhalgh and Dietz (1995) have considered the effects on vaccination programs of using a proportionate mixing matrix, an assortative matrix and a symmetric matrix of WAIFW type.

Acknowledgements

HWH thanks the University of Hawaii for providing support services during his sabbatical leave. The age-interval formulas and estimations for the proportionate mixing activities were done jointly with Vladimir Rouderfer of LaTrobe University in Melbourne, Australia.

References

Adler, F.R. (1992) 'The effects of averaging on the basic reproduction ratio', *Math. Biosci.* **111**, 89–98.

Anderson, R.M. (1988) 'The role of mathematical models in the study of HIV transmission and the epidemiology of AIDS', *J. AIDS* **1**, 241–256.

Anderson, R.M. and May, R.M. (1985a) 'Age-related changes in the rate of disease transmission:Implications for the design of vaccination programmes', *J. Hyg. Camb.* **94**, 365–436.

Anderson, R.M. and May, R.M. (1985c) 'Vaccination and herd immunity to infectious disease', *Nature* **318**, 323–29.

Anderson, R.M. and May, R.M. (1991) *Infectious Diseases of Humans: Dynamics and Control*, Oxford University Press, Oxford.

Anderson, R.M., Medley, G.F., May, R.M. and Johnson, A.M. (1986) 'A preliminary study of the transmission dynamics of the human immunodeficiency virus

(HIV), the causative agent of AIDS', *IMA J. Math. Appl. Med. Biol.* **3**, 229–263.

Becker, N.G. and Angulo, J. (1981) 'On estimating the contagiousness of a disease transmitted person to person', *Math. Biosci.* **54**, 137–154.

Becker, N.G. and Marschner, I.C. (1990) 'The effect of heterogeneity on the spread of disease'. In *Stochastic Processes in Epidemic Theory*, J.P. Gabriel, C. Lefevre and P. Picard (eds.), Lecture Notes in Biomathematics **86**, Springer-Verlag, 90–103.

Blythe, S.P. and Castillo-Chavez, C.C. (1989) 'Like with like preference and sexual mixing models', *Math. Biosci.* **96**, 221–238.

Busenberg, S. and Castillo-Chavez, C.C. (1991) 'A general solution of the problem of mixing of subpopulations and its application to risk- and age-structured models for the spread of AIDS', *IMA J. Math. Appl. Med. Biol.* **8**, 1–29.

Castillo-Chavez, C.C. and Blythe, S.P. (1989) 'Mixing framework for social/sexual behavior. In *Mathematical and Statistical Approaches to AIDS Epidemiology*, C.C. Castillo-Chavez (ed.), Lecture Notes in Biomathematics **83**, Springer-Verlag, 275–285.

Castillo-Chavez, C.C. (ed.) (1989) *Mathematical and Statistical Approaches to AIDS Epidemiology*, Lecture Notes in Biomathematics **83**, Springer-Verlag.

Castillo-Chavez, C.C., Cooke, K.L., Huang, W. and Levin, S. A. (1989) 'On the role of long incubation periods in the dynamics of AIDS Part 2: Multiple group models'. In *Mathematical and Statistical Approaches to AIDS Epidemiology*, C.C. Castillo-Chavez (ed.), Lecture Notes in Biomathematics **83**, Springer-Verlag, 200–217.

Diekmann, O., Heesterbeek, J.A.P. and Metz, J.A.J. (1990) 'On the definition and the computation of the basic reproduction ratio R_0 in models for infectious diseases in heterogeneous populations', *J. Math. Biol.* **28**, 365–382.

Dietz, K. (1975) 'Transmission and control of arboviral diseases'. In *Epidemiology*, SIMS Utah Conference Proceedings, SIAM, Philadelphia, PA, 104–149.

Dietz, K. (1981) 'The evaluation of rubella vaccination strategies'. In *The Mathematical Theory of Dynamics of Biological Populations, Vol II*, Academic Press, 81–97.

Edmunds, W.J., Medley, G.F. and Nokes, D.J. (1995) 'The design of immunization programmes against hepatitis B virus in developing countries', this volume.

Grenfell, B.T. and Anderson, R.M. (1985) 'The estimation of age related rates of infection from case notifications and serological data', *J. Hyg.* **95**, 419–36.

Greenhalgh, D. and Dietz, K. (1995) 'The effect of different mixing patterns on vaccination programs', this volume.

Hasibeder, G. and Dye, C. (1988) 'Population dynamics of mosquito-borne disease: Persistence in a completely heterogeneous environment', *Theor. Pop. Biol.* **33**, 31–53.

Hethcote, H.W. (1978) 'An immunization model for a heterogeneous population', *Theor. Pop. Biol.* **14**, 338–349.

Hethcote, H.W. (1983) 'Measles and rubella in the United States', *Am. J. Epidemiol.* **117**, 2–13.

Hethcote, H.W. (1987) 'Optimal ages of vaccination for measles', *Math. Biosci.* **89**, 29–52.

Hethcote, H.W. (1989) 'Three basic epidemiological models'. In *Applied Mathematical Ecology*, L. Gross, T.G. Hallam and S.A. Levin (eds.), Springer-Verlag, 119–144.

Hethcote, H.W. (1994) 'Modeling AIDS prevention programs in a population of homosexual men'. In *Modeling the AIDS Epidemic: Planning, Policy and Prediction*, E.H. Kaplan and M.L. Brandeau (eds.), Raven Press, New York, 91–107.

Hethcote, H.W. and Van Ark, J.W. (1987) 'Epidemiological models for heterogeneous populations: Proportionate mixing, parameter estimation, and immunization programs', *Math. Biosci.* **84**, 85–118.

Hethcote, H.W. and Van Ark, J.W. (1992a) 'Weak linkage between HIV epidemics in homosexual men and intravenous drug users in New York City'. In *AIDS Epidemiology: Methodological Issues*, N.P. Jewell, K. Dietz and V.T. Farewell (eds.), Birkhauser, 174–208.

Hethcote, H.W. and Van Ark, J.W. (1992b) *Modeling HIV Transmission and AIDS in the United States*, Lecture Notes in Biomathematics **95**, Springer-Verlag.

Hethcote, H.W., Van Ark, J.W. and Karon, J.M. (1991b) 'A simulation model of AIDS in San Francisco. II: Simulations, therapy, and sensitivity analysis', *Math. Biosci.* **106**, 223–247.

Hethcote, H.W., Van Ark, J.W. and Longini, I.M. Jr. (1991a) 'A simulation model of AIDS in San Francisco. I: Model formulation and parameter estimation', *Math. Biosci.* **106**, 203–222.

Hethcote, H.W., Yorke, J.A. and Nold, A. (1992) 'Gonorrhea modeling: Comparison of control methods', *Math. Biosci.* **58**, 93–109.

Hethcote, H.W. and Yorke, J.A. (1984) *Gonorrhea Transmission Dynamics and Control*, Lecture Notes in Biomathematics **56**. Springer-Verlag.

Hoppensteadt, F. (1975) *Mathematical Theories of Populations: Demographics, Genetics and Epidemics*, SIAM, Philadelphia, PA.

Hyman, J.M. and Stanley, E.A. (1988) 'Using mathematical models to understand the AIDS epidemic', *Math. Biosci.* **90**, 415–473.

Hyman, J.M. and Stanley, E.A. (1989) 'The effect of social mixing patterns on the spread of AIDS'. In *Mathematical Approaches to Problems in Resource Management and Epidemiology*, C.C. Castillo-Chavez, S. A. Levin and C. Shoemaker (eds.), Lecture Notes in Biomathematics **81**, Springer-Verlag.

Isham, V. (1988) 'Mathematical modeling of the transmission dynamics of HIV infection and AIDS: A review', *J. R. Stat. Soc. A* **151**, 5–31.

Jacquez, J.A., Simon, C.P., Koopman, J., Sattenspiel, L. and Perry, T. (1988) 'Modeling and the analysis of HIV transmission: The effect of contact patterns', *Math. Biosci.* **92**, 119–99.

Jacquez, J.A., Simon, C.P. and Koopman, J. (1989) 'Structured mixing: Heterogeneous mixing by the definition of activity groups'. In *Mathematical and Statistical Approaches to AIDS Epidemiology*, C.C. Castillo-Chavez (ed.), Lecture Notes in Biomathematics **83**, Springer-Verlag, 301–315.

Kaplan, E.H. and Lee, Y.S. (1990) 'How bad can it get? Bounding worst case epidemic heterogeneous mixing models of HIV/AIDS', *Math. Biosci.* **99**, 157–180.

Kaplan, E.H., Cramton, P.C. and Paltiel, A.D. (1989) 'Nonrandom mixing models of HIV transmission. In *Mathematical and Statistical Approaches to AIDS Epidemiology*, C.C. Castillo-Chavez (ed.), Lecture Notes in Biomathematics **83**, 218–239. Springer-Verlag, 218–239.

Koopman, J.A., Simon, C.P., Jacquez, J.A. and Park, T.S. (1989) 'Selective contact within structured mixing with an application to HIV transmission risk from oral and anal sex'. In *Mathematical and Statistical Approaches to AIDS Epidemiology*, C.C. Castillo-Chavez (ed.), Lecture Notes in Biomathematics **83**, Springer-Verlag, 316–348.

Lajmanovich, A. and Yorke, J.A. (1976) 'A deterministic model for gonorrhea in a nonhomogeneous population', *Math. Biosci.* **28**, 221–236.

Lin, X., Hethcote, H.W. and van den Driessche, P. (1993) 'An epidemiological model for HIV/AIDS with proportional recruitment', *Math. Biosci.* **118**, 181–195.

Longini, I.M., Koopman, J.S., Monto, A.S. and Fox, J.P. (1982) 'Estimating household and community transmission parameters for influenza', *Amer. J. Epidemiol.* **115**, 736–751.

Marschner, I.G. (1992) 'The effect of preferrential mixing on the growth of an epidemic', *Math. Biosci.* **109**, 39–67.

May, R.M. and Anderson, R.M. (1984) 'Spatial heterogeneity and the design of immunization programs', *Math. Biosci.* **72**, 233–266.

May, R.M.and Anderson, R.M. (1987) 'Transmission dynamics of HIV infection', *Nature* **326**, 137–142.

Morris, M. (1995) 'Behavior change and non-homogeneous mixing', this volume.

Nold, A. (1980) 'Heterogeneity in disease transmission modeling', *Math. Biosci.* **52**, 227–40.

Rouderfer, V., Hethcote, H.W. and Becker, N.G. (1994) 'Waning immunity and its effects of vaccination schedules', *Math. Biosci.* **124**, 59–82.

Sattenspiel, L. (1987) 'Population structure and the spread of disease', *Human Biol.* **59**, 411–438.

Schwager, S.J., Castillo-Chavez, C.C. and Hethcote, H.W. (1989) 'Statistical and mathematical approaches in HIV/AIDS modeling: A review'. In *Mathematical and Statistical Approaches to AIDS Epidemiology*, C.C. Castillo-Chavez (ed.), Lecture Notes in Biomathematics **83**, Springer-Verlag, 2-35.

Watson, R.K. (1972) 'On an epidemic in a stratified population', *J. Appl. Prob.* **9**, 659–666.

Discussion

HEESTERBEEK The concept that R_0 for the heterogeneous case is not less than the R_0 for the homogeneous fallacy case may not always apply. In a paper with Klaus Dietz and David Tudor (this volume), we found that heterogeneity due to differences in infectivity decreased R_0.

REPLY This example with the opposite effect of heterogeneity on R_0 is interesting. My observation that heterogeneity does not decrease R_0 is based on several papers which study heterogeneous mixing. Thus it appears that heterogeneous mixing does not decrease R_0, but that other forms of heterogeneity may decrease R_0.

KOOPMAN Your suggestion that the same age dependent contact pattern may apply for many childhood diseases such as measles and chickenpox is questionable. We do not know that their spread is similar. Certainly the probability of transmission, which was not included in your models here, is different for these diseases.

REPLY You are correct that we do not know that these diseases are spread in the same way; I was hypothesizing that the underlying mixing pattern is the same for measles, rubella, mumps and chickenpox. This hypothesis would have to be tested by examining data on these diseases. Of course, the probability of transmission per contact would be different for these diseases and would need to be included explicitly as a parameter in the model as in Rouderfer *et. al.* (1994). The models which we used for gonorrhea and HIV/AIDS did explicitly include parameters for the probabilities of transmission per new sexual partner.

DIETZ In your model for socially-defined groups, you obtained formulas for the basic reproduction number R_0 in terms of the average ages of attack. This may be incorrect since socially-defined groups cannot be used as age groups; they do not consider the progression by aging between groups.

REPLY The formula for the basic reproduction number R_0 is given in terms of the average ages A_i of infection in each of the socially defined groups. These average ages of attack are obtained by incorporating an age structure in each of the socially-defined groups. Thus the socially-defined groups are not considered to be age groups.

Behaviour Change and Non-Homogeneous Mixing

Martina Morris

1 Introduction

Mixing patterns in multi-group populations are now recognized to have an important role in the population dynamics of disease (Hethcote and Yorke 1984, Sattenspiel 1987b, Anderson *et al.* 1990). Initially in response to the resurgence of gonorrhea and later with the rapid growth of the AIDS epidemic, selective mixing has become a major focus for epidemiological modelers. Various methods for summarizing the structure of selective mixing have been proposed (Gupta and Anderson 1989, Blythe *et al.* 1991, Koopman *et al.* 1991, Morris 1991). Simulation studies show that these effects can be both strong and variable (Hyman and Stanley 1988, Haraldsdottir *et al.* 1992, Morris 1995), and that they can bias the estimates of other epidemiological parameters if they are not taken into account (Koopman *et al.* 1991). Analytic expressions for the effect of mixing on the reproductive rate (or number) of a disease and the definition of core groups are beginning to be developed (Diekmann *et al.* 1990, Jacquez *et al.* 1993).

One of the major issues in modeling the mixing patterns of a multi-group population concerns the solution of multiple matching constraints in non-equilibrium populations. Constraints are imposed by the symmetry inherent in contact processes, i.e., if I meet you, then you have to meet me. This is a generalized version of the 'two-sex problem' familiar to demographers. In its classical form this problem arises in life table modeling when births are projected on the basis of two-sex populations. The birth process implies a matching process between the age-structured populations of males and females, and these constraints become complicated when vital dynamics are considered (Pollard 1948, Schoen 1982). In the context of disease transmission, the 'two-sex' problem arises in modeling mixing patterns when the subgroup sizes, contact rates, or selection patterns change over time. The multiple matching constraints that must be satisfied in each case require explicit modeling.

The three sources of change – size, activity and selection – often arise in different contexts but they also interact. Subgroup sizes typically change in response to vital dynamics, e.g., differential birth and death rates, and differential disease-induced mortality. The former is responsible for the so-called 'marriage squeeze' generated by the baby-boom, disrupting the typical pattern of age-matching in marriage (grooms slightly older than brides) as early baby-boom women faced a relative scarcity of older men, and late baby-boom men faced a similar scarcity of younger women (Schoen 1985). Differential disease-induced mortality can raise similar issues. In the case of AIDS, for example, deaths due to disease may change the population age structure (Anderson *et al.* 1988), or the size of risk groups such as gay men or IDUs. This requires some change in the contact patterns of their partners. Changes in contact rates may also arise independently as the result of social and psychological dynamics. The most recent example is the dramatic reduction in unsafe sex reported by gay men since the identification of HIV (Centers for Disease Control 1985, Martin 1987, Becker and Joseph 1988, Winkelstein *et al.* 1988). But similar effects arise in other diseases when disease or quarantine removes an infectious person from general circulation. As with the change in subgroup size, the result is that a group becomes more or less available to its usual partners. The underlying dynamics, however, are different, and this must be recognized in the model. Finally, selection patterns may change independently, apart from (or in addition to) changes in either subgroup size or activity level. This, too, is a social-psychological dynamic. There is anecdotal evidence, for example, that men are choosing substantially younger women as sex partners in some countries in Africa in an attempt to avoid contact with the assumed higher HIV-prevalence among their female peers (Wawer *et al.* 1992).

In the AIDS epidemic, all of these factors are likely to be changing in ways that will have important consequences for the eventual prevalence of the disease, and for the development of effective control strategies. The challenge for epidemiology is that the data necessary to identify and model these changes will almost never be available. Longitudinal network data on patterns of sexual partnering would be needed, and at this point even cross-sectional network data are rare. Network data are difficult, time consuming and expensive to collect. When the topic involves sexual behavior, network methods are also intrusive to the respondent and politically sensitive, so that both funding and permission to collect the data may be hard to obtain (cf. Laumann *et al.* 1992). These obstacles are sufficiently large that appropriate data may never be available in most settings. Methods for estimating the effects of these changes on mixing patterns, and for merging information from multiple sources, may thus be the only realistic option.

The discussion that follows generalizes the modeling framework presented in Morris (1991). Data on sexual partnerships are summarized in a 'contact' or 'mixing' matrix, where the rows and columns represent the subjects' and partners' attributes (e.g., age, gender, sexual preference, marital status, race, etc.), and the cell counts represent pairs of individuals. The object of the mixing model is to predict these counts. If we let $x_{ij}(t)$ denote the observed cell counts at time t, and $m_{ij}(t)$ denote the predicted counts, then the model specifies that

$$m_{ij}(t) = K_{ij}(t)\alpha_{ij}(t) \tag{1.1}$$

where

$$K_{ij}(t) = \frac{N_i(t)N_j(t)}{N(t)}$$

is a term that depends only on the numbers in each subgroup, $N_{(\cdot)}(t)$, and $\alpha_{ij}(t)$ represents the contact and selection preferences of groups i and j. By separating the effects of population size and preferences, this model enables each to vary independently. The resulting contact *rates* (as distinct from *preferences*) will change in response to either or both of the underlying factors. The general loglinear model for $m_{ij}(t)$ can be written as

$$\log(m_{ij}(t)) = \log(K_{ij}(t)) + u(t) + u_{1(i)}(t) + u_{2(j)}(t) + \sum_{s=1}^{S} u_{s(ij)}(t) \tag{1.2}$$

The $K_{ij}(t)$ term is fitted as an offset in the model (Numerical Algorithms Group 1985, Aitkin *et al.* 1989). The remaining u-terms are the loglinear decomposition of the preference term α_{ij}: u is the expected value for the reference category, $u_{1(i)}$ is the marginal effect for row i (and $u_{z(j)}$ for column j) and $u_{s(ij)}$ are the effects of selection factor s on the ijth cell. The marginal effects represent the group-specific contact rate preferences (relative to the reference category u). The selection effects represent the attribute-related preferences. These terms can be interpreted either as odds-ratios, or as simple multiplicative increments (decrements) to the probability of a pair. The general approach taken below is to use data, where possible, to estimate the time-dependent parameters, and to treat the remaining parameters as constant.

For modeling disease transmission, the loglinear parameters can be substituted into the infection rate term, βSI, of a compartmental model (actually $\beta_{ij}S_iI_j$ in the multi-group model) to represent the heterogeneous mixing process. Letting c_i denote the contacts per unit time for group i, π_{ij} denote the probability that this contact is with a member of group j and τ_{ij} denote the per-partnership force of infection from i to j, then

$$
\begin{aligned}
\beta_{ij}(t) &= \frac{c_i\pi_{ij}(t)\tau_{ij}}{N_j} \\
&= \frac{m_{ij}(t)\tau_{ij}}{N_j N_i} \\
&= \frac{\alpha_{ij}(t)\tau_{ij}}{N}
\end{aligned}
\tag{1.3}
$$

2   Modeling changes in sub-population sizes

Methods for dealing with changes in the population profile have been the focus of earlier papers (Blower and McLean 1991, Morris 1991). Such methods may be used in several contexts. One is to update a mixing matrix when changes in subgroup size are known e.g., the change in the population age structure resulting from the baby boom. Data on changes in the population profile are likely to be available, as documenting such changes requires only survey or census estimates of subgroup frequency. Another context in which these methods may be used is to merge data from different sources, e.g., when full network data have been collected from a non-representative sample and the true population profile is known from another sources. Finally, these methods may be used during simulation, to update selection patterns at each step with the current population profile when there is differential disease-induced mortality among the subgroups.

Using the loglinear modeling framework described above, such changes only affect the offset term $K_{ij}(t)$ in equation (1.2). In the absence of corresponding data on change in contact or selection preferences, these may be hypothesized to remain constant. The number of contacts between members of group i and members of group j then varies over time according to the model

$$\log(m_{ij}(t)) = \log(K_{ij}(t)) + \alpha_{ij} \tag{2.1}$$

$$\alpha_{ij} = u + u_{1(i)} + u_{2(j)} + \sum_{s=1}^{S} u_{s(ij)}.$$

As $K_{ij}(t)$ changes, the marginal contact rates will, in general, not be preserved. The model simply specifies that the preferred contact rates for each group do not change. An application of this model will be examined below in conjunction with changing activity preferences.

3   Modeling changes in contact rates

It is not uncommon for simple behavioral data, such as contact rates, to be collected over time. Network data, however, are often collected only at one time point, if at all. When there have been significant changes in contact rates over time, simulating disease transmission will require that the mixing matrix be adjusted. Changes in contact rates present a slightly different modeling problem than changes in group size. With both the subgroup sizes and contact rates known, the margins of the matrix are fixed at each time point. In contrast to the case described above, adjustments to the matrix must now preserve the known marginal totals.

In the absence of data on whether selection patterns are changing in response to the marginal changes, a natural hypothesis is that they remain constant. Changes in contact rates thus index the reference category and marginal effects in equation (1.2) by time, but leave the selection effects constant:

$$\log(m_{ij}(t)) = \log(K_{ij}(t)) + \alpha_{ij}(t) \qquad (3.1)$$

$$\alpha_{ij}(t) = u(t) + u_{1(i)}(t) + u_{2(j)}(t) + \sum_{s=1}^{S} u_{s(ij)}.$$

If contact rates are increasing or decreasing at a constant rate, time can be modeled as a continuous variate, adding a single interaction parameter to the prediction equation for each of the marginal effects. If the trends are not as regular, time may be treated as a discrete variable to represent the observed pattern. In the log-linear context, constant selection preferences are equivalent to assuming that the internal odds-ratios of the matrix do not change.

The effects of changing contact rates are captured in the marginal parameters $u_{1(i)}(t)$ and $u_{2(j)}(t)$ above. If these parameters could be expressed as simple functions of the observed marginal totals, as they can be in standard linear models, the adjustment of the α_{ij} would be a straightforward matter of updating the parameters by substituting the new margins for the old ones. In generalized linear models, however, the marginal parameters are instead multiplicative functions of the fitted m_{ij}, so this approach is not possible.

It is relatively simple to derive the maximum likelihood estimates (MLEs) for the $m_{ij}(t)$, however, and use these to construct the parameter estimates. For a table with known marginal totals and interaction structure (here the observed odds-ratios), the MLEs can be computed using iterative proportional scaling (IPS). This method is also known as the Deming-Stephan algorithm, standardization or 'raking' the cross-tabulated data.

The IPS algorithm updates the cell counts by sequentially multiplying the rows and columns by the ratio of the desired contact rates and the current rates for each group. Letting $m_{ij}^{(k)}$ represent the kth iteration, and $c_{\cdot}^{(*)}$ represent the final desired contact rate,

$$m_{ij}^{(1)} = m_{ij}^{(0)} \frac{c_i^{(*)}}{c_i^{(0)}}$$

$$m_{ij}^{(2)} = m_{ij}^{(1)} \frac{c_j^{(*)}}{c_j^{(1)}}$$

$$m_{ij}^{(3)} = m_{ij}^{(2)} \frac{c_i^{(*)}}{c_i^{(2)}}$$

The first iteration conforms the row margins to the desired contact rate. This will generally change the contact rates for the column margins, so the second iteration conforms the column margins to the desired rate, changing the marginal contact rates for the rows, and the iteration process continues.

It is known that this algorithm always converges (Haberman 1974), and that the resulting estimates are the MLEs of the fitted values under the hypothesis of no change in the interaction structure (Birch 1965). That IPS preserves the interaction structure within the matrix is clear, as the odds-ratios which represent this structure in the loglinear model are unaffected when rows or columns of a matrix are multiplied by an arbitrary constant. The parameters from equation (3.1) can be recovered by fitting the model to the IPS-adjusted matrix.

3.1 Example

In this section we will apply both of the methods above to adjust a matrix of age-matching in sexual partnerships among gay men. The adjustment will compensate for both the decline in the age-group specific prevalence of unsafe sex (a change in group size) and for the reduction in the number of partners among those who continue to report engaging in unsafe sex (a change in contact rates).

The analysis is based on data from the Longitudinal AIDS Impact Project (LAIP), a panel study of gay men in New York City. The study began in 1985 and seven waves of interviews have now been completed. Using structured face-to-face interviews this project has collected a wide range of information on the social and sexual network characteristics of respondents, as well as their serostatus. The original sample of 746 men was selected using a combination of stratified probability sampling, targeted sampling, and snowball sampling. The sample was augmented for the last two waves by a cohort of younger men (18–23 years old) in order to compensate for the age-bias introduced by the panel design. For further information on the sample and data from this project see (Martin and Dean 1990).

For the last two waves of the survey, respondents who reported any anal intercourse without the use of a condom have been asked to report the ages of the men with whom they had anal sex. Insertive and receptive sex were reported separately, and the ages of up to eight partners were recorded. The reported ages were fairly well distributed, with only a small tendency to round to multiples of five. The original age-matching matrix is given in Table 1.

In the prior years of the survey, age-matching information was not collected. Respondents were asked, however, whether they engaged in unsafe anal sex, how frequently, how often they used condoms, and how many partners (new and repeat) they had in that year. Substantial changes in behavior occurred during this time. Two prior time points will be examined here: pre-AIDS and 1985, the first year of the survey. The data on pre-AIDS behavior

Age of insertive partner:	Age of receptive partner:				Total pairs	N	Contact rate
	17-24	25-34	35-44	45-54			
17-24	6	8	2	1	16	15	1.04
25-34	9	38	18	6	72	75	0.95
35-44	3	21	25	7	56	61	0.91
45-54	1	7	7	5	19	18	1.08
Total pairs	19	73	52	19	162		
N	15	75	61	18		169	
Contact rate	1.25	0.97	0.85	1.03			0.96

Table 1. Age-matching matrix for 1990–1991 LAIP data. These data represent an average of the patterns of selection observed in the last two years of the survey, corrected for sampling bias and the tendency for reports of insertive anal sex to be higher than receptive reports.

Behavior	Age Group	Pre-AIDS		1985		1991	
		Ins	Rec	Ins	Rec	Ins	Rec
% reporting unsafe anal sex[1]	18-24	81.3	78.6	81.6	65.0	36.3	29.6
	25-34	91.9	83.6	63.2	59.7	24.4	16.7
	35-44	87.8	77.5	55.6	45.5	21.8	14.9
	45-54	72.6	59.7	53.8	43.8	18.1	14.8
new partners/yr[2]	18-24	9.0 (6)	11.0 (6)	4.5 (3)	3.9 (3)	1.2 (1)	1.1 (1)
	25-34	11.2 (5)	10.5 (5)	4.3 (5)	3.9 (3)	1.1 (1)	1.3 (1)
	35-44	16.5 (7)	15.3 (6)	4.9 (3)	4.0 (3)	1.0 (1)	0.7 (1)
	45-54	9.9 (5)	11.6 (5)	3.8 (3)	4.8 (3)	1.2 (1)	0.9 (1)

[1] Excludes persons in mutually monogamous relationships in 1991
[2] 5% trimmed mean (median), unsafe partners only

Table 2. Changes in risk behavior over time in the LAIP survey.

patterns were collected as retrospective reports in 1985 with questions prefaced by 'In the year before you heard about HIV/AIDS, did you...'. Almost all of the respondents reported hearing about AIDS by 1981. The prevalence of unsafe anal intercourse and the number of new partners reported at each time point is presented in Table 2.

As in every major survey of sexual behavior of gay men in the US, the prevalence of reported unsafe sex in this sample has declined dramatically from the pre-AIDS period. The decline was not, however, the same for each age group: among the three oldest age-groups 15–20% report no unsafe sex in 1991, compared to nearly 40% among the youngest age group. Strong declines can also be observed in the number of new partners among those reporting unsafe sex. Here the 5% trimmed mean number of new partners was over 10 per year in the pre-AIDS era, and has dropped to just under 1 new partner per year in 1991. The reduction is roughly the same for each age group.

One of the primary questions one would like to examine using these data is whether the observed changes in behavior have been sufficient to bring the epidemic below the reproductive threshold. Given the observed heterogeneity in both contact rates and mixing patterns, it is also important to understand what effect these will have on the future of the epidemic.

Simulation is the only way to investigate this question. If all of the necessary parameters were confidently known (including the age-specific HIV prevalence and the distribution of infectivity during the latency period) it would be possible to simulate the path simply from 1991. These parameters are not well known, however, so it is important to assess the adequacy of the model by using it to simulate the initial years of the epidemic and compare the results against some known statistics, such as surveillance data on AIDS incidence among gay men. This means that the 1990–91 mixing matrix in Table 1 will have to be adjusted for changes in the size of the exposed population and contact rates over this period.

These adjustments to the mixing matrix involve both of the methods described above. The original 1991 matrix must first be adjusted for the changes in group size using the $K_{ij}(t)/K_{ij}(91)$ ratio. It must then be further adjusted using IPS to match the changing contact rates. The order of adjustment matters, as the group-size adjustment does not preserve the observed contact rates and must therefore be performed first.

The adjusted matrices for 1985 and the pre-AIDS period are presented in the four tables of Table 3. The first adjustment changes the size of each group (the column labeled 'N'). The second adjustment conforms the marginal contact rates to those observed in each year using IPS. Convergence was obtained after five iterations. Discreteness in the number of persons generates small differences between the final contact rates and the rates observed in the original data.

The loglinear summary parameters for the final matrices are presented in Table 4. The declines in activity were not regular enough that time could be modeled as a continuous variable, so the time effect was modeled instead as a discrete factor. The selection preferences were summarized in a differential assortative bias factor and a diagonal quadrant block. The models were fitted using the statistical package GLIM, the first level of each factor is taken as the reference category and takes the parameter value 1. For the row and column estimates, this is the 18–24 year olds, for the homophily terms it is the off-diagonal cells, and for the block term it is the off-diagonal 4-cell block for each quadrant of the submatrix.

The model above fits the data almost too well, with a residual deviance of 2.45 on 22 degrees of freedom. A simple model of proportional mixing that

Year:

Pre-AIDS (~1980)

1985

STEP 1: Group size adjustment for changes in prevalence of unsafe sex. xii(91) * Kii(t)/Kii(91)

Pre-AIDS (~1980)

Insertive: Partner	Receptive Partner:				Total pairs	N	Contact rate
	17-24	25-34	35-44	45-54			
17-24	6	17	4	1	28	32	0.88
25-34	21	181	87	28	316	339	0.93
35-44	6	98	117	34	255	273	0.93
45-54	2	31	34	23	90	81	1.11
Total pairs	35	327	241	86	689		
N	32	339	273	81		725	
Contact rate	1.10	0.96	0.88	1.06			0.95

1985

Insertive: Partner	Receptive Partner:				Total pairs	N	Contact rate
	17-24	25-34	35-44	45-54			
17-24	8	17	3	2	29	31	0.94
25-34	21	135	59	22	237	250	0.95
35-44	6	66	71	24	168	182	0.92
45-54	2	25	24	20	71	64	1.11
Total pairs	36	243	158	68	505		
N	31	250	182	64		527	
Contact rate	1.17	0.97	0.87	1.06			0.96

STEP 2: IPS adjustment for changing contact rates

Pre-AIDS (~1980)

Insertive Partner	Receptive Partner:				Total pairs	N	Contact rate
	17-24	25-34	35-44	45-54			
17-24	55	161	51	14	281	32	8.80
25-34	207	1875	1360	292	3734	339	11.01
35-44	85	1374	2472	482	4414	273	16.17
45-54	12	229	371	171	783	81	9.67
Total pairs	359	3638	4254	960	9212		
N	32	339	273	81		725	
Contact rate	11.23	10.73	15.58	11.85			12.71

1985

Insertive Partner	Receptive Partner:				Total pairs	N	Contact rate
	17-24	25-34	35-44	45-54			
17-24	30	77	17	8	132	31	4.27
25-34	72	572	280	109	1033	250	4.13
35-44	22	311	378	134	844	182	4.64
45-54	5	76	84	70	235	64	3.67
Total pairs	128	1036	759	322	2245		
N	31	250	182	64		527	
Contact rate	4.13	4.15	4.17	5.03			4.26

Table 3. Constructed age-matching matrices for pre-AIDS and 1985 based on observed matrix for 1990–1991 (in Table 1). Adjustments are made to compensate for changes in group size (step 1) and contact rates (step 2).

Effects:		Exponentiated Parameter for:		
		t=81	t=85	t=91
Main:				
*Reference cat.*u(t):	(t)	6.33*	2.73*	0.85*
Rows $u_{1(i)}(t)$:	insertive 2(t)	2.22	1.82	1.59
	3(t)	2.17	1.47	1.20
	4(t)	1.21	1.03	1.38
Columns $u_{2(j)}(t)$:	receptive 2(t)	1.65	1.88	1.41
	3(t)	1.58	1.35	0.91
	4(t)	1.15	1.51	1.06
Selection $u_{s(ij)}$:		Constant Exponentiated Parameter:		
assortative	1	6.15*		
	2	0.51*		
	3	1.11*		
	4	2.13*		
block	diagonal quadrant	2.08*		

* p < 0.05

Table 4. Loglinear summary parameters for the original 1991, and adjusted 1985 and pre-AIDS matrices.

preserved the time-specific margins would use only 5 fewer parameters (the selection effects at the bottom of the table). The only parameters to reach standard levels of statistical significance are the reference category, which indexes the general decline in contact preferences for each year, and the selection effects. The group-specific differences in contact preferences over time are uniformly insignificant. A more parsimonious model is thus suggested, dropping the preference differentials. This model, however, provides an unacceptable fit (residual deviance of 92.54 on 34 degrees of freedom). An acceptable model will thus need to index at least some of the group-specific differentials. Given the amount of pre-analysis data manipulation, and the small numbers of observations in 1991, significance levels are best treated as a rough guide here. The apparent 'overfitting' of the model in Table 2 may not be a real problem.

Initial simulations using the parameter estimates from Table 2 (calibrated against AIDS surveillance data in New York City for the risk group 'men who have sex with men') suggests that the current patterns of behavior are just on the boundary of reducing the epidemic spread below the reproductive threshold. If these data on behavior are accurate, and the patterns are maintained in the future, then the disease would eventually die out in the absence of other sources of infection (e.g., links with IVDUs). If, on the other hand,

1990

Insertive Partner:	Receptive Partner:				Total pairs	N	Contact rate
	17-24	25-34	35-44	45-54			
17-24	8	7	2	0	18	15	1.19
25-34	6	46	21	3	76	75	1.01
35-44	2	29	24	6	61	61	1.00
45-54	1	9	10	4	25	18	1.38
Total pairs	18	91	57	13	179		
N	15	75	61	18		169	
Contact rate	1.17	1.21	0.94	0.75			1.06

1991

Insertive Partner:	Receptive Partner:				Total pairs	N	Contact rate
	17-24	25-34	35-44	45-54			
17-24	3	13	1	0	17	15	1.16
25-34	9	50	13	7	80	75	1.06
35-44	4	28	25	5	62	61	1.01
45-54	1	10	7	4	22	18	1.20
Total pairs	16	102	46	16	180		
N	15	75	61	18		169	
Contact rate	1.10	1.35	0.75	0.91			1.07

Table 5. 1990 and 1991 mixing matrices from LAIP

respondents have under-reported the number of new partners they have, the result could be quite different. Assuming two new partners per year (instead of the one reported), the disease would instead become endemic, with sero-prevalence levels of about 50% among the exposed population in the oldest group, and about 25% among the youngest (Morris and Dean 1994).

4   Modeling changes in selection preferences

When longitudinal network data are available, loglinear models can be used to examine whether the selection patterns have changed in ways not attributable to changes in group sizes or contact rates. The selection preference parameters in the model can now be indexed by time (equation (1.2)), and various hypotheses may be tested. Again, if the trends over time are monotonically increasing or decreasing, e.g., a rise or fall in the strength of the assortative bias, the time index can be modeled as a continuous variate, with corresponding gains in parsimony.

The LAIP survey has two years of age-matching data, collected in 1990 and 1991. The mixing matrix in Table 1 represented an average of these two years, but they can also be treated as distinct. The two matrices are presented in Table 5. The numbers are small, and a one-year difference in time may be expected to yield little difference in selection effects, but the data do provide an opportunity to test this hypothesis. Neither group sizes nor relative contact rates have changed much between the two years, so a simple model to examine here would be time-dependent uniform assortative bias, indexing only the reference category and a single parameter for assortative mixing by time:

$$\log(m_{ij}(t)) = \log(K_{ij}) + u(t) + u_{1(i)} + u_{2(j)} + u_{(ij)}(t) \qquad t = 1, 2$$

where

$$u_{(ij)}(t) = \begin{cases} \delta & \text{if } i = j \\ 0 & i \neq j. \end{cases}$$

The hypothesis of interest is whether $u_{(ij)}(2)$ is significant, and here it is not. The residual deviance for the model of constant selection effects is 20.38 on 24 degrees of freedom. The reduction in deviance gained by adding the additional parameter for changing selection is a remarkably small 0.27.

Conclusion

Loglinear methods provide a general class of models that are flexible enough to solve many of the important problems in heterogeneous mixing. The multiple matching constraints posed by a non-equilibrium population, whether the changes are due to variation in group sizes, contact rates or selection patterns, can be handled effectively with these methods. The summary parameters are interpretable and easily integrated into the compartmental modeling framework, and the procedures for hypothesis testing make the search for parsimonious models a relatively simple task.

References

Centers for Disease Control (1985) 'Self-Reported Behavioral Change Among Gay and Bisexual Men – San Francisco', *MMWR* **34**, 613–615.

Aitkin, M., Anderson, D., Francis, B. and Hind, B. (1989) *Statistical Modelling in GLIM*, Oxford University Press, Oxford.

Anderson, R.M., Gupta, S. and Ng, W. (1990 'The significance of sexual partner contact networks for the transmission dynamics of HIV', *JAIDS* **3**, 417–429.

Anderson, R.M., May, R.M. and Mclean, A.R. (1988) 'Possible demographic consequences of AIDS in developing countries', *Nature* **332**, 228–234.

Becker, M. and Joseph, J. (1988) 'AIDS and behavioral change to reduce risk: a review', *AJPH* **78**, 394–410.

Birch, M.W. (1965) 'The detection of partial association, II: The general case', *JRSSB* **27**, 111–124.

Blower, S.M. and McLean, A.R. (1991) 'Mixing ecology and epidemiology', *Proc. Roy. Soc.* **245**, 187–192.

Blythe, S., Castillo-Chavez, C., Palmer, J. and Cheng, M. (1991) 'Towards a unified theory of mixing and pair formation', *Math. Biosci.* **107**, 349–407.

Diekmann, O., Hesterbeek, H. and Metz, J.A.J. (1990) 'On the definition and the computation of the basic reproduction ratio R_0 in models for infectious diseases in heterogeneous populations', *J. Math. Biol.* **28**, 365–382.

Gupta, S. and Anderson, R. (1989) 'Networks of sexual contacts: implications for the pattern of spread of HIV', *AIDS* **3**, 807–817.

Haberman, S.J. (1974) *The Analysis of Frequency Data*, University of Chicago Press, Chicago.

Haraldsdottir, S., Gupta, S. and Anderson, R. (1992) 'Preliminary studies of sexual networks in a male homosexual community in Iceland', *JAIDS* **5**, 374–381.

Hethcote, H. and Yorke, J.A. (1984) *Gonorrhea Transmission Dynamics and Control*, Springer Verlag, Berlin.

Hyman, J. and Stanley, E. (1988) 'Using mathematical models to understand the AIDS epidemic', *Math. Biosci.* **90**, 415–473.

Jacquez, J., Simon, C. and Koopman, J. (1995) 'Core groups and the R_0s for subgroups in heterogeneous SIS and SI models'. In *Epidemic Models: their Structure and Relation to Data*, D. Mollison (ed.). Cambridge University Press, Cambridge, 279–301.

Koopman, J., Longini, I., Jacquez, J., Simon, C., Ostrow, D., Martin, B. and Woodcock, D. (1991) 'Assessing risk factors for transmission', *Am. J. Epidemiol.* **133**, 1199–1209.

Laumann, E.O., Gagnon, J.H. and Michael, R.T. (1992) 'A political history of the national sex survey of adults'. Paper presented at the Annual Meetings of the American Sociological Association, August 1992.

Martin, J.L. (1987) 'The impact of AIDS on gay male sexual behavior patterns in NYC', *AJPH* **77**, 578–581.

Martin, J.L. and Dean, L. (1990) 'Development of a community sample of gay men for an epidemiologic study of AIDS', *Am. Beh. Sci.* **33**, 546–561.

Morris, M. (1991) 'A log-linear modeling framework for selective mixing', *Math. Biosci.* **107**, 349–377.

Morris, M. (1995) 'Data driven network models for the spread of infectious disease'. In *Epidemic Models: their Structure and Relation to Data*, D. Mollison (ed.), Cambridge University Press, Cambridge, 302–322.

Morris, M. and Dean, L. (1995) 'The effects of sexual behavior change on long-term HIV seroprevalence among homosexual men', *Am. J. Epidemiol.* **140**, 217–32.

Numerical Algorithms Group (1985) *Glim 3.77 Reference Manual*, Oxford University Press, Oxford.

Pollard, A. H. (1948) 'The measurement of reproductivity', *J. Inst. Act.* **74**, 288–305.

Sattenspiel, L. (1987b) 'Population structure and the spread of disease', *Hum. Biol.* **59**, 411–438.

Schoen, R. (1982) 'Generalizing the life table model to incorporate interactions between the sexes'. In *Multidimensional Mathematical Demography*, K.C. Land and A. Rogers (eds.), Academic Press, 385–443.

Schoen, R. (1985) 'The impact of the marriage squeeze in five western countries', *Soc. and Soc. Res.* **70**, 8–19.

Winkelstein, W., Wiley, J., Padian, N., Samuel, M., Shiboski, S., Ascher, M. and Levy, J. (1988) 'The San Francisco men's health study: continued decline in HIV seroconversion rates among homosexual/bisexual men. *Am. J. Pub. Health* **78**, 1472–1474.

Sources and Use of Empirical Observations to Characterise Networks of Sexual Behaviour

Anne M. Johnson

1 Introduction

Models of the transmission dynamics of sexually acquired infections have recently turned greater attention to the importance of sexual mixing patterns and sexual networks in the spread of such diseases (Hethcote and Yorke 1984, Ramstedt *et al.* 1992, Haraldsdottir *et al.* 1992). Apart from the theoretical problems of constructing models which can adequately characterise the complexity of human sexual partnership formation, there remain practical problems in obtaining sufficiently robust empirical data to measure parameters of interest for use by modellers. This paper addresses some aspects of empirical measurement and discusses the validity of some basic parameter estimates commonly used in models of sexually transmitted disease (STD) transmission, particularly where they are used to demonstrate quantitative rather than qualitative considerations.

Key parameters of interest in deterministic models include the population 'rate of partner change' and its variance, the probability of transmission per sexual partnership (or per act of intercourse) and the duration of infectiousness of the organism under consideration (Hethcote and Yorke 1984, Anderson and May 1988).

Recent studies of sexual behaviour (Johnson *et al.* 1992, ACSF investigators 1992, Catania *et al.* 1992, MMWR 1988) have emphasised the marked heterogeneity in sexual behaviour in human communities as measured by numbers of sexual partners in different time intervals. These distributions suggest that models need to take account not only of simple population means, but also to consider stratification of the population into high- and low-activity classes (Hethcote and Yorke 1984). This can, in part, be achieved by considering the demographic correlates of variability in sexual behaviour. These include, for example, varying effects in different cultures of age cohort, life-course, gender, marital and socio-economic status (Johnson *et al.* 1992).

For the purposes of studying sexual mixing, it becomes equally important to answer the question 'who mixes with whom' and to identify the behavioural characteristics of partnerships within a population as well as of individuals in cross-sectional surveys. Relevant characteristics of current partnerships include patterns of age and gender mixing; comparative experience of each member of the partnership (assortative or disassortative mixing); the prevalence of other risk behaviours relevant to the transmission of the organism under study (e.g. homosexuality and injecting drug use in the transmission of HIV); and the characterisation of specific behaviours, e.g. unprotected vaginal intercourse, condom use and anal intercourse, which may influence transmission probabilities.

2   Sampling methods for parameter measurement

Possible sampling frames for parameter measurement include general population samples; samples of patients with defined STDs; individuals with high risk behaviours; and sampling of so-called 'core groups'. The last are those who contribute disproportionately to the spread of STDs in a population and typically might include populations such as prostitutes and their clients. General population samples which can be demonstrated to be representative (e.g. through response rate and demographic characteristics) have the advantage that they are able to define the overall behavioural characteristics of the population. They may be inefficient in terms of sampling for purposes of 'core-group' studies because they include very large numbers of people who are primarily monogamous and who are at low risk of STD acquisition. All the remaining strategies, although arguably increasing sampling efficiency, are in general limited by their lack of representativeness either because they recruit volunteer samples or because they depend on patient attendance at particular health service outlets. Methodological approaches to measurement within defined population groups include surveys of individual behaviour, the use of self-reports of partners' behaviours and demographic attributes and the use of contact tracing, using reports from both members of a partnership. The advantages and pitfalls of these methods are discussed in greater detail below drawing examples from specific studies.

Sampling strategies for general population studies include quota sampling using age, sex and social classes quotas to construct a 'representative' sample; and random sampling frames using electoral, other population registers, household or telephone numbers. Attempts to improve sampling efficiency by selecting those with more active sexual lifestyles have been attempted. Researchers in France used filter questions to systematically over-sample those with a high activity lifestyle (ACSF investigators 1992). These methods are, however, highly dependent on the sensitivity of filter questions in selecting those at highest risk. Work from the British survey indicates that there may be rather different rates of reporting higher risk lifestyles through self-completion rather than face-to-face interviews and that repeated questioning may lead to greater disclosure (Johnson *et al.* 1994).

In estimating parameters relevant to models, careful account must be taken of sample size, sampling error, response rate, potential response bias and that appropriate weighting strategies are used in relation to the sampling method.

3 Some problems of measurement

As with all aspects of self-reported behavioural data, researchers face problems of memory error, veracity and comprehensibility of question format. All require considerable attention in the design phase and assessment of data validity in analysis (Wellings *et al.* 1990). Such problems are not trivial and much remains to be learnt of the optimal methods for collection of relevant data. Measurement instruments need to pay careful attention to definitions, question format, comprehensibility and comparability between populations. Interviewers require training and standardisation of interview techniques, while respondents may be influenced by the situation, by the problems of recall bias and by the potential problems of veracity in reporting a sensitive subject (Wadsworth and Johnson 1991).

Most mathematical models require at a minimum some measure of the distribution of numbers of reported partners in a given time interval in a population. The definition of such an apparently simple concept may lead to quite wide variability in parameter estimates dependent on the exact definition used. For example, in the British National Survey of Sexual Attitudes and Lifestyles (Johnson *et al.* 1994), for the purposes of analysis a heterosexual partner is defined as someone of the opposite sex with whom the respondent has had vaginal or anal intercourse or oro-genital contact. This can be contrasted with the definition of a partner used in Project SIGMA, a volunteer sample of gay men, in which a sexual partner is defined as follows: 'A sexual partner is any person with whom you had sexual contact where the aim was orgasm for one or both of you' (Hunt *et al.* 1991). Project SIGMA distinguishes a *penetrative* sexual partner as someone with whom the respondent has had anal or vaginal intercourse. Using these different definitions, very diverse results are obtained for the median and mean of the distribution of numbers of partners in different time intervals. For example, Project SIGMA measured a mean of 279 lifetime sexual partners in a sample of homosexual and bisexual men (with a median of 38) while in striking contrast, the mean lifetime numbers of *penetrative* sexual partners was 79, with a median of only 7. Similar differences occurred for shorter time intervals, demonstrating that unless precise definitions are used for parameter estimates relevant to the transmission dynamics of the organism under question, quite erroneous measures of the case reproduction rate may arise.

A common parameter used in mathematical models is the rate of sexual partner change per unit time. This remains, however, a largely theoretical construct. In many instances it is derived, arguably incorrectly, from sexual behaviour survey data by calculating the rate of partner change by subtraction using the numbers of partners reported over a series of well-defined time intervals. This method reflects a process of disacquisition rather than acquisition of partners, and as pointed out by Blower *et al.* (1990), does not measure the true rate of partner change. Empirical epidemiological studies of STDs in general demonstrate the relationship between increasing number of partners in a defined time interval and the probability of infection, rather than the 'rate of change' although the latter is generally used in models (Winkelstein *et al.* 1987). The practical implication of using partner acquisition per unit time in modelling exercises is that different partnership patterns can result in similar 'rates of partner change' (Figure 1). Three different cases are presented, indicating that individuals with relatively large number of partners over a given time interval may have low rates of partner change if some or all of these partnerships are concurrent. Similarly, where a process of subtraction is used to measure the 'rate of partner change', an erroneous value may arise for the true rate of partner change (Figure 2). In the situation described in Figure 2, the rate of partner change by subtraction gives a figure higher than that for the true rate of new partner acquisition. The 'effective' rate of partner change may be higher than in a situation of serial monogamy when an individual with a series of concurrent relationships experiences a new partnership with an individual who introduces an STD to the index case. Each of the concurrent partners would effectively become a new partner with respect to potential STD transmission. Thus, the 'effective rate of partner change' in situations of concurrent partnerships is higher than the simple rate of new partner acquisition.

However, there are considerable difficulties in collecting detailed time-related data relevant to studying partnership networks. Surveys have attempted to collect such data. The National Survey of Sexual Attitudes and Lifestyle, for example, collected detailed information on the last three partners in the last five years including the time of commencement and ending of the relationship, the age of the partner and the type of partnership. This question was the one with the highest rate of non-completion, largely due to the difficulties individuals encountered in remembering precise dates and details, a problem which was more common amongst those with large numbers of partners (Johnson *et al.* 1993, Chapter 5). Knox *et al.* (1993) used a similar approach to collect details of the last 10 partners and again reported high rates of non-completion. Error rates are thus liable to be the greatest amongst those with the most sexually varied lifestyles and those who are of the greatest interest for the purposes of network studies.

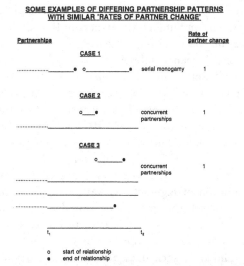

Figure 1. Some examples of differing partnership patterns with similar 'rates of partner change'.

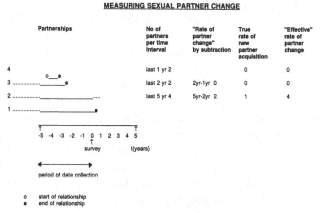

Figure 2. Measuring sexual partner change.

4 Data from surveys

Cross-sectional surveys provide only limited data about sexual networks, although they allow assessment of the variability in sexual behaviour in the population and provide information about sampling strategies for those with highest risk lifestyles. The British sexual lifestyle survey (Johnson *et al.* 1992) was drawn from a random sample of the British population aged 16–59, with a sample size of 18,876 individuals. The data indicate that variability in the number of partners in different time intervals is highly dependent on current age. For example, the mean number of partners in the last five years for men aged 16–24 was 4.2, but only 1.3 for those aged 45–59. In addition, account needs to be taken of the gender differences in models. Virtually all surveys show quite marked differences in the numbers of partners reported by men and women, with men consistently reporting more partners than women. In the British survey, the mean number of partners reported in the last five years for men was 2.6, but only 1.5 for women. Other surveys have found discrepancies of a larger magnitude. This discrepancy has generated a considerable literature on the subject (Smith 1992, Johnson *et al.* 1990, Wadsworth *et al.* 1993, Morris 1993). Mixing outside the sampled population; age mixing; under-representation of high-activity women, such as prostitutes; and the time period over which the mean is measured may account for some of the discrepancy. However, the differences may also be related to social influences leading men to over-report, women to under-report, or both. Further research into the validity of such data are required, particularly where parameter values are used for quantitative models. The extreme skewness of the number of partners in defined time intervals indicates that the mean of the distribution is unstable, the variance extremely high and the accuracy of reporting likely to be the most suspect amongst those with very large number of partners. Indeed, in survey data of this kind, there is evidence in the upper centiles of the distribution that many individuals round figures to tens or hundreds. While differences between men and women and the accuracy of recall can be improved by using shorter time periods, in heterosexual populations the variability in numbers of partners over periods of one year is frequently insufficient to represent the degree of variation in the population. For example, despite the age-related variability in partners over a five year period for women, little variability is seen in the mean over a one year period (Johnson *et al.* 1992). A compromise between accuracy of recall and representing the variability in sexual behaviour may best be achieved by use of five year estimates. Lifetime estimates are inherently inaccurate, both due to recall bias and due to the varying length of sexual history amongst different respondents.

Some models take little account of stratification of the population by age, an important facet in view of the marked variability in levels of activity in different age classes, a factor which relates not only to ageing but also to changes over historical time (age cohort effects). Models may also need to consider other key influences such as marital status on variability in sexual lifestyle relevant to mixing patterns. For example, the British survey demonstrated that the adjusted odds ratio of reporting two or more partners in the last year was of the order of 10 for single, widowed, separated and divorced men and women when compared with the married, after controlling for age, social class and age at first intercourse. Mixing models need to also consider compartments for other demographic variables in addition to age.

Cross-sectional surveys can also provide information relevant to patterns of age mixing in the population. It has been suggested that this is an important determinant of the transmission of the epidemiology of STDs in some African countries where women become infected with HIV and other STDs at a much earlier age than men (Quinn *et al.* 1986). The same is to some extent true in UK populations (Catchpole 1992). Data from the British survey show that men tend to mix with younger women, a tendency which increases with increasing age (Johnson *et al.* 1994, Chapter 5). Similarly, survey data can provide information about the timing of partnerships, in turn informing the extent to which partnerships are serially monogamous or concurrent. In many societies, the pattern of concurrent and serially monogamous relationships may be very important in STD transmission. Concurrent partnerships relevant to STD transmission may occur where men take commercial contacts at the same time as maintaining a relationship with a regular partner, as well as situations in which individuals have two or more long term relationships.

5 Sampling networks to understand the epidemiology of STD transmission

Surveys of sexual behaviour give some indication of the possible existence of a 'core' group for STD transmission. 1% of men who reported the greatest numbers of partners in the last five years in the British sample reported 16% of all partnerships. The equivalent figure for women was 12% in the same time period (Johnson *et al.* 1992). It is amongst individuals in this upper 1–5% of the distribution that the greatest risk of STD may be expected. The British survey showed a very strong relationship between reported number of homosexual and heterosexual partners and the probability of attendance at an STD clinic, which rose to over 15% of those reporting 5 or more partners in the last five years. Thus, for the purposes of studying core networks, it is inefficient to start from the basis of total population samples because of the high rate of monogamy amongst the general population.

An alternative strategy is to study those with a defined sexually transmitted disease and their partners, provided that recruitment of a representative sample of those with the disease in question is feasible. This is likely to be easier in populations where STD services are used by all sectors of the population and where they account for the majority of STD diagnoses in the country. These criteria are fulfilled for the UK and some other European and Scandinavian countries, but are not in the USA or in many developing countries. The defined STD needs to be one of relatively high prevalence and one which is symptomatic at least in one gender. This reduces the potential bias of recruiting individuals who attend medical services on suspicion of infection, in which social factors may influence probability of attendance. Finally, the condition should be one for which contact tracing is both ethical and beneficial to partners. Gonorrhoea and chlamydia are obvious potential candidates, but HIV is problematic under these criteria. Alternatively, individuals with a defined STD may be recruited by population screening.

A third strategy is to sample those with a defined behaviour. Strategies which have been used have, for example, been samples of homosexual men who report anal intercourse. The obvious difficulty with such an approach is that sample representativeness, as with any convenience sample, may be poor. For example, comparisons between sample structure in volunteer samples of gay men and those derived from national population surveys indicate that general population samples recruit a high proportion of men who have had transient homosexual experience. Prostitutes are another population clearly worthy of study, but difficulties arise in recruiting clients and in completing partnership networks.

A fourth strategy is to define those demographic characteristics associated with high risk sexual lifestyles. A suitable population derived from the British survey data might, for example, be young single men and women who also demonstrate other health risk-related behaviours, such as smoking and high alcohol consumption (Johnson *et al.* 1993). Thus far, relatively few networks studies have been carried out in detail to trace the transmission of sexually transmitted diseases. Interpretation of such networks is complex and a major problem within them is that networks are frequently incomplete. For example, Haraldsdottir *et al.* (1992) examined networks of activity amongst a group of homosexual HIV carriers and their sexual partners. Although at first sight such networks may appear to have key individuals involved in the transmission of infection, it is frequently impossible to interview in detail all the contacts of index cases, potentially giving a false impression of the simplicity of the network. A further problem of studying networks is that data may frequently rely on index cases reporting the behaviours of their partners, which for the reasons discussed above may be inherently inaccurate. The sampling of index cases may be potentially biased towards particularly compliant individuals, while the sampling of partners may be biased, either towards the under-sampling of casual partners or the over-sampling of recent partners. For example, Ramstedt *et al.* (1992) attempted to define patterns of mixing by screening women for chlamydia infection, contact tracing their male partners and asking both partners about the number of partnerships in the last six months. Such studies may be biased by the types of partners identified, while collecting data over the last six months may be inadequate to represent the true variability in sexual lifestyle. For example, nearly half the sample pairs reported only one partner in the last six months, indicating that either there was error in reporting or that the six month period was too short to describe adequately the source of infection in the partnership because of the lengthy infectious period of asymptomatic chlamydia.

6 Homosexual and heterosexual networks

Differences also occur in understanding sexual mixing in homosexual versus heterosexual networks. Although an obvious point, it can be argued that heterosexual populations are by definition examples of disassortative mixing. Half the population (women) is only able to mix with the other half of the population (men) whereas in homosexual populations there is much greater opportunity for mixing since all individuals can mix with one another. In effect, for a population of a given size, the total number of possible partnerships is higher in a homosexual population and the choice of partnerships is greater. This allows for denser networks and potentially rapid rates of transmission within a community.

7 Conclusion

Increased attention on the study of sexual lifestyles, in response to the AIDS epidemic, has improved the quantity and quality of empirical data available for deriving parameter estimates for mathematical models of STD. This includes survey data, focussed studies of individuals at high risk of infection and most recently network studies.

All have their methodological pitfalls, but all can contribute to improve the understanding of STD epidemiology. Greater attention to the detail of empirical data needs to be paid when parameter estimates are used in theoretical models. This might be better achieved by greater dialogue between modellers and empirical epidemiologists.

References

ACSF investigators (1992) 'AIDS and sexual behaviour in France', *Nature* **360**, 407–409.

Anderson, R.M. and May, R.M. (1988) 'Epidemiological parameters of HIV transmission', *Nature* **333**, 514–519.

Blower, S.M., Anderson, R.M. and Wallace, P. (1990) 'Log-linear models, sexual behaviour and HIV. Epidemiological implications of heterosexual transmission', *JAIDS* **3**, 763–772.

Catania, J.A., Coates, T.J., Stall, R., Turner, H., Peterson, J., Hearst, N., *et al.* (1992) 'Prevalence of AIDS-related risk factors and condom use in the United States', *Science* **258**, 1101–1106.

Catchpole, M. (1992) 'Sexually transmitted diseases in England and Wales: 1981–1990', *Communic. Dis. Rep.* **2**, R1–R12.

Haraldsdottir, S., Gupta, S. and Anderson, R.M. (1992) 'Preliminary studies of sexual networks in a male homosexual community in Iceland', *JAIDS* **5**, 374–381.

Hethcote, H.W. and Yorke, J.A. (1984) *Gonorrhoea: transmission dynamics and control*, Lecture Notes in Biomathematics, **56**, 1–105.

Hunt, A.J., Davies, P.M., Weatherburn, P., Coxon, A.P. and McManus, T.J. (1991) 'Sexual partners, penetrative sexual partners and HIV risk', *AIDS* **5**, 723–728.

Johnson, A.M., Wadsworth, J., Field, J., Wellings, K. and Anderson, R.M. (1990) ' Surveying sexual lifestyles', (letter), *Nature* **343**, 109.

Johnson, A.M., Wadsworth, J., Wellings, K., Bradshaw, S. and Field, J. (1992) 'Sexual behaviour and HIV risk', *Nature* **360**, 410–412.

Johnson, A.M., Wadsworth, J., Wellings, K. and Field, J. (1994) *Sexual Attitudes and Lifestyles*, Blackwell Scientific, Oxford.

Knox, E.G., Macarthur, C. and Simons, K.J. (1993) *Sexual behaviour and AIDS in Britain*, HMSO, Birmingham.

MMWR (1988) 'Number of sex partners and potential risk of sexual exposure to human immunodeficiency virus', *MMWR* **37**, 565–568.

Morris, M. (1993) 'Telling tails explain the discrepancy in sexual partner reports', *Nature* **365**, 437–440.

Quinn, T.C., Mann, J.M., Curran, J.W. and Piot, P. (1986) 'AIDS in Africa: an epidemiologic paradigm', *Science* **234**, 955–963.

Ramstedt, K., Giesecke, J., Forssman, L. and Granath, F. (1991) 'Choice of sexual partner according to rate of partner and social class of the partners', *Int. J. STD and AIDS* **2**, 428–431.

Smith, T.W. (1992) 'A methodological analysis of the sexual behaviour questions on the general social surveys', *J. Offic. Statist.* **8**, 309–325.

Wadsworth, J., Wellings, K., Johnson, A.M. and Field, J. (1993) 'Sexual behaviour', *BMJ* **306**, 582–583.

Wadsworth, J. and Johnson, A.M. (1991) 'Measuring sexual behaviour', *J. Roy. Statist. Soc. A* **154**, 367–370.

Wellings, K., Field, J., Wadsworth, J., Johnson, A.M., Anderson, R.M. and Bradshaw, S.A. (1990) 'Sexual lifestyles under scrutiny', *Nature* **348**, 276–278.

Winkelstein, W., Lyman, D.M., Padian, N., Grant, R., Samuel, M. and Wiley, J.A. et al. (1987) 'Sexual practices and risk of infection by the human immunodeficiency virus', *JAMA* **257**, 321–325.

Invited Discussion

Sally Blower

We have had three very interesting and very different papers this morning. So to be fair, I thought that I would raise for discussion three issues that are problems for both the data collectors and the transmission modellers.

The first problem is how to classify individuals into risk groups on the basis of their reported sexual behaviour. An individual's sexual behaviour is not a stable, easily measurable characteristic like gender or age. Furthermore, it cannot be viewed in isolation, because it involves the formation of partnerships and consequently is affected by the behaviour of others in the population. It may be extremely difficult to decide how to characterize an individual on the basis of reported risk behaviour at any one time; for example, should this be regarded as a constant or as a random variable (so that the reported behaviour at any moment is an observation on an underlying stochastic process)? Deciding upon a suitable classification scheme may require an analysis of the variability of the risk behaviour of each individual over a long period of time. It may be more appropriate to characterize this by averaging over a period of several years, rather than a particular, short time interval. It has been shown that the behaviour of individuals with high levels of sexual activity tends to be highly variable over time. Hence if individuals are characterised by their behaviour in a short time interval, then low activity individuals will generally be correctly classified (because of their low variability), but high-activity individuals may be misclassified. Deciding exactly how to characterise sexual risk groups in order to avoid misclassification and also to ensure that the size of the high risk group can be estimated accurately is therefore a problem for both the data collectors and the modellers.

The second problem is that both empiricists and modellers need to determine how individual risk behaviour changes over time. The real-world mechanisms for this are unknown. Generally a pattern of changing behaviour is observed in a population and a process producing this pattern is assumed. However, many different processes within individuals can give the same pattern. Consequently, it is essential to conduct longitudinal surveys to assess the temporal trends in sexual behaviour. Ideally such surveys would collect linked HIV serostatus and risk behaviour data. Such cohort studies of injecting drug users and gay men have been in progress since the early eighties. However, it is also necessary to monitor the more general population. A mechanistic analysis of risk behaviour change in two cohorts of gay men has recently been completed, and this shows that it is not possible to deduce the process simply by examination of the static pattern. The results suggest that

263

behaviour changes are time-independent and may be modelled as a homo-geneous one-step Markov process. The results illustrate that behaviour is a dynamic process and that it should not be viewed simply as a means by which individuals in high risk groups cascade into low risk groups and then remain there. It is important to carry out similar analyses on other longitudinal data sets in order to see whether such results hold for other risk groups and in other geographic locations. Such work is needed in order (1) that current and future incidence rates and seroprevalence patterns may be understood and predicted, (2) that intervention strategies can be adequately evaluated, and (3) that appropriate vaccination campaigns can be devised.

The third problem is an example of the 'chicken and the egg' syndrome: should we collect data and then develop models (and have the modellers complain that the 'wrong' data has been collected), or should we develop models and then collect data (and have the data-collectors complain that the models are 'wrong'). Epidemiologists, biostatisticians and modellers all have different priorities: data collection, risk factor and pattern identification and transmission dynamics. Obviously some continuous level of interaction between these groups would be most beneficial to everyone. Therefore, it is essential to begin joint studies that involve epidemiologists, biostatisticians and modellers. Maybe such an approach would make everyone hold hands, smile and produce something novel.

Invited Discussion

Günther Hasibeder

Comments on Heterogeneity Aspects in Mathematical Epidemiology

To begin with I remark generally upon two important aspects of communication in mathematical epidemiology, nomenclature and interpretation of formulae (Sections 1 and 2), and then upon the tension between simple and sophisticated models (Section 3). Finally possible quantitative and qualitative effects of heterogeneity on the basic reproduction ratio in epidemic models are discussed (Section 4).

1 Nomenclature

Mathematical epidemiology is a scientific field where interdisciplinary collaboration is essential and, as part of this, communication between mathematicians and non-mathematicians (biologists, epidemiologists, etc.) is most important. One prerequisite for efficient and fruitful communication – in particular with people who are not specialists in mathematical epidemiology – is a joint nomenclature which tries to avoid using verbal expressions in ambiguous or misleading ways. But unfortunately there seems to persist some confusion about this, not only between persons who are specialists in different scientific fields, but occasionally even within fields.

One example of expressions in epidemiology which are quite misleading, but can be easily avoided, is *random mixing* and *non-random mixing*. Both terms assume that an infection is transmitted through contacts which are made at random (even if the mathematical model does not contain explicitly a stochastic formulation, but some deterministic counterpart). But whereas the first of these two terms intends to express that the population mixes homogeneously, and thus even contacts between individuals of distinct subpopulations are made uniformly, the latter particularly expresses that this is not the case. Since both types of mixing patterns involve random contacts, these two inappropriate verbal expressions should not be used. Instead of *random mixing*, both *uniform mixing* and *homogeneous mixing* are suitable; *non-random mixing* is appropriately replaced by *non-uniform, heterogeneous,* or *non-homogeneous mixing*.

Another source of confusion is the use of the word *rate* for purposes other than declaring some quantity to be meant *per unit time*. It has now become widely accepted that R_0 is called *basic reproduction number*, or *basic reproduction ratio*, as insistently motivated by Diekmann *et al.* (1990), but not *basic reproduction rate*. However, in the biological literature the terms *prevalence rate* and *incidence rate* can still be found, intending to express prevalence and incidence as proportions, e.g. of the total population, rather than absolute numbers of cases. This is not appropriate, as has been expounded also by Elandt-Johnson (1975)[1]. I suggest using – wherever possible and unambiguous – the expressions *prevalence* and *incidence* both for numbers and proportions. If an explicit verbal distinction between numbers and proportions is required, the terms *absolute prevalence* and *absolute incidence* can characterize numbers, whereas *relative prevalence* and *relative incidence* (or perhaps *prevalence proportion* and *incidence proportion*) would designate the corresponding relative quantities.

2   Interpretation of formulae

A related aspect of mathematical epidemiology which, for similar reasons, should be treated with more care, is the interpretation of formulae. I will illustrate this by means of the well-known formula

$$R_0 = 1 + \frac{L}{A}$$

which Herb Hethcote mentioned in his talk. This formula refers to the simple SIR model with vital dynamics and provides a link between the basic reproduction ratio R_0 and the endemic equilibrium, assuming the death rate μ and the force of infection λ are both age-independent. $L = \mu^{-1}$ is the 'average lifetime', and frequently

$$A = \lambda^{-1}$$

is interpreted as 'average age at infection' (e.g. Dietz and Schenzle 1985). But this usual interpretation of A in the above formula is not correct and quite misleading: In fact λ^{-1} would be the 'average age at infection of fictitious individuals who never die', but this interpretation is cumbersome and not very useful.

Therefore it seems highly justified to replace the above R_0 formula, although it has become very popular, by

$$R_0 = \frac{L}{A},$$

but with

$$A = (\lambda + \mu)^{-1}$$

which now really is the 'average age at infection (of all individuals who are infected during their lifetime)'.

---

[1] Thanks to Jim Koopman for letting me know this reference.

3 Simple versus sophisticated models

This workshop section on 'heterogeneity' seems to be an appropriate opportunity to emphasize that epidemic models, as all mathematical models, should be as simple as possible, but as detailed and sophisticated as required for the purpose for which they are designed!

This refers to the question of how much detail about population heterogeneity a model should contain, but also, e.g., to the question of deterministic and stochastic models. I consider deterministic models as usually very appropriate for large populations when prevalence is near the endemic equilibrium, and reasonable far from outbreak; but stochastic models seem to be more appropriate for the outbreak situation, or in the endemic situation when group sizes of a heterogeneous population are small.

An epidemic model should be as simple as possible, in accordance with its intended purpose; but this also puts corresponding constraints on the extent to which it can be interpreted. When listening to the talks and discussions at this workshop, and also at previous workshops within this *Epidemic Models* research programme, I frequently observed that there seems to exist the widespread temptation to ask more detailed questions than relatively simple models can answer. In analysing such a model, and interpreting results, one always has to keep in mind the intended purpose of the model, and must not exceed it!

4 Heterogeneity effects on the basic reproduction ratio R_0

Does heterogeneity bring dramatic changes to R_0? Dye and Hasibeder (1986) analysed a data set of mosquito biting rates on men and observed, for a vector-transmitted disease, that heterogeneity would increase R_0 only by about 10–30%. This moderate quantitative effect can be nicely demonstrated with a simple numerical example. Assume that the hosts consist of two subpopulations which are equal in number, and that hosts in one of these groups are bitten two, three, or four times as frequently as hosts in the other group. Then R_0, always considering a constant host population *average* of bite numbers per day, is only 11%, 25%, or 36%, respectively, higher than in the corresponding homogeneous model.

I guess that the increase in R_0 due to heterogeneity is, for many epidemic models, quite restricted by the 'reasonableness' of the assumptions. Therefore by means of numerical exploration of the heterogeneity factor, which we get from the model, an estimate (or even upper estimate) of the effect of heterogeneity on R_0 could be obtained. In quite a few cases this could indicate that it is unnecessary to sample extremely detailed data, and thus considerable amounts of time and cost could be saved. It would then be required to estimate only the 'homogeneous' R_0 and to multiply this by the maximum 'reasonable' heterogeneity factor.

However, this method of estimating the heterogeneity effects on R_0 might not be sufficient in some cases, when small changes in R_0 could lead to enormous qualitative or quantitative consequences. This is obvious when R_0 is near the threshold value 1. But it might be less obvious when R_0 is high: then the success of a vaccination campaign, if a considerable proportion of vaccination failures has to be taken into account, could quite sensitively depend on R_0 and hence also on heterogeneity.

Herb Hethcote in his talk explained that when a population, which is actually heterogeneous, is falsely assumed to be homogeneous, this can affect estimates obtained from data on the population. The rule of thumb he mentioned is that the estimate of the basic reproduction ratio obtained under the 'homogeneous fallacy' is lower than the actual R_0 for the heterogeneous population. I would like to suggest that this rule of thumb should be applied cautiously: I suspect that if, for example, R_0 is not estimated from model parameters, but from equilibrium prevalences, this rule does not apply in general.

References

Diekmann, O., Heesterbeek, J.A.P. and Metz, J.A.J. (1990) 'On the definition and the computation of the basic reproduction ratio R_0 in models for infectious diseases in heterogeneous populations', *J. Math. Biol.* **28**, 365–382.

Dietz, K. and Schenzle, D. (1985) 'Proportionate mixing models for age-dependent infection transmission', *J. Math. Biol.* **22**, 117–120.

Dye, C. and Hasibeder, G. (1986) 'Population dynamics of mosquito-borne disease: effects of flies which bite some people more frequently than others', *Trans. Roy. Soc. Trop. Med. Hyg.* **80**, 69–77.

Elandt-Johnson, R.C. (1975) 'Definition of rates: some remarks on their use and misuse', *Am. J. Epidemiol.* **102**, 267–271.

Response from Martina Morris

The discussants raise a number of interesting points. I will restrict my response to the issues of risk-group classification and behavioral change.

Classifying individuals on risk behaviors is a difficult task, as Dr. Blower points out, due both to measurement error and behavioral change. Perhaps more fundamentally, it is important note that a 'risk group' is not defined exclusively by individual behavior. If risk can be roughly defined by the magnitude of the infection rate term (βSI) in the compartmental model, this term comprises both individual-level behavior (the contact rate) and mixing structure. A contact rate of 100/yr is risky only if an individual is likely to come into contact with an infected partner: given the high prevalence of HIV among gay men, for example, contact rates of even 1/yr would be risky. Such levels would probably not be sufficient to place most non-IVDU heterosexuals into a 'risk group'. Risk is as much a function of the mixing structure, therefore, as it is of individual behavior.

It is also worth asking whether behaviorally-based risk groups are the most useful to measure, model and track. Consider the dynamics of selective mixing, for example. We know little to nothing about the degree of assortative bias in behavior matching, and this severely constrains our ability to model 'core group' behavior (Morris 1993). Partner selection is, however, more likely to be driven by demographic attributes (e.g., race-, age- and gender-matching) than by behavior-matching. People do not wear their past and present behaviors visibly, so the impact of these behaviors on selection can only be indirect. For the same reason, intervention is also more easily targeted at demographic subgroups than at behavioral groups: they are more easily defined, measured and reached. Patterns of behavioral change, finally, are age-, gender- and race-dependent; not determined by these attributes, but also not random with respect to them. For disease modeling, then, the choice of classification group ultimately depends on the purpose of the exercise. Behavioral categories are a natural choice if the purpose is to identify the disproportionate contribution of highly-active individuals, e.g., Hethcote and Yorke (1984). For surveillance and intervention purposes, on the other hand, demographic categories capture much of the behavioral variance and may provide more useful information.

The issue of behavioral change raised by Dr. Blower is an important one, and is linked to the effect of mixing on the reproductive number, R_0, raised by Dr. Hasibeder. When individual attributes change, natural bridges are formed between groups that may otherwise be weakly linked: paired and single, safe- and unsafe-sex practicers, and different age groups are some examples. As people move between (or among) these groups, they effectively strengthen the transmission between them. In some cases, this can lead to the counterintuitive result that selective mixing raises, rather than lowers the transmission of infection (Morris 1995), as noted by Dr. Hasibeder. This has an analogy in spatial epidemic modeling in the distinction between 'nearest-neighbor' models, where an individual's geographic location is a permanent attribute which limits contact, and models with distance-dependent contact distributions, where geographic location can change (Mollison 1977). The velocity of an epidemic is much higher in the latter. Analytic formulations for the effects of heterogeneous mixing on the reproductive threshold have not yet addressed the impact of changing attributes. This is an important area for future research, and one that is likely to bring together models for physical and social space.

Both discussants refer to the importance of, and problems accompanying, interdisciplinary efforts in this field. This is an appropriate point to thank the organizers of this workshop, and the Newton Institute program of which it was a part. Both have contributed a unique and sustained environment for interdisciplinary collaboration. The organizers, Professors Isham and Mollison, and Drs. Grenfell and Medley are to be congratulated.

References

Hethcote, H. and Yorke, J.A. (1984) *Gonorrhea Transmission Dynamics and Control* Springer Verlag, Berlin.

Mollison, D.M. (1977) 'Spatial contact models for ecological and epidemic spread', *J. Roy. Statist. Soc. Ser. B* **39**, 283–326.

Morris, M. (1993) 'Telling tails explain the discrepancy in sexual partner reports', *Nature* **365**, 437–440.

Morris, M. (1995) 'Data driven network models for the spread of infectious disease'. In *Epidemic Models: their structure and relation to data*, D. Mollison (ed.), Cambridge University Press, Cambridge, 302–322.

Per-contact Probabilities of Heterosexual Transmission of HIV Estimated from Partner Study Data

A.M. Downs and I. De Vincenzi

Introduction

The probability with which the human immunodeficiency virus (HIV) is transmitted from an infected to a susceptible individual during the course of one or more unprotected sexual contacts plays an important role in models of the AIDS epidemic. Several studies found no association between the number of contacts with a given partner and transmission, and some modellers have therefore preferred to use transmission rates per partnership rather than per contact. However, an analysis of data from the California Partners' Study (Padian *et al.* 1990) indicated the presence of an association, although not consistent with a constant probability of transmission per contact. Similar data from a European study have been analyzed to investigate further the relationship between the number of unprotected sexual contacts and the probability of transmission of HIV.

Methods

Data on 563 HIV-infected subjects (index cases) and their stable heterosexual partners were collected at study entry (between March 1987 and March 1991) and at 6-monthly intervals thereafter (European Study Group on Heterosexual Transmission of HIV 1992). For each couple, the number of unprotected sexual contacts was estimated using the reported frequency of contacts and of condom use, both before and after any reported change in behaviour, together with an estimate of the length of the period during which the partner was at risk. This latter was determined as the duration of the relationship prior to the date of HIV test of the partner and from either the date of infection of the index case, when known (rarely the case), or January 1982 (or one of several alternative dates). Following Kaplan (1990) and Jewell and Shiboski (1990), dependence of the partner's HIV status on the number of unprotected contacts was assessed non-parametrically by isotonic regression using the pool adjacent violators algorithm (Ayer *et al.* 1955). Per-contact transmission rates were estimated by maximum likelihood fitting of a Bernoulli model, assuming constant infectivity per contact. Male to female (M-F) and female to male (F-M) transmission rates were estimated separately.

Results

A total of 525 couples (377 M-F, 148 F-M) with at least one unprotected contact since January 1982 were included in the analysis. Based on the partner's HIV status at study entry, the results of the non-parametric analysis were as follows:

Male to female		Female to male	
no. contacts	pr.[HIV+]	no. contacts	pr.[HIV+]
<10	0.10 (1/10)	<11	0.00 (0/6)
13–77	0.18 (11/62)	17–462	0.07 (7/106)
79–1433	0.20 (59/292)	475–900	0.18 (4/22)
1447–2515	0.23 (3/13)	910–1991	0.36 (5/14)

Similar results were obtained when the earliest date considered for potentially infective contacts was either January 1981 or January 1983. Using the Bernoulli model, estimates of per-contact transmission rates (95% confidence intervals) were 0.00054 (0.00029–0.00068) for M-F and 0.00035 (0.00020–0.00055) for F-M transmission respectively. The M-F and F-M estimates were not significantly different ($0.05 < p < 0.1$, likelihood ratio test). In comparison with the non-parametric estimates, the simple Bernoulli model appears, at least for M-F transmission, considerably to under-estimate the risk of transmission after very few contacts and to over-estimate the risk associated with a large number of contacts. This effect was much less marked in the case of F-M transmission. Analysis of 121 initially discordant couples who continued to have unprotected sexual contacts (maximum 450 contacts) gave higher per-contact estimates of 0.0015 (0.0007–0.0028) and 0.0009 (0.0000–0.0021) for M-F and F-M transmission respectively.

Discussion

Our results support the conclusion of Padian *et al.* (1990) that the number of unprotected sexual contacts with an HIV-infected person is indeed associated with the probability of transmission, but that this association is not well described by a model assuming constant per-contact infectivity. All estimates of per-contact transmission probabilities should therefore be interpreted with caution. Our estimates of around 0.0005 based on data at study entry are lower than that of Jewell and Shiboski (1990) (M-F: 0.001) and also than our estimates based on the follow-up data (around 0.001). The latter difference may be related to more advanced stages of infection in the index cases, but may also reflect the more accurate estimates of the number of at-risk contacts. The poor fit of the Bernoulli model is almost certainly due to heterogeneities in transmission, both between couples and, within couples, over time (as a function of disease stage in the index case). More complex models taking into account such effects are being developed.

References

Ayer, M., Brunk, H.D., Ewing, G.M.*et al.* (1955) 'An empirical distribution function for sampling with incomplete information', *Ann. Math. Statist.* **26**, 641–647.

European Study Group on Heterosexual Transmission of HIV (1992) 'Comparison of female to male and male to female transmission of HIV in 563 stable couples', *BMJ* **304**, 809–813.

Jewell, N.P. and Shiboski, S.C. (1990) 'Statistical analysis of HIV infectivity based on partner studies', *Biometrics* **46**, 1133–1150.

Kaplan, E.H. (1990) 'Modeling HIV infectivity: must sex acts be counted?', *JAIDS* **3**, 55–61.

Padian, N.S., Shiboski, S.C. and Jewell, N.P. (1990) 'The effect of number of exposures on the risk of heterosexual HIV transmission', *J. Infect. Dis.* **161**, 883–887.

Heterosexual Spread of HIV with Biased Sexual Partner Selection

J.M. Hyman and E.A. Stanley

We use a deterministic model to study heterosexual HIV transmission. We focus on questions related to sexual partner selection across risk levels and the sensitivity of the model to the differences in infectivity between men and women. We neglect transmission into this purely heterosexual subpopulation from people who have been infected through other means, such as intravenous drug use or sex between men. As well, we neglect age, migration, and many other important features of the epidemic.

Modeling studies have shown that the AIDS epidemic is very sensitive to both the biological aspects of HIV infection and the human behaviors that spread HIV. They have demonstrated that the epidemic is sensitive to subtle features of the biology of HIV and human behavior, including the distribution of times from infection to AIDS, changes in infectiousness with duration of infection, and the distribution of partner acquisition-rates in the population (Hyman and Stanley 1989).

The male and female at-risk populations are divided into uninfected people, those infected with HIV but who have not yet developed AIDS, and the infecteds that have progressed to AIDS. We assume that the major characteristic that affects the probability of infection is the partner-acquisition rate, and distribute each of these populations according to a risk variable which determines this rate. NonAIDS infecteds are also distributed according to their duration of infection, and AIDS cases are distributed according to the duration of time since their diagnosis. People mature into a given risk group. They may change behavior, switching from one risk group to another. Before the introduction of HIV, there was a balance between this constant maturation rate into each risk group, flows between the groups, and the constant rate per individual of retirement or death out of the population.

We assume that all contacts between a specific pair of individuals can be treated as a single event. The transmission rate depends on the sex and duration of infection of the infected partner. Infected people develop AIDS at a rate that depends on the length of time they have been infected, but is assumed to be independent of sex and risk. AIDS cases are assumed to be sexually inactive, and to die at a rate that depends on the time since they were diagnosed. Since the number of partners must be the same for both sexes, partner acquisition rates change over time. Therefore, we distribute the two populations according to a risk variable which is proportional at any time to the partner acquisition rate.

With the subscripts M and F refering to males and females, respectively, we define

variables

t	time (years)
τ	duration of infection
α	duration of AIDS
r	risk
$U_i(t,r)$	uninfecteds, distributed by risk
$I_i(t,r,\tau)$	nonAIDS infecteds, distributed by risk and duration of infection
$A_i(t,r,\alpha)$	AIDS cases, distributed by risk and duration of AIDS
$N_i(t,r)$	total number of sexually active individuals, distributed by risk: $N_i(t,r) = U_i(t,r) + \int I_i(t,r,\tau)d\tau$

parameters

μ	per person rate of leaving the sexually active population
$U_{io}(r)$	equilibrium distribution of the uninfected populations in the absence of HIV
$i_i(\tau)$	probability of infection per contact with an infected person of sex i who has been infected a time τ
$c_i(r,r')$	increased probability of transmission due to multiple contacts between a person of sex i and risk r with one of sex j and risk r'
$\gamma_i(\tau)$	per person rate of developing AIDS for those infected τ years ago
$\delta_i(\alpha)$	per person death rate due to AIDS for those diagnosed α years ago
$\zeta_i(r,s)$	per person rate of changing behavior from risk r to risk s
$\lambda_i[t,r;U,I]$	per person rate of infection for an uninfected of sex i and risk r
$r_i[t,r;N]$	partner acquisition rate for a person of sex i and risk r
$\rho_i[t,r,s;N]ds$	probability that the partner (of a person of sex i and risk r) has risk in $(s, s+ds)$.

Based on our assumptions, we have the following equations for the changes in the populations:

$$\frac{\partial U_i(t,r)}{\partial t} = \mu(U_{io}(r) - U_i(t,r)) + \int_0^\infty (\zeta_i(s,r)U_i(t,s)$$
$$-\zeta_i(r,s)U_i(t,r))ds - \lambda_i[t,r;U,I]U_i(t,r) \quad (1a)$$

$$I_i(t,r,0) = \lambda_i[t,r;U,I]U_i(t,r) \quad (1b)$$

$$\frac{\partial I_i(t,r,\tau)}{\partial t} + \frac{\partial I_i(t,r,\tau)}{\partial t} = \int_0^\infty (\zeta_i(s,r)I_i(t,s,\tau) - \zeta_i(r,s)I_i(t,r,\tau))ds$$
$$-(\gamma_i(\tau) + \mu)I_i(t,r,\tau), \quad (1c)$$

$$A_i(t,r,0) = \int_0^\infty \gamma_i(\tau)I_i(t,r,\tau)d\tau, \quad (1d)$$

$$\frac{\partial A_i(t,r,\alpha)}{\partial t} + \frac{\partial A_i(t,r,\alpha)}{\partial \alpha} = \int_0^\infty (\zeta_i(s,r)A_i(t,s,\alpha) - \zeta_i(r,s)A_i(t,r,\alpha))ds$$
$$-(\delta_i(\alpha) + \mu)A_i(t,r,\alpha). \quad (1e)$$

The per partner probability of transmission, λ_i, is a product of the partner acquisition rates, r_i, and the probability of infection per partner. The probability of infection from a new partner depends on the risk level of the partner, which is determined by ρ_i, and the probability of infection by a partner from that risk group, integrated over all possible risk groups of the partner:

$$\lambda_i[t,r;N] = r_i(t,r)\int \rho_i[t,r,x;N]c_i(r,x)\int_0^\infty i_j(\tau)\frac{I_j(t,x,\tau)}{N_j(t,x)}\,d\tau dx. \quad (2)$$

We ensure that the total number of female partners that men have per year equals the number of male partners that women have per year by taking

$$r_i(t,r) = R_i[t;N]r, \text{ for } i \in \{M,F\}, \quad (3)$$

with

$$R_i(t) = \left[\int_0^\infty rN_j(t,r)dr\right]^{1/2}\left[\int_0^\infty rN_i(t,r)dr\right]^{-1/2}, \text{ for } i \neq j. \quad (4)$$

The mixing function, ρ_i, must satisfy a set of constraints. In our simulations, we explored how different types of mixing affect the epidemic. We did this by comparing the results from random partner choice to biased mixing created by using two different algorithms, described in Hyman and Stanley (1994).

We have done a series of numerical simulations of the above model, comparing different scenarios. The results of these simulations are described in Hyman and Stanley (1994): here we provide a brief review of the more interesting aspects. In all simulations, we have taken all of the parameters to be the same for both sexes, except the infectivity and the distribution over risk. Also, we took $\mu = 0.02\text{yrs}^{-1}$, $\gamma_i(\tau) = 0.004\tau^{1.4}$, $\zeta_i(r,s) = 0$, a small number of initial infecteds and AIDS cases, uniformly distributed in risk, and

$$\delta_i(\alpha) = D'(\alpha)/(1 - D(\alpha)), \quad D(\alpha) = \exp\left\{\frac{-0.075\alpha}{1 + 0.05\alpha}\right\}. \quad (5)$$

We assume that an individual of sex i who develops AIDS τ_A units of time after infection has an infectivity $i_{iA}(\tau/\tau_A)$ at τ time units after infection. In Hyman and Stanley (1994) we show that this assumption gives an average infectivity $i_i(\tau)$ of the people of sex i infected for τ units of time:

$$i_i(\tau) = [1 - C(\tau)]^{-1}\int_\tau^\infty i_{iA}\left(\frac{\tau}{\tau_A}\right)\frac{dC}{d\tau}(\tau_A)d\tau_A. \quad (6)$$

We took $i_{iA}(x) = \beta_i i_L(x)$, where $i_L(x)$ is a piecewise linear function that connects the points $\{(0,0), (0.013,0), (0.05,1), (0.088,0.4), (0.625,0.4), (1,1)\}$ with straight lines. Thus we assumed that there is a sharp peak in infectiousness shortly after infection, followed by a long non-infectious period, and then a rise shortly before the start of AIDS. This gives a mean value for $i(\tau)$ of $0.06\beta_i$.

We then did some sensitivity studies in the remaining parameters. We first set up a baseline scenario, in which $c_i(r,s) = 1 + 19e^{-0.05(r+s)}$, $\beta_M = 0.1$, $\beta_F = 0.025$, and the initial population distribution is

$$N_{i0}(r) = \frac{(n_i - 1)}{2a_i} \frac{(1 + (n_i + 1)r/a_i)}{(1 + r/a_i)^{n_i+1}}, \qquad (7)$$

with $n_i = 3$ and a_i chosen so that the mean risk is 3 partners/yr. We took the initial mixing to be such that women were paired primarily to men of the same risk as themselves, but high-risk men were paired about half the time with high-risk and half with low-risk women (this is possible because the number of high-risk men is so small that the fraction of low-risk women paired to a high-risk man is small). This gave an epidemic which grew initially, then saturated and appeared to be heading toward an equilibrium, with a smaller population than initially. About one and a half times as many women were infected as men. Also, while the epidemic in men spread from high- to low-risk with time, in women the epidemic appeared early in low-risk women.

Compared to this baseline, random mixing gave a much less rapid epidemic early on and a larger one later (in fact, random mixing gave an exponentially growing epidemic for the first few years, while the baseline scenario grew polynomially in time). Different relative infectivities changed the ratio of female to male infections, in a nonlinear fashion. Changing the initial distribution of men so that $n_i = 4$ set up mixing in which men were more likely to pair only with women of the same risk as themselves than in the baseline scenario, having the opposite effect from random mixing. Finally, changing the muliplicative factor $c_i(r,s)$ to the constant value of 10 had a radical effect on the epidemic shape, vastly increasing the intial speed of spread and decreasing the later spread.

References

Hyman, J.M. and Stanley, E.A. (1989) 'The effect of social mixing patterns on the spread of HIV'. In *Mathematical Approaches to Ecological and Environmental Problem Solving*, Lecture Notes in Biomathematics **81**, Springer-Verlag, New York, 190–219.

Hyman, J.M. and Stanley, E.A. (1994) 'A risk-based heterosexual model for the AIDS epidemic with biased sexual partner selection'. In *Modeling the AIDS Epidemic*, E. Kaplan and M. Brandeau (eds.), Raven Press, New York, 331–363.

Dynamic Simulation of Sexual Partner Networks: which Network Properties are Important in Sexually Transmitted Disease (STD) Epidemiology?

G.P. Garnett and J. Swinton

Conventional deterministic models of infection spread through populations aggregate individuals into compartments and study the dynamics of the resulting simplified system (Anderson and May 1991, Hethcote and Van Ark 1992). In this paper we explore whether knowledge of contact networks at an individual level can add to our epidemiological understanding in the particular setting of STDs. In the case of STDs the limited number and well defined nature of sexual contacts between people allows the description of the networks along which an STD can spread (Klovdahl et al. 1992, 1994). To this end a simple model describing the sexual behaviour of individuals is developed which generates sexual partner networks. The spread of a sexually transmitted disease (STD) through the population is simulated, and the characteristics of the network are related to the resultant spread of the STD. The model constructed contains many assumptions about the mechanisms controlling the sexual partnership formation behaviour, which are varied to generate a large range of possible networks. A central aim of this work is the development of the model as a tool to assist in the analysis of behavioural data. From simulations the parameters which are most influential in STD epidemiology can be identified. Samples can be taken from this network in a way which mirrors methods of sampling used in behavioural research.

The model

Individuals within the population, which can be varied in size, are treated as discrete entities with particular characteristics related to their sexual behaviour. Currently these include: sex; desired number of sexual partners per unit of time; desired duration of sexual partnerships; and a preference function for choosing sexual partners on the basis of *their* desired number of partners. At each time step it is determined from these characteristics whether an individual requires a new partner. A stochastic process in which the individual's preference is accounted for then determines whether or not a sexual partnership is formed. Once formed a record is kept of the duration of the sexual partnership, which is terminated after the minimum of the two desired lengths of sexual partnerships has been reached. To prevent the continual reformation of the same sexual partnerships amongst the members of the population with the highest levels of sexual activity a refractory period is maintained before the reformation of a sexual partnership is allowed. By following these rules a dynamic graph of sexual partnerships is formed. An additional characteristic of individuals in the model is whether or not they are infected with 'gonorrhoea', and if they are, for how long they have been infected. Once the graph (or network) has moved away from the initial conditions a gonorrhoea epidemic can be seeded in randomly assigned hosts. Gonococcal infection is transmitted through the network by a stochastic process where there is a specific transmission probability per unit of time from men to women and from women to men. After a set duration the individual recovers from infection. Following the spread of infection in the model we can determine: (1) whether gonorrhoea establishes itself within the population; (2) the rate at which the infection progresses through the population and (3) the endemic prevalence of the infection. These epidemiological properties of the dynamic sexual partner network can then be compared with parameters describing the characteristics of the graph. All sexual partnerships are assumed to involve the same intensity of connection, an assumption we will relax in future work.

Parameters describing the sexual partner networks

Statistics for the sexual partner network are of two types. The first are measures of the full bipartite graph, which describe the properties of the population as a whole. These statistics can be those generally used in other modelling approaches such as the mean number of sexual partners, its variance, or mixing between groups, or they can be those only definable in networks, such as the number of monogamous partnerships, the number of isolated groups or components, and the size of these groups (Scott 1991). These variables can be compared with the simulated prevalence of an STD in the population. The second type of statistic is that relating to the individual, for example centrality. A variety of measures for the centrality of an individual have been proposed. Here we use the simplest. One such measure is the number of sexual partnerships an individual has divided by the possible number. Another is one which also looks at the degree of adjacent points. This is effectively looking at the number of partners at path length 2. The path length can be increased to 3 and 4 etc., and the effect that the position of the individual within the network has on the likelihood of infection can be measured.

Preliminary results suggest that inclusion of the structure of the network beyond descriptions commonly used in other approaches to modelling is of more importance in assessing the risk of infection in individuals than in the epidemiology of infection in the whole population. In particular, the number of sexual partners of an individual's sexual partners was most frequently the best predictor of infection in an individual. This supports the central importance of patterns of mixing in STD epidemiology (Garnett and Anderson 1993). At a population level the mean number of sexual partners, the variance in numbers of sexual partners and the pattern of mixing were most influential. Other network statistics used correlated very closely to these three measures. However, the amount of subdivision of the population into isolated groups did play a role in how widely spread a simulated STD was. Thus, the size and number of components does appear to be epidemiologically important.

The results outlined here are based upon a limited number of simulations. Future work will include a full mathematical description of the model and a full sensitivity analysis. The analysis of the relationship between the properties of networks and the spread of an STD is a first stage in developing the model framework as a tool for understanding behavioural and epidemiological data. Further work will compare the properties of the network models with more traditional compartmental STD models.

References

Anderson, R.M. and May, R.M. (1991) *Infectious diseases of humans: dynamics and control*, Oxford University Press, Oxford.

Garnett, G.P. and Anderson, R.M. (1993) 'Contact tracing and the estimation of sexual mixing patterns: the epidemiology of gonococcal infections', *Sex. Transm. Dis.* **20**, 181–191.

Hethcote, H.W. and Van Ark, J.W. (1992) 'Modeling HIV transmission and AIDS in the United States', *Lecture Notes in Biomathematics* **95**, 1–234.

Klovdahl, A.S., Potterat, J.J., Woodhouse, D.E., Muth, J.B., Muth, S.Q. and Darrow, W.W. (1992) 'HIV infection in an urban social network: a progress report', *Bull. Methodol.Sociol.* **36**, 24–33.

Klovdahl, A.S., Potterat, J.J., Woodhouse, D.E., Muth, J.B., Muth, S.Q. and Darrow, W.W. (1994) 'Social networks and infectious disease: the Colorado Springs study', *Soc. Sci. Med.* **38**, 79–88

Scott, J. (1991) *Social network analysis*, Sage, Beverly Hills, CA.

The Spread of an STD on a Dynamic Network of Sexual Contacts

Mirjam Kretzschmar

The fact that AIDS is mainly a sexually transmitted disease has brought human sexual behaviour into the focus of attention and with it the underlying social structure of the population. The problem of how to incorporate the determinants of the sexual contact structure into a mathematical model of disease transmission has been one of the central questions in AIDS-modelling in recent years. While most of this work up to now has been based on the methodology of differential equations, lately there has been some interest in so-called network models. The basic idea of the network approach is that a population and its sexual contact structure can be described by a graph, where the vertices represent individuals and the edges existing sexual relations.

A simulation model based on the network approach has been developed in Kretzschmar *et al.* (1990,1994). The model describes a stochastic pair formation and dissolution process in a heterosexual population. Infection can be transmitted in contacts between an infected and a susceptible individual. A major problem in analyzing results from network simulations is the question of what are the appropriate quantities to measure and compare. I have chosen, amongst others, to look at the degree distribution of the 'cumulative' network over a given time of observation, because this can be determined with a certain accuracy in sociological surveys. One can then study how the number of infected individuals in the course of the epidemic depends on the mean and variance of this degree distribution.

The following topics are discussed:

1. Comparability of simulation results with results from deterministic models. To show how simulation results relate to results from deterministic modelling I compare them with pair formation models and with multigroup mixing models. This also serves as a reference point for simulation results from more complex situations.

2. A comparison between 'serial monogamy' and 'polygamy'. In heterosexual populations one finds that even if individuals accumulate many partners over a certain time span, they mostly have only one partner at a time. This has been termed 'serial monogamy'. I compare this situation with that when individuals can have more than one partner at a time ('polygamy').

3. A model with two types of pairs: 'steady' and 'casual'. Survey data shows that there is a quite clear distinction between longlasting steady relationships and casual sexpartners. This can also be seen in a life course

perspective. Before or between steady relationships individuals go through 'experimental' phases in which they have a number of casual partners. What are the effects on network structure and disease transmission?

4. Heterogeneity of the population and partner preferences. Partner choice can depend on many variables, among others demographic variables like age, but also psychosocial variables which are difficult to quantify. How do different types of heterogeneity and preference functions influence the network structure?

References

Kretzschmar M., Reinking D.P., Brouwers H., Zessen G. van, Jager J.C. (1990) 'Network models: from paradigm to mathematical tool'. In *Modeling the AIDS Epidemic*, E.H. Kaplan and M. Brandeau (eds.), Raven Press, New York.

Kretzschmar M., Reinking D.P., Zessen G. van, Brouwers H., Jager J.C. (1994) 'The basic reproduction ratio R_0 for a sexually transmitted disease in a pair formation model with two types of pairs', *Math. Biosc.* **124**, 181–205.

Network Measures for Epidemiology

Michael Altmann

There has been considerable recent interest in expanding traditional mass action models for disease transmission to include selectivity and clustering in the contact process. One approach has been to stratify the population according to one or more population characteristics and then to model the effect of these characteristics on contact patterns. The contact rate between two members with known attributes is described by a mixing matrix or kernel function. The usual approach is to consider a parameterized family of mixing matrices and ask how important epidemiological outcomes are affected by these parameters.

In contrast, we have taken the contact network as the primary unit of observation. Networks are modeled as weighted graphs (static and undirected in the studies reported here). Because a complete description of a network entails a very large amount of information, our goal was find summary statistics that were effective predictors of the speed at which a disease would propagate through the network. The approach was to generate random networks, compute summary statistics, simulate a disease spreading through the network, and then examine the relationship between the statistics and epidemiologically significant outcomes. These simulation studies are preliminary, indicating the direction of ongoing research, and ask more questions than they answer.

Networks were generated using two different probability models, producing clustering by different mechanisms. The first model assumes that spatial proximity is a major consideration in network formation. Each individual in the population is assigned a random location in a square region and is assigned a circular territory of radius r in which it seeks contacts. Links are formed between individuals with overlapping territories with a probability α and this formation is independent from link to link (in contrast to our second model). Although this model uses characteristics (spatial location and territory size) to generate the network, the analysis ignored these.

The second model assumes that the network is a random graph. The graph is assumed to be 'Markov' in the sense that edges are dependent if they share a node. Furthermore the population is assumed to be homogeneous, so the probability distribution can be described by a log-linear function

$$P(G) = \frac{1}{Z} \exp(\rho R + \sum_k \sigma_k S_k + \tau T).$$

Here R is the number of edges in the graph G, S_k is the number of stars with k edges and T is the number of triangles. The number Z is a normalizing

283

constant. Samples from this probability model were generated using the Metropolis algorithm.

A very large number of graph theoretic statistics (e.g. diameter, density, thickness, etc) have been developed to summarize features of a network and potentially could be used as predictors of epidemic spread. In our studies, we restricted attention to the number of complete subgraphs of each size. These clique counts are well studied in theoretical work and can be estimated from social network data.

Three sets of experiments were conducted. In the first, the spatial model was used to generate 60 networks, each with 1000 nodes, and with 4000, 5000, or 6000 edges. The number of triangles in the networks varied from 300 to 7000. For each network, a stochastic SIR epidemic process was then simulated and the average (over the 1000 nodes) infection time and the fraction of the population ever infected were recorded. As expected, the number of edges was the primary predictor of epidemic speed and intensity. Near the threshold for large epidemics, speed and intensity were well described by the function $a_1 R + a_2 T / R^4$ with certain constants a_1 and a_2. The form of this can be explained by considering the scaling of R and T as functions of α.

In the second experiment, the spatial model was used to generate networks with 1000 nodes, 4000 edges, and between 300 and 7000 triangles. In all, 150 networks were generated at 20 different levels of spatial localization. An SIR epidemic was simulated 6 times in each network. The number of triangles was found to have a significant effect on both the speed and intensity of the epidemic. At one extreme, networks with no spatial localization had an effective R_0 of 3 and 95% of the population became infected. Networks at the other extreme, with 7000 triangles, took three times as long to propagate an epidemic and were roughly at threshold. This suggests that a twenty-fold increase in the number of triangles corresponded to a threefold decrease in R_0, or equivalently about a threefold decrease in the effective transmissibility of the disease.

The third experiment used Markov random graphs to determine whether the effects of triangle density on epidemic speed and intensity were peculiar to spatially generated networks, or reflected a universal relationship. The difficulty involved in generating large Markov random graphs led us to use networks with 100 nodes. A positive value for τ was used to generate a high density of triangles. At the highest densities, a negative σ_2 value was needed in order to avoid degenerate graphs consisting of a single clique. Again, an SIR process was simulated on each network.

As in the second experiment, the number of triangles had a large impact on the epidemic intensity. Increasing the number of triangles from 70 to 2000 decreased the epidemic intensity from 95% to 0, which may be represented as decreasing the effective R_0 from 3 to 1. However, in this experiment there was a slight positive relationship between the number of triangles in a network and the speed of epidemics propagating through the network.

We hypothesize the following explanation for the different effect of triangle density on epidemic speed observed with the two models. A Markov graph with many triangles easily breaks apart under the random deletion of edges (thus the low epidemic intensity), but has as small a diameter as an unstructured network (thus the fast epidemics). By contrast, the most spatially localized networks have large diameters – roughly the distance across the square, leading to slower epidemics. This suggests that different features of a graph must be considered when predicting the speed of an epidemic, the final fraction infected, and the critical level of intervention necessary to bring the network below the epidemic threshold.

Spatial Heterogeneity and the Spread of Infectious Diseases

L. Sattenspiel

Numerous factors influence the likelihood of contact between susceptible and infectious people, including participation in different social activities, cultural barriers such as membership of particular ethnic groups with associated customs, or separation due to geographic distance. These factors guarantee that contact among individuals within a population is distinctly nonrandom. Results from several theoretical studies show that nonrandom mixing among subgroups has many consequences for the outcome of epidemic spread, including affecting the time at which a disease is introduced into different subgroups and the speed of propagation and severity of an epidemic.

Most recent models for the spread of infectious diseases in human populations incorporate nonrandom patterns of mixing across subgroups and include a parameter for contact between groups that depends on the subgroups from which the susceptible and infective individuals derive. This parameter represents only the end result of the mixing process, leaving implicit the mechanism by which contact occurs. Here we describe a model that explicitly incorporates the mechanism for contact among individuals from different subgroups. Contact between individuals occurs as a result of the mobility of participants across either geographic or social space[1]. Because it is simpler to visualize, we limit our discussion here to geographic mobility. Models for behavioral mobility are straightforward adaptations of this process (e.g. Sattenspiel and Castillo-Chavez 1990, Jacquez *et al.* 1989).

Consider a population that is distributed among n regions. Individuals from region i leave the region at a rate σ_i per unit time. These visitors are then distributed among the $n - 1$ destinations with probabilities ν_{ij} to each destination j. A person who has traveled from region i to region j returns to region i at a rate ρ_{ij}. The travel patterns among groups are represented by a mobility matrix with the following elements

$$
m_{ij} = \begin{cases} \dfrac{\sigma_i \nu_{ij}}{\rho_{ij}\left(1 + \sigma_i \sum_{k \neq i} \dfrac{\nu_{ik}}{\rho_{ik}}\right)} & \text{if } j \neq i \\[20pt] \dfrac{1}{\left(1 + \sigma_i \sum_{k \neq i} \dfrac{\nu_{ik}}{\rho_{ik}}\right)} & \text{if } j = i \,. \end{cases}
$$

---

[1]The model to be described below applies only when the mobility process is at equilibrium. A more general model which does not assume this equilibrium is presented in Sattenspiel and Dietz (1995).

The terms in this matrix give the prevalence of people in region j who are permanent residents of region i.

Because the transmission of disease involves two people, both of whom can and often do travel, the mobility mechanism operates simultaneously on these two people. The maathematical formulation of this joint process results in a term, $\sum_k m_{ik} m_{jk}$, which describes the process by which two individuals, one from region i and one from region j, come into contact with one another in some region k. This formulation is combined with standard epidemic models to give a model to describe the spread of infectious diseases among different subpopulations in geographic and/or social space.

This formulation has two primary advantages over other models for epidemic spread in structured populations. First, it explicitly models the mechanism by which contact occurs among individuals over geographic or social space. Second, because of this, transmission and contact rates can vary not only with intrinsic characteristics of susceptibles and infectives, but also with location of contact.

We give here an example of incorporating the mobility process into a model for the spread of measles on the Caribbean island of Dominica. Although the model is highly complex, most of the parameters can be estimated from easily collected data. For example, data on daily activities and short-term travel patterns on the island have been collected for estimation of the mobility matrix (Sattenspiel and Powell 1993). Weekly incidences by health district of a 1984 measles epidemic on the island are also available.

The mathematical model for measles transmission on Dominica divides the population into seven districts, each of which is further divided into three age classes; infants (b: 0–2 years), primary school age (s: 2–12 years), and adults (a: > 12). Three kinds of mobility relevant to measles transmission are considered – general travel of adults; general travel of children (c), which is assumed to follow patterns representative of adults, but which is adjusted by age; and school-related travel, which is biassed toward those districts with significant educational features. The contact rates for the three ages classes are as follows:

Contacts of district i infants visiting district k	$=$	family contact with infected child	$+$	family contact with infected adult

$$(\tau_{bijk}) \quad = \quad m_{cik} m_{cjk} \left[\frac{I_{bjk} + I_{sjk}}{N_k^*} \right] \quad + \quad m_{cik} m_{ajk} \left[\frac{I_{ajk}}{N_k^*} \right]$$

Contacts of   = family contact with infected child
district i school-age   + family contact with infected adult
visiting district k + school contact with infected school child

$$(\tau_{sijk}) = m_{cik}m_{cjk}\left[\frac{I_{bjk} + I_{sjk}}{N_k^*}\right] + m_{cik}m_{ajk}\left[\frac{I_{ajk}}{N_k^*}\right] + m_{sik}m_{sjk}\left[\frac{I_{sjk}}{N_{sk}^*}\right]$$

Contacts of district i adults visiting district k		family contact with infected child		family contact with infected adult

$$(\tau_{aijk}) \quad = \quad m_{aik}m_{cjk}\left[\frac{I_{bjk} + I_{sjk}}{N_k^*}\right] \quad + \quad m_{aik}m_{ajk}\left[\frac{I_{ajk}}{N_k^*}\right]$$

The complete measles transmission model is:

$$\frac{dS_{bi}}{dt} = b_i N_i - \sum_{j=1}^{7}\sum_{k=1}^{7}\beta_{ijk}\tau_{bijk}c_b S_{bi} - (d_b + \alpha_b)S_{bi}$$

$$\frac{dS_{si}}{dt} = \alpha_b S_{bi} - \sum_{j=1}^{7}\sum_{k=1}^{7}\beta_{ijk}\tau_{sijk}c_s S_{si} - (d_s + \alpha_s)S_{si}$$

$$\frac{dS_{ai}}{dt} = \alpha_s S_{si} - \sum_{j=1}^{7}\sum_{k=1}^{7}\beta_{ijk}\tau_{aijk}c_a S_{ai} - d_a S_{ai}$$

$$\frac{dI_{bi}}{dt} = \sum_{j=1}^{7}\sum_{k=1}^{7}\beta_{ijk}\tau_{bijk}c_b S_{bi} - (d_b + \gamma + \alpha_b)I_{bi}$$

$$\frac{dI_{si}}{dt} = \alpha_b I_{bi} + \sum_{j=1}^{7}\sum_{k=1}^{7}\beta_{ijk}\tau_{sijk}c_s S_{si} - (d_s + \gamma + \alpha_s)I_{si}$$

$$\frac{dI_{ai}}{dt} = \alpha_s I_{si} + \sum_{j=1}^{7}\sum_{k=1}^{7}\beta_{ijk}\tau_{aijk}c_a S_{ai} - (d_a + \gamma)I_{ai}$$

$$\frac{dR_{bi}}{dt} = \gamma I_{bi} - (d_b + \alpha_b)R_{bi}$$

$$\frac{dR_{si}}{dt} = \gamma I_{si} + \alpha_b R_{bi} - (d_s + \alpha_s)R_{si}$$

$$\frac{dR_{ai}}{dt} = \gamma I_{ai} + \alpha_s R_{si} - d_a R_{ai}$$

where $S_{(b,s,a)i}$, $I_{(b,s,a)i}$, and $R_{(b,s,a)i}$ are the number of susceptible, infective, and recovered individuals, respectively, of a particular age class in district i (N_i is the number of residents of district i), N_k^* is the number of people actually present in district k at time t, N_{sk}^* is the number of school children actually present in district k at time t, m_{cik} is the prevalence of children from district i in district k for family-related activities, m_{sik} is the prevalence of children from district i who are in district k for school-related activities, m_{aik} is the prevalence of adults from district i in district k, β_{ijk} is the fraction of contacts between a susceptible from district i and an infective from district j that occur in district k and that result in transmission of the virus, $c_{(b,s,a)}$ is the average number of contacts made by a person in a particular age class, b_i is the crude birth rate, $d_{(b,s,a)}$ is the death rate of individuals from district i for a particular age class, α_b is the rate at which infants transfer to school age, α_s is the rate at which school age children become adults, γ is the recovery rate from measles.

References

Jacquez, J.A., Simon, C.P. and Koopman, J. (1989) 'Structured mixing: heterogeneous mixing by the definition of activity groups'. In *Mathematical and Statistical Approaches to AIDS Epidemiology*, C. Castillo-Chavez (ed.), Springer-Verlag, Berlin 301–315.

Sattenspiel, L. and Castillo-Chavez, C. (1990) 'Environmental context, social interactions, and the spread of HIV', *Am. J. Hum. Biol.* 2, 397–417.

Sattenspiel, L. and Dietz, K. (1995) 'A structured epidemic model incorporating geographic mobility among regions', *Math. Biosci.*, in press.

Sattenspiel, L. and Powell, C. (1993) 'Geographic spread of measles on the island of Dominica, West Indies', *Hum. Biol.* 65, 107–129.

Data Analysis for Estimating Risk Factor Effects using Transmission Models

J. Koopman

A major activity of both academic and governmental epidemiologists involves ascertaining the environmental contaminations, personal behaviors, biological factors, and other risk factors whose control will lead to the control of disease risks. Almost always the data analytic models used in this task are consistent with linear models of the causal process leading to disease. One of their basic assumptions is thus that the outcomes in one study subject are independent of the outcomes in other study subjects.

Infection transmission between humans is inconsistent with these linear model forms. Some particular consequences of this inconsistency explain why epidemiologists have been so unsuccessful in defining the modes of transmission of many infectious agents. Model inconsistencies also explain the poor performance of epidemiological methods in determining the relative importance of different factors contributing to infection risk at both an individual and a population level. It will be demonstrated how most of the effect of risk factors which increase transmission risk will not be detected by the usual analytic methods of epidemiology. This inadequacy of standard methods occurs even when contact patterns are random. It will be further demonstrated how non-random contact patterns can create additional difficulties for the detection of secondary risk factors.

Standard analytic models in epidemiology assume that causal actions occur directly on individuals. Thus their basic parameters are unlike those in transmission models which relate to interactions between individuals. The paradigm jump from cause acting directly on individuals to cause acting on interactions between individuals is a big one for epidemiologists. The paradigm jump would be facilitated if a data collection and analysis framework existed based on transmission models. Some approaches to developing that framework will be discussed.

Causal effects of risk factors affecting transmission may be at four levels:

1. upon the susceptibility of individuals;

2. upon the contagiousness of individuals;

3. upon individual encounters with environments where direct or indirect contact between individuals can be established;

4. upon the establishment of potentially transmitting contacts within those environments.

Causal effects on susceptibility come closest to fitting into the standard individual effects paradigm of epidemiology. But even there, they fit the standard paradigm only where susceptibility effects are all or none. Even all or none susceptibility effects will be misperceived using the standard epidemiological paradigm because of the indirect effects created by transmission dynamics of changing the susceptibility of other individuals.

The above four types of causal effects can be parameterized within transmission models. The first two types of cause affect transmission probabilities and the last two affect contact patterns. To relate data on epidemiological risk factors to the parameters of transmission models, the risk factors should be conceptualized as generating one or more of the above four types of causal effects. Structured and selective mixing models provide a framework for doing this with regard to the last two types of causal effects.

The usual data collected in an epidemiological investigation of risk factors will have deficiencies with regard to its use within the framework of a transmission model. These deficiencies are of the following types:

1. inadequate information on individuals is obtained (this is especially true with regard to factors that may be affecting contagiousness);

2. inadequate information on interactions between individuals and/or the determinants of those interactions will be obtained (only in the case of sexually transmitted diseases is there now a major effort by epidemiologists to collect this sort of data);

3. the sampling frames of the investigations may not allow for adequate modelling of contacts within a population.

Despite these deficiencies, it is proposed that models using available data can be a first step toward eventually getting better data. The attempts of the Michigan HIV Modelling group to assess the effects of stage of infection and type of sex acts on HIV transmission probabilities will be discussed in this context.

Homosexual Role Behaviour and the Spread of HIV

Hans van Druten, Godfried van Griensven and Jan Hendriks

Introduction

In general, little attention is given to homosexual role behaviour as a factor in the sexual transmission of HIV. Models that include variations in sexual behaviour are usually restricted to heterogeneity in sexual partner-change and the manner in which subpopulations mix. Following Trichopoulos *et al.* (1988), Wiley and Herschkorn (1989), van Griensven *et al.* (1990), we lay emphasis on homosexual role behaviour (role separation) as a factor influencing the spread of HIV in homosexual populations. If there are large differences between the risks of receptive and insertive anal intercourse, with the latter carrying only minimal risk, then one may expect that changes in role behaviour distributions influence the spread of HIV. As pointed out by Trichopoulos *et al.* (1988), role separation is expected to reduce the spread of HIV since those who are practicing insertive intercourse would be at low risk and those practicing receptive intercourse would not be at very high risk because of the low prevalence of HIV among their sexual partners.

Based on this conjecture Wiley and Herschkorn (1989) constructed a theoretical model for exploring the effect of differentiation of roles in anal intercourse on the size of AIDS epidemics in homosexual populations. Under the assumption of no risk associated with insertive anal intercourse it was shown that epidemic intensity increases with increasing size of the dual-role (both insertive and receptive) subpopulation. Their paper, however, was not concerned with the analysis of specific data. Recently van Griensven *et al.* (1990) and van Zessen and van Griensven (1992) provided empirical evidence, using data from the first two cycles of the Amsterdam cohort, that homosexual role behaviour is a factor in the spread of HIV. The data were further analysed by van Druten *et al.* (1992) using a role separation mixing model.

Here we report on further modelling based on Markov chain theory using 8 cycles of data collection in the period 1984–1988. First a short summary is given of some main elements of the role separation mixing model.

Role separation mixing model

Using two cycles of data collection of the Amsterdam cohort – data on homo-sexual role behaviour and HIV prevalence in 1984–1985 – a role separation mixing model has been developed. The men are classified into four sexual subgroups:

1. no anal intercourse;

2. anal insertive only;

3. anal receptive only;

4. both insertive and receptive (dual-role behaviour).

These subgroups are associated with different levels of acquiring HIV infection. As long as sexual role behaviour is constant, say in time period (t_1, t_2), one can define κ_{ij}^m to be the mean number of partners in group j in time period (t_1, t_2) of persons in group i; the superscript m refers to the role of the partner in sexual anal intercourse ($m = i$: partners are insertive; $m = r$: partners are receptive). The sexual mixing matrix associated with anal intercourse has 8 parameters, 4 with partner-type insertive ($m = i$) and 4 with partner-type receptive ($m = r$). The parameters are not independent, receptive and insertive partners should match; this results in 4 side conditions. The Amsterdam cohort data provides estimates of 4 model related parameters (linear combinations of κ_{ij}^m). In a closed cohort these estimates should obey the law of conservation of sex. A difficult problem is the determination of the contact matrix κ_{ij}^m. Actually the contact matrix κ_{ij}^m is not identifiable from the cohort data without an additional assumption. Using the assumption of proportionate random mixing and Least Squares estimates of the data related parameters (subject to the law of conservation of sex) a solution was obtained. Furthermore a sensitivity analysis was employed. The results indicated that without validation of the type of mixing it will be difficult to determine the contact matrix. A provisional estimate was obtained for the probability of HIV transmission from an infected insertive partner (in subgroup 2 or 4) to a receptive susceptible in subgroup 4. Assuming a closed cohort this probability assumes a value between 1 and 5% per partnership. The results supported the conjecture that there are differences between the risks of receptive and insertive anal intercourse, with the latter carrying the smaller risk. It was shown that role behaviour and the changes therein should be taken into account when modelling the spread of HIV. Figure 1 shows the main routes of HIV transmission in the role separation mixing model.

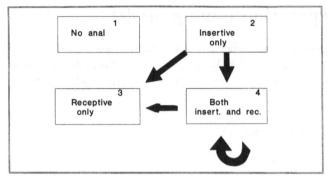

Figure 1: Role separation mixing model: main routes of HIV transmission

Role behaviour and the spread of HIV

Recently we have studied changes in homosexual role behaviour in the Amsterdam cohort over a period of 8 cycles of data collection, in the period 1984–1988. It appears that Markov chain theory can be used to predict homosexual role behaviour and that changes in sexual role behaviour can to a large extent explain the spread of HIV in role specific subgroups. Changes in role behaviour at connected cycles can be studied by turnover (transition) matrices $T(t)$, $t = 1, \ldots, 7$.

Let the turnover matrix $T(t) = (T_{ij}(t))$ at the connected cycles $t, t + 1$, be defined so that $T_{ij}(t)$ is the proportion of men classified in subgroup i at cycle t who are classified into subgroup j at cycle $t+1$ ($i, j = 1, \ldots, 4$). From the definition of $T_{ij}(t)$, it follows immediately that

$$\sum_j T_{ij}(t) = 1, \quad (i = 1, \ldots, 4).$$

The 7 turnover matrices $T(t)$, ($t = 1, \ldots, 7$), are remarkably similar. This suggests that we may use homogeneous Markov chain theory to predict the changes in the role behaviour distributions. The state space is the set of role behaviour options (no anal, insertive only, receptive only, dual-role behaviour). Whenever the process is in state i, there is a fixed probability T_{ij} that it will be next in state j. For a Markov chain, the conditional probability distribution of any future state depends only on the present state. The process is characterized by the initial probability distribution of being in state i ($i = 1, \ldots, 4$) and the matrix $T = (T_{ij})$ of transition probabilities. In the application we focussed on two particular questions:

(a) can the initial turnover matrix $T(1)$, measured at the connected cycles 1–2, predict the role behaviour distributions at the subsequent cycles;

(b) is the limiting role behaviour distribution (Markov equilibrium) stable?[1]

For an (irreducible ergodic) Markov chain the limiting probabilities can be derived from the nth power, T^n, of the transition matrix T. As n approaches infinity, $\lim T_{ij}^n$ exists and is independent of the initial state i ($i = 1, \ldots, 4$). Therefore let

$$\pi_j = \lim_{n \to \infty} T_{ij}^n \quad (j = 1, \ldots, 4), \text{ and } \pi = \begin{bmatrix} \pi_1 \\ \pi_2 \\ \pi_3 \\ \pi_4 \end{bmatrix},$$

then π is the unique solution of the matrix equation,

$$\pi = T^{tr} \pi .$$

Thus π is the eigenvector which corresponds with the eigenvalue 1 of the transpose of the transition matrix T.

Markov equilibrium appears not to be a moving target and the initial turnover matrix $T(1)$, predicts rather well the role behaviour distributions in the years 1984–1988.

HIV prevalence in the four subgroups in the Amsterdam cohort in 1984–1988 is a result of:

(a) HIV infections before and during the period of observation;

(b) changes in role behaviour;

(c) loss to follow-up.

The effect of changes in role behaviour on the spread of HIV in role specific subgroups is determined by the 7 turnover matrices $T(t)$, $t = 1, \ldots, 7$. Let $x(t)$ and $y(t)$ be the vectors describing the numbers of HIV-negative and HIV-positive men in the four subgroups at cycle t. Let, in the absence of new HIV infections in period 1984–1988, $x_e(t+1)$ and $y_e(t+1)$ be the vectors describing the classification of men in the four subgroups at cycle $t + 1$ (classification based on turnover matrix $T(t)$ and no seroconversions between cycle t and $t + 1$). We then have ($t = 1, \ldots, 7$),

$$x_e(t + 1) = T^{tr}(t)x(t) \text{ and } y_e(t + 1) = T^{tr}(t)y(t) .$$

The values of $y_e(t+1)$ relative to $n_e(t+1)$, i.e. the 'expected' HIV prevalence rates in the four subgroups at cycle $t+1$ ($t = 1, \ldots, 7$), were compared with the observed rates. The predicted and the observed rates show similar patterns of HIV prevalence, although the levels of HIV prevalence observed in subgroups 3 and 4 are higher than expected. This excess cannot be explained by loss

---

[1]Stable in an epidemiological sense

to follow-up, and suggests that the highest risk of HIV infection is associated with receptive and dual-role behaviour. Further research is necessary, but at present it seems justified to say that Markov chain theory and role separation mixing models may be tools for studying change in homosexual role behaviour and the effects on the spread of HIV in role specific subgroups.

References

van Druten, J.A.M., van Griensven, G.J.P. and Hendriks, J.C.M. (1992) 'Homo-sexual role separation: implications for analysing and modelling the spread of HIV', *J. Sex Res.* **29**(4), 477–499.

van Griensven, G.J.P., de Vroome, E.M.M., Veugelers, P. and Coutinho, R.A. (1990) 'Heterogeneity and fluctuations in homosexual behaviour: implications for modelling the AIDS epidemic'. In *Abstracts, Sixth International Conference on AIDS*, Volume 1, San Francisco, 20–24 June, 1990, abstract no. Th.C.112, 161.

Trichopoulos, D., Sparos, L. and Petridou, E. (1988) 'Homosexual role separation and spread of AIDS', *Lancet*, ii, 966.

Wiley, J.A. and Herschkorn, S.J. (1989) 'Homosexual role separation and AIDS epidemics: insights from elementary models', *J. Sex Res.* **26**, 434–449.

van Zessen, G.J., and van Griensven, G.J.P. (1992) 'Heterogeneous mixing models, homosexual role separation and consistency over time'. In *AIDS Impact Assess-ment Modelling and Scenario Analysis. Proceedings of the 3rd EC Workshop on AIDS Modelling and Scenario Analysis 1989*, J.C. Jager and E.J. Ruitenberg (eds.), Elsevier, Amsterdam, 203–210.

Homogeneity Tests for Groupings of AIDS Patient Classifications

Daphne Smith and Lynne Billard

Classifications for identifying AIDS cases can take many forms depending often on the use for which the data were assembled. These can include geographical, gender, behavioural, racial and risk factor classifications, with or without further subgroupings within these broader classes. Of interest herein is the modelling of the number of cases over time by traditional autoregressive-moving average time series models for purposes of short term forecasting. One question then to be answered is whether or not some or all of these classifications can be grouped homogeneously.

Our attention is focussed on AIDS reported cases for the United States as reported by the Centers for Disease Control (CDC 1992), using those cases meeting the CDC definition of AIDS. The observed data values refer to the month and year in which the AIDS disease was first diagnosed. Cases diagnosed before 1982 have been recorded as cumulative totals through December 1981. Cases diagnosed from January 1982 through June 1991 are recorded as the number of cases in a given month. In this study, patients are classified according to specific CDC classifications, viz., homosexual males, bisexual males, heterosexual males, intravenous (IV) drug use and male homosexual/bisexual contact, IV drug use (female and heterosexual males), haemophilia/coagulation disorder, recipient of transfusion of blood products or tissue, white males, black males, hispanic males, total males, white females, black females, hispanic females, and total females. Thus, the aim of the analysis is to consider which of these patient classifications can be identified by a common time series model. To achieve this, a time series model is fitted to each classification. Then, groups of these classifications are proposed. A test of homogeneity for the models within each group is applied using the test statistic developed for such purposes in Basawa *et al.* (1984).

To illustrate the method, let us suppose the underlying model for the classifications in a particular group is a first order moving average process, MA(1), that is, the observation value, after suitable transformation if necessary, for month i, in the jth classification, satisfies

$$Y_{i,j} = Z_{i,j} - \theta_j Z_{i-1,j} \quad i = 1, ..., n_j, \; j = 1, ..., m,$$

where $Z_{i,j}$ are independent normally distributed error terms with mean zero and variance σ^2.

The null hypothesis is that the m classifications follow the same model, $H_0 : \theta_1 = \ldots = \theta_m = \theta_{H_0}$, against the alternative hypothesis that at least one θ_j is different. The likelihood ratio statistic for testing H_0 is defined by

$$Q = -2\log\{L(\hat{\beta}_{H_0})/L(\hat{\beta})\}$$

where $L(\beta)$ is the likelihood function based on all m data sets, $\hat{\beta}$ is the maximum likelihood estimator of $\beta = (\theta_1, \ldots, \theta_m, \sigma^2)$ and $\hat{\beta}_{H_0}$ is the maximum likelihood estimator of β restricted by H_0.

The likelihood function $L(\beta)$ is

$$L(\beta) = \prod_{j=1}^{m} L_j(\theta_j)$$

where

$$
\begin{aligned}
L_j(\theta_j) &= (2\pi)^{-n_j/2} \exp\{-\frac{1}{2}\sum_{i=1}^{n_j} Y_{i,j}^2\} \\
&= (2\pi)^{-n_j/2} \exp\{-\frac{1}{2}\sum_{i=1}^{n_j}(Z_{i,j} - \theta_j Z_{i-1,j})\} \\
&= \text{constant} \times \exp\{-\frac{1}{2}S_j(\theta_j)\}.
\end{aligned}
$$

The unresricted maximum likelihood estimator of θ_j, $\hat{\theta}_j$, is obtained by solving the equation

$$\frac{\partial}{\partial \theta_j} S_j(\theta_j) = 0, j = 1, \ldots, m.$$

Likewise, the restricted (by H_0) likelihood function $L(\beta_{H_0})$ is

$$
\begin{aligned}
L(\beta_{H_0}) &= (2\pi)^{-n/2} \exp\{-\frac{1}{2}\sum_{j=1}^{m}\sum_{i=1}^{n_j} Y_{i,j}^2\} \\
&= \text{constant} \times \exp\{-\frac{1}{2}\sum_{j=1}^{m} S_j(\theta_{H_0})\}
\end{aligned}
$$

and hence, the restricted maximum likelihood estimator of $\beta = \beta_{H_0} = (\theta_{H_0}, \ldots, \theta_{H_0}), \hat{\beta}_{H_0}$, is found by solving

$$\sum_{j=1}^{m} \frac{d}{d\beta} S_j(\beta) = 0.$$

Therefore, the likelihood ratio test statistic Q becomes

$$Q = \sum_{j=1}^{m}\{S_j(\hat{\theta}_{H_0}) - S_j(\hat{\theta}_j)\}.$$

Under H_0, the limiting distribution of Q is that of a chi-square distribution with $(m-1)$ degrees of freedom.

For example, suppose we have a grouping of females by race, viz., white, black, or hispanic. After the data for each of these three series are suitably transformed, differencing is applied to achieve a stationary process. In this case, if $X_{i,j}$ is the total number of female AIDS cases at the end of month i for the jth race, $i = 1, \ldots, 115$, $j = 1, 2, 3$, then

$$Y_{i,j} = \nabla^2 \log X_{i,j} \ , \qquad \nabla W_i = W_i - W_{i-1},$$

formed a stationary process. Examining plots of the resultant autocorrelation functions and partial autocorrelation functions suggested that the $\{Y_{i,j}\}$ followed a moving average process of order one.

When the theory is applied to these data, the maximum likelihood estimates of θ_j are found to be

$$
\begin{array}{lr}
\text{white females} & \hat{\theta}_1 = 0.889 \\
\text{black females} & \hat{\theta}_2 = 0.847 \\
\text{hispanic females} & \hat{\theta}_3 = 0.912
\end{array}
$$

and the (restricted) estimate of θ_j under H_0 is

$$\hat{\theta}_1 = \hat{\theta}_2 = \hat{\theta}_3 = \hat{\theta} = 0.883.$$

The test statistic is

$$Q = 2.757,$$

to be compared with $\chi^2_2(5\%) = 5.99$. Therefore, based on this analysis, all three racial classifications for females can be grouped homogeneously and modelled by the same time series model with the common parameter θ; thus parsimony has been achieved.

Similar results pertained when considering the heterosexual male population by racial classification. Again, after a log transformation and twice differencing to obtain stationarity, a MA(1) model obtained for each racial class. Thence, the respective maximum likelihood estimates are

$$
\begin{array}{lr}
\text{white heterosexual males} & \hat{\theta}_1 = 0.418 \\
\text{black heterosexual males} & \hat{\theta}_2 = 0.862 \\
\text{hispanic heterosexual males} & \hat{\theta}_3 = 0.784
\end{array}
$$

with the restricted (under H_0) estimate of θ_j being

$$\hat{\theta}_1 = \hat{\theta}_2 = \hat{\theta}_3 = \hat{\theta} = 0.755$$

and test statistic $Q = 4.767$, which again supports the hypothesis that all three racial groups follow a common model.

In contrast, when males were classified according to reported behavioural category, viz., homosexual, bisexual, heterosexual, we found that (after the same transformations as before, i.e., log and twice differencing) homosexual and bisexual males were modelled by a mixed autoregressive moving average process ARMA(1,1) while heterosexuals were modelled as a pure MA(1) process. To apply the test of homogeneity here, it is necessary to 'add' the first order autoregressive parameter, so that the test is being applied to $m = 3$ models each of which follows the same order ARMA(1,1) process. Thus, the maximum likelihood estimates were accordingly found to be, respectively,

$$\begin{aligned}
\text{homosexual males} \quad &\hat{\phi}_1 = 0.286, \ \hat{\theta}_1 = 0.462 \\
\text{bisexual males} \quad &\hat{\phi}_2 = -0.327, \ \hat{\theta}_2 = 0.794 \\
\text{heterosexual males} \quad &\hat{\phi}_3 = 0.000, \ \hat{\theta}_3 = 0.686.
\end{aligned}$$

The test statistic $Q = 16.75$ which when compared with $\chi^2_4(1\%) = 13.28$ clearly indicates that the three models are not homogeneous.

As a final example, when looking at racial classifications for all males (regardless of behavioural category), we see that (after again the same transformations as before) white males are modelled by a MA(2) process (with $\hat{\theta}_1 = 0.286$, $\hat{\theta}_2 = 0.462$), black males are modelled by a MA(1) process (with $\hat{\theta}_1 = 0.745$), hispanic males are modelled by an AR(2) process (with $\hat{\phi}_1 = -0.887$, $\hat{\phi}_2 = -0.509$) and other racial groups by a MA(1) process (with $\hat{\theta}_1 = 0.926$). Since the model autogressive order p and moving average order q are not consistent for each racial group, this test statistic Q cannot be applied (since such a test is a test of homogeneity of parameter values, which naturally presupposes common p and q values).

Clearly, other groups of classifications can be tested for homogeneity using these same methods.

References

Basawa, I.V., Billard, L. and Srinivasan, R. (1984) 'Large sample tests of homogeneity for time series models', *Biometrika* **71**, 203–206.

Centers for Disease Control (1992) *AIDS Public Information Data Set*, Division of HIV/AIDS.

Risk Factors for Heterosexual Transmission of HIV

Katherine L. Fielding

Partner studies of heterosexual transmission of HIV have observed tranmissions after relatively few sexual contacts and couples who have remained discordant, with respect to HIV, whilst considered to be at high risk over prolonged periods, suggesting huge variation between individuals in whether a contact seroconverts. This paper is based on a longitudinal partner study which aims to identify behavioural and biological factors which influence heterosexual transmission of HIV. The index case (the first infected) is defined as a patient who is HIV positive whilst the contact partner is a person of the opposite sex who has had a sexual relationship with the index case. In Edinburgh, from October 1987 to the beginning of June 1992, one-hundred and twenty couples have been recruited where the contact's risk of infection is only through heterosexual intercourse with his/her index case. At recruitment, 24 couples (20%) were concordant with respect to HIV and since recruitment one contact has seroconverted. At the initial interview the contact is asked about her/his past sexual practices and contraceptive use and counselled about safer sex. Follow-up interviews of negative contacts take place to reassess these behavioural data and their HIV status. Biological data on the index is also available as the majority of cases are in clinical care.

Three factors which might influence heterosexual transmission of HIV are to be assessed:

- behavioural aspects of the couple,

- infectivity of the index,

- susceptibility of contact.

Behavioural data are required to confirm that the virus has an 'opportunity' to transmit. Virological and immunological factors form the basis for assessing the infectivity of the index and susceptibility of the contact. HLA type, secretor status and cervical abnormalities (if contact is female) are all thought to be associated with the susceptibility of the contact to HIV. Interest also lies in evaluating whether infectivity of the index case changes with the disease course of HIV infection. Evidence suggests that infectivity peaks close to the time of seroconversion and around the time of onset of symptoms and diagnosis of AIDS (Ho *et al.* 1989). There is also some evidence that HIV positive cases with low CD4 counts and p24 antigenaemia are more infectious (MRC 1992). Immunological data collected on the index case includes CD4 counts and p24 antigen. It is anticipated that these data will be used to model infectivity of the index cases in the Edinburgh cohort. However, at present, a time dependent risk score (based on sex, age, CD4%, total lymphocyte count, WBC and IgA) has been calculated, describing the health of the index, and will be used as a proxy for infectivity. Using these data a behavioural and biological profile of each couple can be constructed, in yearly blocks, over the period the contact is at risk of infection. Data corresponding to yearly blocks are required due to time dependence of some factors associated with transmission, for example, changes in behaviour of the couple such as contraceptive methods and health of the index case.

The seroconversion dates of the index cases and the contacts (if appropriate) are not known precisely, but only to within a seroconversion interval defined by the last negative and first positive test. Thus, some couple/year data cannot be determined with certainty as occurring pre- or post-seroconversion for either index or contact. This is overcome by generating a year of seroconversion for the index and contact (if appropriate) using knowledge of the HIV infection curve in Edinburgh; from these data the profile of a couple, in yearly blocks, can be constructed. This process is repeated so that many data sets are constructed, allowing for the uncertainity of the actual year the index and contact (if appropriate) seroconverts; these data sets are then analysed.

A fully appropriate analysis of these data should be based on a random effects generalized linear model therefore allowing for repeated years within couples. The linear logistic model with Gaussian random effects will be used where the interest lies in the the probability of transmission in a particular year, that is logit(contact of couple i seroconverts in year j) which is a linear function of the covariates x_{ijk} where i identifies the couple and j identifies the year of risk of infection. As b_i relates to couple i the contact effect will be confounded with the index effect. Since some index cases provide more than one contact it would be necessary to have two random effects, one associated with the contact and the other with the index, to overcome this problem and this is a possibility for future analyses. Other outcome variables are of interest, such as 'protected intercourse against HIV' defined as condom use as a proportion of non-abstinent time, in a particular year. Future work will extend this outcome to an ordered categorical variable.

We adopt a quasi-likelihood method based on generalized estimating equations (Zeger and Liang 1986). Using a 'population-averaged' approach we consider the marginal expectation of the response and specify a 'working' correlation matrix for the vector of responses. A related method, based on multi-level models, will also be examined using ML3 software and will allow a comparison of results. For further details of this work, see Fielding *et al.* (1995).

References

Fielding, K.L., Brettle, K.P., Gore, S.M., O'Brien, F., Wyld, R., Robertson, J.R., and Weightman, R. (1995) 'Heterosexual transmission of HIV analysed by generalised estimating equations', *Stat. Med.*, to appear.

Ho, D.D., Moudgil, T. and Alam, M. (1989) 'Quantitation of Human Immunodeficiency Virus Type I in the Blood of Infected Persons', *New Eng. J. Med.* **321**, 1621–1625.

MRC (1992) *Summary of the 2nd MRC AIDS Epidemiology Workshop; Proceedings and Conclusions, Section 2.*

Zeger, S.L., and Liang, K. (1986) 'Longitudinal Data Analysis for Discrete and Continuous Outcomes', *Biometrics* **42**, 121–130.

The Effect of Behavioural Change on the Prediction of R_0 in the Transmission of AIDS

David Tudor, Klaus Dietz and Hans Heesterbeek

Diekmann *et al.* (1991) developed a model for calculating R_0 for a multi-state disease including pair formation and dissolution. This model is analogous to a model of Blythe and Anderson (1988) and Jacquez *et al.* (1988) which did not include pair formation. The model in Diekmann *et al.* (1991) is a generalization of the model of Diekmann *et al.* (1990). In the sequel to Diekmann *et al.* (1991), Dietz *et al.* (1993) investigated the effects of variable HIV-infectivity. This paper will summarize the model and results of Dietz *et al.* (1993) and will present further results obtained with the same model.

We assume four stages of HIV-infection, three pre-AIDS, and the final stage, AIDS. The parameters incorporated in the model are:

θ_i transition rate from infection state i to infection state $i +$ 1. $\theta_1 = 4.0$ per year; $\theta_2 = \theta_3 = 0.2$ per year;

$p_i(k)$ probability of infection by an infective of sex k in infection state i.

μ_0 death rate of susceptibles (both sexes).

μ_i death rate of infected individuals in infection state i. $\mu_i = 0.02$ per year ($i \neq 4$); $\mu_4 = 0.5$ per year.

$\rho_i(k)$ partner acquisition rate of an individual of sex k in infection state i.

σ break-up rate
    We pick σ as a function of ρ to guarantee that the total expected number of contacts is 500 for the infectious period.

s_{ij} probability that an infected individual in state i remains sexually active after separating from a partner in infection state j.
    The effect of s will be demonstrated in the sequel.

β sexual contact rate.
    $\beta = 100$ per year in the numerical calculations.

q probability per contact of use of condoms.
    We take $q = 0$ for the calculations.

The pairings considered are (note $[\cdot]$ indicates male and $(\cdot)$ female, the numbers refer to the stage of HIV infection and + or − means seropositive or seronegative):

For the male index case:

$$
\begin{array}{cccc}
[+1] & [+2] & [+3] & [+4] \\
[+1](-) & [+2](-) & [+3](-) & [+4](-) \\
[+1](+1) & [+2](+1) & [+3](+1) & [+4](+1) \\
[+1](+2) & [+2](+2) & [+3](+2) & [+4](+2) \\
[+1](+3) & [+2](+3) & [+3](+3) & [+4](+3) \\
[+1](+4) & [+2](+4) & [+3](+4) & [+4](+4)
\end{array}
$$

The analogous cases with the square and round brackets exchanged for the female index case is also included in the model, but not presented here.

In Dietz *et al.* (1993) the matrix of transition probabilities between the pairing states taking the parameters above into account was presented as a matrix G, so that $-G^{-1}$ gives the waiting times in each of the pairing states. Then the multi-type branching process represented by the matrix M of secondary cases of males produced by females, respectively, secondary cases of females produced by males, is given by

$$
\begin{pmatrix} 0 & M_2 \\ M_1 & 0 \end{pmatrix}
$$

where M_1 describes the secondary male cases generated by a female, and M_2 describes the secondary female cases generated by a male.

By the theory of multi-type branching processes (result of Diekmann *et al.* (1991)), R_0 is given by the Perron-Frobenius (PF) eigenvalue of M, and the components of the corresponding eigenvector, $\boldsymbol{v}$, give the probabilities, respectively, of starting in the following states (collectively exhaustive list of starting possibilities):

$$
\begin{array}{lll}
1:[+1](+1) & 2:[+1](+2) & 3:[+1](+3) \\
4:(+1)[+1] & 5:(+1)[+2] & 6:(+1)[+3]
\end{array}
$$

Next, we want to calculate the number of partners and the number of contacts after infection. For the number of partners, we dot the vector $\boldsymbol{v}$ with the vector whose components are:

1: to 3: the sum of the time spent in infection-pair state $[+1]$, $[+2]$, $[+3]$ after starting in the infection-pair state $[+1](+i)$, where i is the component 1 to 3, respectively.

4: to 6: the sum of the time spent in infection-pair state $(+1)$, $(+2)$, $(+3)$ after starting in the infection-pair state $(+1)[+i]$, where i is the component 4 to 6, respectively.

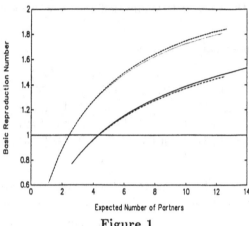

Expected Number of Partners

Figure 1

This dot product is then multiplied by ρ, the rate of acquisition of new partners.

To calculate the number of contacts within established partnerships, we multiply β, the contact rate within partnerships by the dot product of v with the vector of sums of times spent in partnerships. The total number of contacts is the sum of the two calculations from this and the previous paragraph.

The first graphics (see Figure 1) using this model compare the expected number of partners (after infection) versus R_0 for variable infectivity $p_i(k)$. Keeping the average infectivity constant, the four cases considered are:

I: sex dependent, time dependent: $p_1(1) = 0.05$, $p_2(1) = 0.001$, $p_3(1) = 0.01$, $p_4(k) = 0$, $p_1(2) = 0.025$, $p_2(2) = 0.0005$, $p_3(2) = 0.005$.

II: sex independent, time dependent: $p_1 = 0.0354$, $p_2 = 0.0007$, $p_3 = 0.0071$.

III: sex dependent, time independent: $p_{men} = 0.00654$, $p_{women} = 0.00327$.

IV: sex independent, time independent: all $p_i = 0.00462$.

Figure 1 shows the relationship: $R_0(I) \leq R_0(II) \leq R_0(III) \leq R_0(IV)$.

Other (not previously reported) results:

- R_1, the basic reproduction ratio for men is the PF eigenvalue of M_1.

- R_2, the basic reproduction ratio for women is the PF eigenvalue of M_2.

- $R_0 = \sqrt{R_1 \cdot R_2}$.

- The variable s has a considerable effect on the the predictions of R_0 as a function of the expected number of partners (see Figure 2).

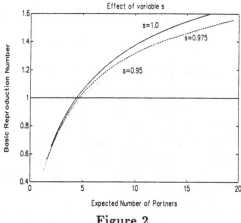

Figure 2

- In other calculations not presented here, distinguishing q_0, the probability of condom use at the first contact, from q, the probability of condom use on subsequent contacts was shown to have a negligible effect.

References

Blythe, S.P. and Anderson, R.M. (1988) 'Variable infectiousness in HIV transmission models', *IMA J. Math. Appl. Med. Biol.* **5**, 181–200.

Diekmann, O., Dietz, K. and Heesterbeek, J.A.P. (1991) 'The basic reproduction ratio for sexually transmitted diseases I: theoretical considerations', *Math. Biosci.* **107**, 325–339.

Diekmann, O., Heesterbeek, J.A.P. and Metz, J.A.J. (1990) 'On the definition and the calculation of the basic reproduction ratio R_0 in models for infectious diseases in heterogeneous populations', *J. Math. Biol.* **28**, 365–382.

Dietz, K., Heesterbeek, J.A.P. and Tudor, D.W. (1993) 'The basic reproduction ratio for sexually transmitted diseases II: effects of varaible HIV-infectivity', *Math. Biosci.* **117**, 35–48.

Jacquez, J.A., Simon, C.P., Koopman, J., Sattenspiel, L. and Perry, T. (1988) 'Modeling and analysing HIV transmission: the effect of contact patterns', *Math. Biosci.* **92**, 119–199.

The Saturating Contact Rate in Epidemic Models

J.A.P. Heesterbeek and J.A.J. Metz

We consider a population of density n (i.e. n individuals per unit area). Suppose the individuals in this population have some specified kind of pairwise contacts of some given average duration. We want to know what the average fraction of the population is that is engaged in a contact at any given time (in other words, the fraction of the time that will be taken up by contacts for any given individual), and we denote this fraction by $c(n)$.

The following reasonable properties of the function $c(\cdot)$ are usually assumed in the literature (see, for example, Thieme (1992)): $c(n) > 0$ for all $n > 0$; $c(n)$ is non-decreasing in n; $c(n)$ is linear for small n and constant for very large n. Of course many functional forms can be suggested to satisfy these properties. Dietz (1992) suggested the form $c(n) = \frac{an}{b+cn}$ as a convenient phenomenological description (this is the famous Holling disc equation from a submodel of a predator that searches and 'handles' prey). In predator-prey population dynamics this functional response is derived by an argument that assumes a predator lives in an abundance of prey and is time-limited from catching more and more prey by the fact that it needs to eat once in a while the prey it has already caught. If the prey density is increased further and further the number of prey actually caught per predator will saturate because of this time-limitation (Holling 1966). In the context of epidemiology, however, where predator and prey are replaced by infected and susceptible individuals, this argument is incomplete because now both individuals taking part in a contact are time-limited. In Heesterbeek and Metz (1993) we give a derivation, based on mechanistic assumptions about the contact process, of the function $c(\cdot)$ taking this into account.

Let $x(t)$ denote the density of single individuals at time t (i.e. those individuals that are, at time t, not engaged in a contact of the specified kind). Two single individuals can form a (social) complex (in which the contacts will take place) with some probability per unit of time ρ and such a complex can break up into two singles with some probability per unit of time σ. So, the average complex duration is $1/\sigma$. The density of complexes at time t is denoted by $k(t)$, so we have a conservation equation $x(t) + 2k(t) = n(t)$. We assume that the temporary complexes are formed between individuals according to law of mass-action kinetics. Our key assumption is that the complexes are only short lived, as compared to the time-scale on which the demographic processess occur.

The above assumptions lead to the following system of differential equations that describe the changes in x and k,

$$\frac{dx}{dt} = -\rho x^2 + 2\sigma k, \qquad \frac{dk}{dt} = \frac{1}{2}\rho x^2 - \sigma k$$

because one single individual contributes one half to a complex, and one complex gives two single individuals when it dissolves. Note that births and deaths do not appear in these equations as a result of our key assumption about the time-scales at which the various processes occur; n is constant on the time-scale of complex formation and dissociation (one can make this argument mathematically precise; for details see Heesterbeek and Metz (1993)). If we look at the (quasi) steady state of this simple system, we find

$$\bar{k} = \frac{1}{2}\theta\bar{x}^2$$

where $\theta := \rho/\sigma$, which together with the conservation equation $\bar{x} + 2\bar{k} = n$ leads to the (quasi) steady state density $\bar{k} = c(n)n$ with

$$c(n) = \frac{2\theta n}{1 + 2\theta n + \sqrt{1 + 4\theta n}} \tag{1}$$

The function $c(\cdot)$ can easily be seen to have the properties listed in the second paragraph.

When we want to apply this reasoning to epidemic models, we are, in the simplest case, interested in two types of single individuals, susceptibles and infectives. Of the three possible types of complexes formed, only the complexes involving an infective and a susceptible are important for the transmission rate that describes the number of new cases arising per unit of time per unit area. If we let β describe the transmission rate constant within a susceptible/infective complex, and we denote the (quasi) steady state density of these complexes by $\bar{k}_{12}$, then the transmission rate is $\beta\bar{k}_{12}$. We allow the rates of complex formation and dissociation to depend on the type of complex and introduce ρ_{lj}, σ_{lj} (with the obvious interpretations). In general, one cannot give an explicit expression for $\bar{k}_{12}$ but in the special case that

$$\frac{\rho_{lj}}{\sigma_{lj}} = \theta, \text{ for all } l, j$$

we obtain

$$\beta\bar{k}_{12} = \frac{2\theta n\beta}{1 + 2\theta n + \sqrt{1 + 4\theta n}}\frac{si}{n} = \beta c(n)s\frac{i}{n} \tag{2}$$

where s and i are the densities of susceptible and infective individuals, respectively (counting both the single individuals and those involved in a complex), and where $c(n)$ is given by (1), as in the single-type case (see Heesterbeek and Metz (1993) for details, the general result and other special cases).

Instead of generalising the above approach, let us look at a special case of (2). If the contacts between individuals were instantaneous and governed by mass-action kinetics, the transmission rate would be given by $\hat{\beta}si$, where $\hat{\beta}$ is the transmission rate constant, since by definition of the mass-action law (originating in chemical reaction kinetics) the collision rate of two types of molecule is proportional to the product of the concentrations of the molecule-types (which translates into the product of the densities of susceptible and infective individuals in the epidemiological context). If contacts are instantaneous, their average duration is zero. Therefore, the transmission rate $\hat{\beta}si$ should be obtained as a special case of (2) if we let the average complex duration $\frac{1}{\sigma}$ tend to zero (i.e. let $\sigma \to \infty$). First note that letting σ tend to infinity, implies that $\theta \to 0$ if ρ remains fixed. Second, if the complex duration tends to zero and if we do not adjust the transmission rate constant β, then the infection probability per contact will also tend to zero. This can easily be seen directly from the probability p of transmission of infection per complex,

$$p = \int_0^\infty (1 - e^{-\beta t})\sigma e^{-\sigma t}dt, \tag{3}$$

where the first expression under the integral-sign is the probability that transmission occurs within the first t time-units of the existence of the complex, and the second term is the probability density function for complex duration. Calculating p leads to

$$p = \frac{\beta}{\beta + \sigma} = \frac{\beta/\sigma}{\beta/\sigma + 1}$$

One now sees that the correct procedure in letting $\sigma \to \infty$ is to let $\beta \to \infty$ so as to keep the average infection probability p per complex fixed. This is the same as assuming that $\beta/\sigma = b$, a constant. By rewriting (2) and taking limits, the instantaneous mass-action expression is now obtained,

$$\lim_{\substack{\sigma,\beta \to \infty \\ \beta/\sigma = b}} \frac{2\rho bn}{1 + 2\theta n + \sqrt{1 + 4\theta n}} \frac{si}{n} = 2\rho bns\frac{i}{n} = \hat{\beta}si$$

with $\hat{\beta} := 2\rho\beta/\sigma$.

References

Dietz, K. (1982) 'Overall population patterns in the transmission cycle of infectious disease agents'. In *Population Biology of Infectious Diseases*, R.M. Anderson and R.M. May (ed.), Springer, 87–102.

Heesterbeek, J.A.P. and Metz, J.A.J (1993) 'The saturating contact rate in marriage and epidemic models', *J. Math. Biol.* **31**, 529–539.

Holling, C.S. (1966) 'The functional response of invertebrate predators to prey density', *Mem. Ent. Soc. Canada* **48**.

Thieme, H.R. (1992) 'Epidemic and demographic interaction in the spread of potentially fatal diseases in growing populations', *Math. Biosci.* **111**, 99–130.

A Liapunov Function Approach to Computing R_0

Carl P. Simon, John A. Jacquez, and James S. Koopman

The basic reproduction number R_0 plays a central role in mathematical models of the spread of communicable diseases. It is usually defined as 'the number of disease transmitting contacts by an average infective, during the course of his or her infection, in a population of susceptibles.' With this definition, it is clear that the disease will die out if and only if $R_0 < 1$. In simple models, R_0 appears as the product of the average number c of contacts per person per period, the probability β that a contact transmits infection, and the average length D of the infectious period.

In a simple differential equation SIS model in a homogeneous population, let X be the number of susceptibles, Y the number of infectives and $N = X + Y$ the size of the population. Let α be the average rate at which infecteds recover, so that the average duration of the infection is $D = 1/\alpha$. Then, the dynamics for Y is given by: $\dot{Y} = c\beta X(Y/N) - \alpha Y$, or after factoring out αY and replacing $c\beta(1/\alpha)$ by R_0:

$$\dot{Y} = \alpha Y \left(R_0 \frac{X}{N} - 1 \right). \tag{1}$$

Of course, $X/N \le 1$. If $R_0 \le 1$, then $R_0(X/N) - 1 < 0$ for $Y > 0$, and $\dot{Y} < 0$. It follows that the solution $Y(t)$ will be monotone decreasing to $Y = 0$. On the other hand, if $R_0 > 1$, then for $Y(0)$ small enough, $R_0(X(0)/N) - 1 > 0$, $\dot{Y} > 0$; and so $Y(t)$ increases away from 0. In the first case, the disease free equilibrium is globally asymptotically stable; in the second case, it is unstable. Finally, if (X^*, Y^*) is an *endemic* equilibrium for (1), with $Y^* > 0$, then (1) implies that

$$\frac{X^*}{N} = \frac{1}{R_0} \quad \text{and} \quad \frac{Y^*}{N} = 1 - \frac{1}{R_0}. \tag{2}$$

This analysis illustrates the many roles that the basic reproduction number plays. Mathematically, it gives a criterion for the local stability of the disease-free equilibrium $Y = 0$ of the model. In this role, it also describes the initial rate of the spread of the disease; see Jacquez and Simon (1990). Epidemiologically, R_0 provides a threshold for disease takeoff; and somewhat surprisingly, when $Y = 0$ is unstable, it even carries important information (2) about the endemic equilibrium.

The goal of this note is to illustrate that similar results hold for much more complex models, by surprisingly similar techniques. The function $V(X, Y) = Y$ plays the role of a *Liapunov function* for the disease free equilibrium of the above system. In general, a function V defined on the state space S of a dynamical system $\dot{\mathbf{x}} = F(\mathbf{x})$ is a Liapunov function for an equilibrium $\mathbf{x}^*$ in S if

(a) $\mathbf{x}^*$ is a minimizer of V, and

(b) V is decreasing on orbits of the dynamical system. Condition (b) can be rewritten as:

$$0 > \frac{d}{dt} V(\mathbf{x}(t)) = \nabla V(\mathbf{x}(t)) \cdot \dot{\mathbf{x}}(t) = \nabla V(\mathbf{x}) \cdot F(\mathbf{x}) \equiv \dot{V}(\mathbf{x});$$

so it can be checked without solving the system.

If V is a Liapunov function for $\mathbf{x}^*$, then $\mathbf{x}^*$ is a locally asymptotically stable equilibrium of $\dot{\mathbf{x}} = F(\mathbf{x})$. If conditions (a) and (b) hold globally, then $\mathbf{x}^*$ is a globally asymptotically stable equilibrium. The intuition is clear: '$\dot{V} < 0$' means that solutions of $\dot{\mathbf{x}} = F(\mathbf{x})$ move to lower and lower level sets of V toward the point that minimizes V. If Condition (b) is replaced by '$\dot{V}(\mathbf{x}) > 0$ for all $\mathbf{x}$ in a punctured neighborhood of $\mathbf{x}^*$ in S,' then $\mathbf{x}^*$ is an unstable equilibrium of $\dot{\mathbf{x}} = F(\mathbf{x})$.

We complicate the above model in a number of illustrative ways to bring it closer to a model of the spread of HIV. In particular, we add stages of disease (Y_1, Y_2, Y_3, with stage-to-stage transfer rate k), stage-dependent transmissibilities β_i, background death rate μ, rate of recruitment U into the susceptible population, and disease-related death. The resulting dynamic is

$$\dot{X} = -\frac{cX(\sum_i \beta_i Y_i)}{N} + U - \mu X \qquad \dot{Y}_1 = \frac{cX(\sum_i \beta_i Y_i)}{N} - \mu Y_1 - k Y_1 \tag{3}$$

$$\dot{Y}_2 = k Y_1 - \mu Y_2 - k Y_2 \qquad\qquad \dot{Y}_3 = k Y_2 - \mu Y_3 - k Y_3.$$

We look for a Liapunov function of the form $V(X_1, \ldots, X_n, Y_1, \ldots, Y_n) = \sum_i a_i Y_i$, with the a_i's to be chosen. For such a V, $\dot{V} = \sum a_i \dot{Y}_i$ equals:

$$\frac{a_1 c X}{N} \left(\sum_i \beta_i Y_i \right) - [a_1(\mu + k) - a_2 k] Y_1 - [a_2(\mu + k) - a_3 k] Y_2$$

$$- [a_3(\mu + k)] Y_3. \tag{4}$$

If we can choose the a_i's so that the bracketed coefficient of Y_i in (4) equals β_i, we will be able to factor $\sum_i \beta_i Y_i$ from expression (4). Specifically setting

$$a_3 = \frac{\beta_3}{\mu + k}, \qquad a_2 = \frac{1}{\mu + k} \left[\beta_2 + \beta_3 \frac{k}{\mu + k} \right],$$

$$a_1 = \frac{1}{\mu + k} \left[\beta_1 + \frac{\beta_2 k}{\mu + k} + \frac{\beta_3 k^2}{(\mu + k)^2} \right],$$

(4) can be rewritten as:

$$\dot{V} = \left(\frac{a_1 cX}{N} - 1\right) \left(\sum_i \beta_i Y_i\right). \tag{5}$$

Compare (5) with (1). Let $R_0 \equiv a_1 c = \dfrac{1}{\mu + k} \left[\beta_1 + \dfrac{\beta_2 k}{\mu + k} + \dfrac{\beta_3 k^2}{(\mu + k)^2}\right] \cdot c$, an expression of the form $D \cdot \bar{\beta} \cdot c$. Since (5) can be written as

$$\dot{V} = \left(R_0 \frac{X}{N} - 1\right) \left(\sum_i \beta_i Y_i\right),$$

we conclude that, if $R_0 < 1$, the disease free equilibrium $Y_0 = 0$ is a globally asymptotically stable equilibrium for system (3). If $R_0 > 1$, then Y_0 is unstable. Furthermore, as we show in Jacquez *et al.* (1991), if one changes coordinate systems from (X, Y_1, Y_2, Y_3) to (N, V, Y_2, Y_3), system (3) becomes nearly linear. In this case, one can use N, V, Y_2, Y_3 to construct a Liapunov function for the *endemic* equilibrium (X^e, Y^e), thus yielding a rare proof of the global stability of the endemic equilibrium for the case $R_0 > 1$.

This method works in much greater generality, including models with sub-populations and with rather complex mixing patterns (e.g., proportional or preferred mixing), and in models that keep track of *fractions* of the population in each state. See Jacquez *et al.* (1991), Simon and Jacquez (1992) for details. The advantages of this approach include:

(1) a straightforward method for calculating R_0 or at least of some endemicity threshold of the system, and

(2) a simple proof of the global stability of the disease-free equilibrium when $R_0 \leq 1$.

References

Jacquez J.A. and Simon C.P. (1990) 'AIDS: the epidemiological significance of two different mean rates of partner change', *IMA J. Math. Appl. Med. Biol.* **7**, 27–32.

Jacquez J.A., Simon C.P. and Koopman J.S. (1991) 'The reproduction number in deterministic models of contagious diseases', *Comm. Theoret. Biol.* **2**, 159–209.

Simon C.P. and Jacquez J.A. (1992) 'Reproduction numbers and stability of equilibria of SI models for heterogeneous populations', *J. Appl. Math.* **52**, 541–576.

Discussion

MORRIS One aspect that was not considered by Simon's paper is the possibility of individuals changing their behavior, for example, moving from high activity groups to lower activity groups. The next step in the construction of such models should be to allow individuals to change their behavior.

REPLY I strongly agree. We have been including such behavior change in the models we are using to estimate transmission probabilities, but not yet in the models we are analyzing mathematically.

SWINTON Simon has shown that for a wide variety of mixing patterns, there is a globally stable point. In physical problems, the appropriate Liapunov function can usually be interpreted as a conserved quantity that can be related to the system. Can Simon offer any interpretation of his Liapunov function in the same way?

REPLY Yes, the Liapunov function we present can be considered as the total number of infectious contacts (at each t).

GREENHALGH Has Simon tried extending these results to different models, for example, looking at SIS models, introducing incubation periods or more general models?

REPLY We have, especially focusing on more general mixing patterns. However, we have not tried this Liapunov function approach in models that include incubation periods.

Stochastic Models for the Eradication of Poliomyelitis: Minimum Population Size for Polio Virus Persistence

M. Eichner, K.P. Hadeler and K. Dietz

Introduction

In small communities there are usually only few infectious individuals. If they contact too few susceptibles, this might lead to local extinction. On the other hand, if they contact too many susceptibles, they give rise to too many secondary infections. This reduces the number of susceptibles, which may eventually also lead to extinction. In order for long term persistence of the infection to be likely, the population must exceed a minimum size. If there is a long infectious period (e.g. for leprosy, tuberculosis and HIV it lasts for years), the infection can persist even in small populations. High contact rates cause a better 'exploitation' of the population, but they also bear the risk of causing large epidemics which in turn can cause local extinction. Human birth and death rates define the population turnover and therefore also influence the persistence of infectious diseases. It is the aim of this study to determine the minimum population size that is necessary for the persistence of polio virus infection by using stochastic simulations.

Methods

The computer models are stochastic. The sequence of epidemiological events is generated by a Markov process. The type of the event (birth, death of a susceptible, infection, loss of infectivity) is assigned according to a multinomial distribution which depends on the state of the population (number of susceptible and infectious individuals; see Appendix for details). If the event is a birth, the number of susceptibles is increased by one. If it is an infection, the number of susceptibles is decreased by one and the number of infectives is increased by one.

The population is forced to retain constant size (birth rate = death rate; mean life expectancy = 45 years for a developing country and 75 years for an industrialised one). Newborn infants are susceptible. The non-structured population is homogeneously mixing. The structured population consists of subpopulations of equal size. Each individual has the same average number of contacts which is independent of the size of the population or subpopulation. Most of the contacts occur within his or her own subpopulation (where homogeneous mixing is assumed) and only a small constant fraction is shared with individuals of other subpopulations (preferred mixing model). The basic reproduction number of the underlying deterministic model is assumed to be 12 for a developing country and 5 for an industrialised one. This means that a single infectious person would on average cause 12 (or 5) secondary infections in a completely susceptible population (these numbers are derived from age-specific antibody data published by Fox *et al.* (1957), Gear and Measroch (1952), Gelfand and Miller (1956), Gelfand *et al.* (1957), Paul *et al.* (1952a,b), and others; a summary of estimation procedures ⦿ given by Dietz (1993)). This estimate of the basic reproduction number leads to an estimate of 144.3 (60.1) potentially infectious contacts per year. If an infectious individual contacts a susceptible one, the latter immediately becomes infectious without a latent period. The average duration of the infectious period is one month (Gelfand *et al.* 1957, Marine *et al.* 1962). Infectivity is lost at a constant rate and the individual becomes completely and permanently immune.

All simulations start at the endemic equilibrium of the underlying deterministic SIR model (see Appendix) and are terminated after a fixed period of time or after extinction of the polio virus has occurred.

Results

Minimum population size of an unstructured population

Starting from the endemic equilibrium of the underlying deterministic model, stochastic processes cause fluctuations which soon lead to minor epidemics (Figure 1 shows an example of a simulation run). These in turn often cause larger epidemics and can finally lead to spontaneous extinction. If the infection is able to persist, the fluctuations lead to oscillations with an average duration of 3.45 years (calculated from a simulation over 10,000 years; parameter values as given in Figure 1). This is slightly less than that of the deterministic model (3.67 years; see Anderson and May (1991), Dietz (1976)).

To estimate the 'minimum' population size 500–1,000 simulation runs are performed for each population size. Figure 2a refers to the epidemiological situation as it may be found in a developing country. Polio virus infection cannot persist in towns of 20,000–50,000 inhabitants, but long term persistence becomes likely for populations of at least 100,000 inhabitants. For populations of 150,000 spontaneous extinctions are very rarely observed even within the period of 100 years. In contrast to this, a population of 200,000 inhabitants in an industrialised country is still too small (Figure 2b).

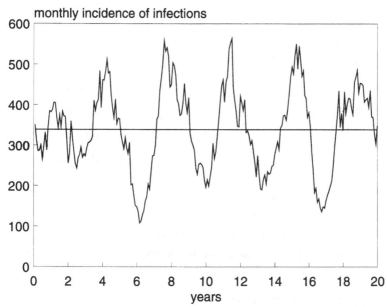

Figure 1. Example simulation of the monthly incidence of wild virus infection. PARAMETER VALUES: population size = 200,000; loss rate of infectivity = 12 per year; birth rate = death rate = 1/45 per year; the simulation starts at the endemic equilibrium of the corresponding deterministic model.

Populations of more than 500,000 inhabitants are necessary for long term persistence of poliomyelitis infection. The simulations for developing and industrialised countries differ in the life expectancy of the human population and in the basic reproduction number of the infection. To gain more insight into the observed differences, two further combinations are examined: A country with low life expectancy (45 years) but good hygiene ($R_0 = 5$) and a country with high life expectancy (75 years) but bad hygiene ($R_0 = 12$). The results of all combinations are summarised in Figure 3 for a population of 100,000 inhabitants. Improving the hygiene (R_0 changed from 12 to 5) at constant life expectancy has less impact on virus persistence than improving the life expectancy (from 45 to 75 years) at constant hygienic conditions.

After an initial period of five years the persistence curves show an exponential decline with a constant extinction rate (which is estimated by a linear least-square fit to the logarithms of the persistence curves). Figures 4a–c plot the average duration of persistence (= 1/extinction rate). The average duration of persistence increases in an approximately exponential manner as the population size or the basic reproduction number is increased (Figures 4a–b) and it strongly decreases with increasing life expectancy (Figure 4c).

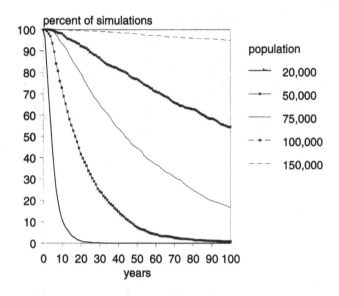

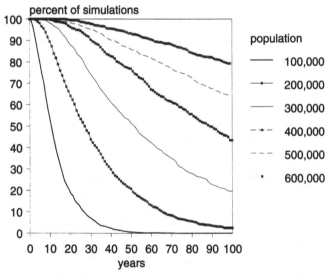

Figures 2a–b. Persistence of polio virus infection in an unstructured population (this can be regarded as an analogue to the survival function in demography). **(a)** Population with low life expectancy ($L = 45$ years) and hygienic standards ($R_0 = 12$). **(b)** Population with high life expectancy ($L = 75$ years) and hygienic standards ($R_0 = 5$).

PARAMETER VALUES: loss rate of infectivity $= 12$ per year; birth rate $=$ death rate $= 1/L$; all simulations start at the endemic equilibrium of the corresponding deterministic model; 1,000 simulations for each population size.

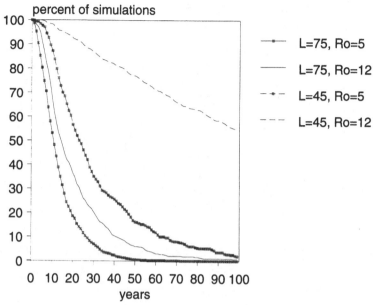

Figure 3. Persistence of polio virus infection in an unstructured population. Comparison of the impact of life expectancy (L) and basic reproduction number (R_0) on persistence. PARAMETER VALUES: loss rate of infectivity = 12 per year; birth rate = death rate = $1/L$; population size = 100,000; all simulations start at the endemic equilibrium of the corresponding deterministic model; 500 simulations for ($R_0 = 5$, $L = 75$) and for ($R_0 = 12$, $L = 45$) and otherwise 1,000 simulations each.

Minimum population size for a structured population

In reality a population of some 100,000 individuals can hardly be regarded as homogeneously mixing. Groups of inhabitants are always separated to some extent (socially and spatially). This separation slows down the spread of the infection, but it also decrease the risk of devastating epidemics. The total population size is now set to 100,000. 95% of the contacts of each individual remain within his own subpopulation while the remaining 5% are homogeneously distributed over all other subpopulations. The other parameter values are that of a developing country. The ability of the infection to persist in a population decreases with increasing number of subpopulations (Figure 5). If the number of subpopulations is kept constant but the fraction of contacts with individuals of other subpopulations increases (that is, if the separation becomes weaker), virus persistence improves (Figure 6).

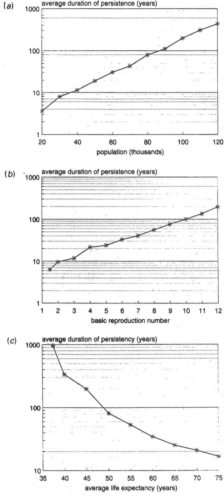

Figures 4a–c. Average duration of polio virus persistence (= 1/extinction rate) by (a) population size, (b) basic reproduction number and (c) life expectancy. The extinction rates are calculated by least-square fits to the logarithms of the extinction dates between 5 and 50 years after the start of the simulation (except for life expectancies < 45 years in (c), where the interval between 10 and 100 years is evaluated).

BASIC PARAMETER SET: population size = 100,000; life expectancy L = 45 years; basic reproduction number = 12; in (a)–(c) one of these parameters is varied while the other two are kept constant.

OTHER PARAMETER VALUES: birth rate = death rate = $1/L$; loss rate of infectivity = 12 per year; all simulations start at the endemic equilibrium of the corresponding deterministic model; 500 simulations for each set of parameter values.

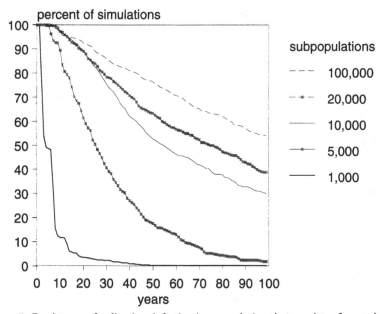

Figure 5. Persistence of polio virus infection in a population that consists of a number of equally sized subpopulations.

PARAMETER VALUES: total population size = 100,000; basic reproduction number = 12; 95% of the contacts of each individual remain within his or her own subpopulation; loss rate of infectivity = 12 per year; birth rate = death rate = 1/45 per year; all simulations start at the endemic equilibrium of the corresponding deterministic model; 500 simulations each (the result for '1 ∗ 100,000' is taken from Figure 2a).

Discussion

Severe poliomyelitis epidemics frequently occurred within the last two centuries in Europe and North-America (Bertenius 1947, Cohen 1987, Paul 1955), whereas epidemics have only rarely been reported from developing countries. This can only be partially attributed to underreporting (Freyche and Nielsen 1955, Gear 1955). The simulation model presented above largely oversimplifies reality, but it mirrors the most striking differences between developing and industrialised countries: The minimum population size is larger than half a million inhabitants for industrialised countries (Figure 2a). Polio virus infection, therefore, cannot persist in most European cities and towns. After local extinction, the population is free of polio virus infections until a pool of newborn susceptibles forms and the infection is reintroduced successfully. If a structured population is considered instead of a single homogeneously mixing population, the minimum size becomes even larger. Even a group of neighbouring towns, therefore, is usually not sufficiently large for polio

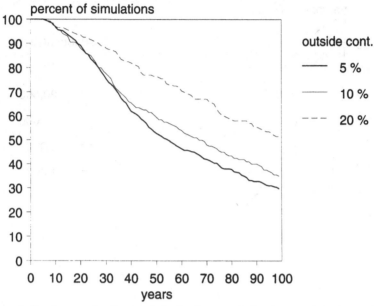

Figure 6. Persistence of polio virus infection in a population that consists of ten subpopulations of 10,000 inhabitants each.

PARAMETER VALUES: basic reproduction number = 12; 80–95% of the contacts of each individual remain within his or her own subpopulation; loss rate of infectivity = 12 per year; birth rate = death rate = 1/45 per year; all simulations start at the endemic equilibrium of the corresponding deterministic model; 200 simulations each.

virus infection to persist. Also, there is a marked seasonal variation in polio virus transmission in zones with temperate and cold climates (Armstrong 1950, Bradley *et al.* 1952, Hemmes *et al.* 1962, Nathanson 1984, Nathanson and Martin 1979, Spicer 1959, Yorke *et al.* 1979). Seasonality increases the minimum population size (Schenzle and Dietz 1987). The minimum population size is much smaller in developing countries (Figure 2a). The smaller minimum population size and the year-round transmission of the infection contribute greatly to its persistence in developing countries. With respect to the plan for world-wide eradication it is of highest importance to cover every region with vaccination. If a region of only 50,000 to 100,000 inhabitants is neglected or refuses to participate in the vaccination program, this may enable the infection to persist for decades (Figure 2a) and to provide a source of infection in adjacent regions.

It has been assumed that the increasing hygienic standards in Northern Europe were the cause of the first appearance of epidemics, while the low hygienic standard of developing countries was assumed to be the main cause of the endemic behaviour of polio in these countries (Olin 1952, Paul 1955).

According to the simulation results, the higher population turnover has a much larger impact on the persistence of infection than the mere improvement of hygienic standards (Figure 3). In a population with large birth and death rates many (susceptible) newborns are introduced per unit of time while older (mostly immune) individuals die early. As a result of this rapid population turnover, infection can persist even in relatively small populations.

Acknowledgements

Martin Eichner received financial support from Evangelisches Studienwerk eV, Haus Villigst, Schwerte. Klaus Dietz and Martin Eichner acknowledge the support by the Prudential Fellowship during their stay at the Isaac Newon Institute. Klaus Dietz thanks the University of Tübingen for granting leave of absence.

Appendix

Simulation procedure

The length of time until a given state of the system is changed by a birth, a death of a susceptible, an infection or a loss of infectivity is calculated in the following way: The time the system stays in a state has an exponential distribution with the parameter equal to the sum of all the rates leaving this state (ξ = birth + death rate of a susceptible + rate of transfer of one susceptible to become infectious + rate of loss of infectivity). The cumulative distribution function of the time T for remaining in this state is given by $P(T \leq t) = 1 - e^{-\xi t}$. If r is a uniformly distributed random number in the interval $[0, 1]$, then

$$t = -\frac{\ln(r)}{\xi}$$

is a realisation of the waiting time T. When the actual waiting time t is known, it must be decided what type of transition (birth, death, ...) takes place at time t: All possible transitions are arranged in an arbitrary order and 'cumulative rates' are calculated by adding the single rates and dividing the sums by ξ. A new random number, with uniform distribution over $[0, 1]$, is taken and the first transition in the order, whose 'cumulative rate' is larger than this random number, is performed (Karlin 1966, Kendall 1950). Because the per capita birth rate equals the death rate, the population size would remain approximately constant in the simulations. It is therefore assumed that the population size is constant over time. As a consequence of this assumption, the recruitment rate and the total death rate remain constant over time and the immunes are not traced in the simulations. Deaths of

infectious individuals are neglected (during their relatively short infectious
period) which has nearly no influence on the course of the simulations, but
largely reduces the time needed for the simulations.

Endemic equilibrium of the model without vaccination

The endemic equilibrium without vaccination is given by (see Dietz 1975,
Hethcote 1974)

$$\begin{pmatrix} S \\ I \\ R \end{pmatrix} = \begin{pmatrix} N/R_0 \\ N\mu(R_0 - 1)/\beta \\ N - S - I \end{pmatrix}.$$

Here, S denotes the number of susceptibles, I the number of infectious and
R the number of immunes. $S + I + R = N$ is the total size of the population.
Birth rate and death rate are equal to μ. $R_0 = \beta/(\gamma + \mu)$ is the basic
reproduction number, β is the rate of contacts that are sufficiently close for
virus transmission and γ is the loss rate of infectivity. The equilibrium formula
can also be applied to the structured population: N then has to be interpreted
as the subpopulation size and β as the total contact rate (sum of contacts
inside and outside the subpopulation per unit of time).

References

Anderson, R.M. and May, R.M. (1991) *Infectious Diseases of Humans. Dynamics and Contol*, Oxford University Press, Oxford, New York, Tokyo.

Armstrong, C. (1950) 'Seasonal distribution of poliomyelitis', *Am. J. Pub. Health and the Nations Health* 40, 1296-304.

Bertenius, B.S. (1947) 'On the problem of poliomyelitis. An epidemiological-statistical study', *Acta Pathol. Microbiol. Scan. Supplementum* LXVIII.

Bradley, W.H., Richmond, A.E., Thomson, D. (1952) 'Patterns of incidence of poliomyelitis in England and Wales, 1912-1950'. In *Poliomyelitis. Papers and Discussions Presented at the Second International Poliomyelitis Conference*, Lippincott, Philadelphia, London, Montreal, 408-11.

Cohen, H.H. (1987) 'Sabin and Salk poliovirus vaccine: vice versa', *Acta Leiden.* 56, 65-83.

Dietz, K. (1975) 'Transmission and control of arbovirus diseases'. In *Epidemiology*, D. Ludwig and K.L. Cooke (eds.), SIAM, Philadelphia, PA, 104-21.

Dietz, K. (1976) 'The incidence of infectious diseases under the influence of seasonal fluctuations'. In Lecture Notes in Biomathematics 11, 1-15.

Dietz, K. (1993) 'The estimation of the basic reproduction number for infectious diseases', *Stat. Meth. Med. Res.* 2, 23-41.

Fox, J.P., Gelfand, H.M., LeBlanc, D.R. and Conwell, D.P. (1957) 'Studies on the development of natural immunity to poliomyelitis in Louisiana. I. Overall plan, methods and observations as to patterns of seroimmunity in the study group', *Am. J. Hyg.* **65**, 344–66.

Freyche, M.-J. and Nielsen, J. (1955) 'Incidence of poliomyelitis since 1920'. In *WHO Monograph* **26**, 59–106.

Gear, J.H.S. (1955) 'Poliomyelitis in the under-developed world'. In *WHO Monograph* **26**, 31–58.

Gear, J.H.S. and Measroch, V. (1952) 'Poliomyelitis in Southern Africa'. In *Poliomyelitis. Papers and Discussions Presented at the Second International Poliomyelitis Conference*, Lippincott, Philadelphia, London, Montreal, 437–41.

Gelfand, H.M., LeBlanc, D.R., Fox, J.P. and Conwell, D.P. (1957) 'Studies on the development of natural immunity to poliomyelitis in Louisiana. II. Description and analysis of episodes of infection observed in study group households', *American Journal of Hygiene* **65**, 367–85.

Gelfand, H.M. and Miller, M.J. (1956) 'Poliomyelitis in Liberia. Prevalence of the disease, sero-immunity resulting from subclinical infection, and indications for prophylactic vaccination', *Am. J. Trop. Med. Hyg.* **5**, 791–6.

Hemmes, J.H., Winkler, K.C. and Kool, S.M. (1962) 'Virus survival as a seasonal factor in influenza and poliomyelitis', *Ant. van Leeuwenhoek J. Microbiol.* **28**, 221–33.

Hethcote, H.W. (1974) *Asymptotic behavior and stability in epidemic models*, Lecture Notes in Biomathematics **2**, 83–92.

Karlin, S. (1966) *A First Course in Stochastic Processes*, Academic Press, New York, London.

Kendall, D.G. (1950) 'An artificial realization of a simple "birth-and-death" process', *J. Roy. Statist.l Soc.* **12**, 116–9.

Marine, W.M., Chin, T.D.Y., Gravelle, C.R. (1962) 'Limitation of fecal and pharyngeal poliovirus excretion in Salk-vaccinated children. A family study during a type 1 poliomyelitis epidemic', *Am. J. Hyg.* **76**, 173–95.

Nathanson, N. (1984) 'Epidemiologic aspects of poliomyelitis eradication', *Rev. Inf. Dis.* **6**, *Supplement* **2**, 308–12.

Nathanson, N., Martin, J.R. (1979) 'The epidemiology of poliomyelitis: enigmas surrounding its appearance, epidemicity and disappearance', *Am. J. Epidemiol.* **110**, 672–92.

Olin, G. (1952) 'The epidemiologic pattern of poliomyelitis in Sweden from 1905 to 1950'. In *Poliomyelitis. Papers and Discussions Presented at the Second International Poliomyelitis Conference*, Lippincott, Philadelphia, London, Montreal, 367–75.

Paul, J.R. (1955) 'Epidemiology of poliomyelitis'. In *WHO Monograph* **26**, 9–29.

Paul, J.R., Horstmann, D.M. (1955) 'A survey of poliomyelitis virus antibodies in French Morocco', *Am. J. Trop. Med. Hyg.* **4**, 512–24.

Paul, J.R., Melnick, J.L., Barnett, V.H. and Goldblum, N. (1952a) 'A survey of neutralizing antibodies to polomyelitis virus in Cairo, Egypt', *Am. J. Hyg.* **55**, 402–13.

Paul, J.R., Melnick, J.L. and Riordan, J.T. (1952b) 'Comparative neutralizing antibody patterns to Lansing (type 2) poliomyelitis virus in different populations', *Am. J. Hyg.* **56**, 232–51.

Schenzle, D. and Dietz, K. (1987) 'Critical population sizes for endemic virus transmission'. In *Räumliche Persistenz und Diffusion von Krankheiten*, W. Fricke and E. Hinz (eds.), Selbstverlag des Geographischen Instituts der Universität Heidelberg, 31–42.

Spicer, C.C. (1959) 'Influence of some meteorological factors in the incidence of poliomyelitis', *Brit. J. Prev. Soc. Med.* **13**, 139–44.

Yorke, J.A., Nathanson, N., Pianigiani, G. and Martin, J. (1979) 'Seasonality and the requirements for perpetuation and eradication of viruses in populations', *Am. J. Epidemiol.* **109**, 103–23.

Discussion

NOKES Has Eichner taken into account the fact that polio virus may remain infective in the environment for some time? This could be incorporated either by extending the infectious period of individuals beyond that derived from clinical data, or, better, by altering the rate of infection function to include some background transmission. This effect may substantially alter the times to extinction, and decrease the minimum population size required to sustain the infection.

REPLY Extinction of an infection becomes less likely if the infectious agent can persist within the environment and so can form a source of infection. I have found not much evidence in the recent literature that this in the case with polio virus. The model is, therefore, entirely based on transmission by direct contacts.

EDMUNDS Eichner's assumption of a constant population size is obviously not realistic for either developing countries, nor for now developed countries during the first half of this century.

REPLY The intention of my model is to examine the influence of some basic parameters (such as the population turnover and the basic reproduction number) on the minimum population size for persistence of polio virus infection. Starting with this simple approach, more realistic examinations can be performed that take into consideration age-dependent contact rates and an age-structured population of non-constant size. The demographic effects can be incorporated into the homogeneous version of the model. Then persistent distributions (stable age distributions with exponentially growing population) have to be studied instead of stationary distributions.

BOLKER I have three points for Eichner's presentation. First, the amplitude of the oscillations can be heavily influenced by the initial conditions chosen.

Second, has he compared the model results to observed data in terms of frequency and amplitude of the oscillations? Third, the model contains no seasonal forcing at present, but this would make a great difference to the character of the oscillatory behaviour.

REPLY   The simulations start at the endemic equilibrium of the underlying deterministic model. The amplitude of the oscillations seem to be an intrinsic property of the model. The frequency of the oscillations resembles that of the deterministic SIR model. Annual fluctuations (as have frequently been observed in cold and temperate countries) can be obtained by adding a small factor to the contact rate.

NÅSELL   There is a real need for stochastic models of the type presented by Eichner. One approach which is worth considering is to study two aspects separately: the quasi-stationary distribution of the model conditioning on non-absorbtion (i.e. non-extinction), and the distribution of times to extinction.

VAN DRUTEN**   Eichner has simulated the appearance of new infection of polio in a population. By linking new infections with case notifications of poliomyelitis it is possible to estimate the probability of getting acute poliomyelitis after infection. My first question is have you attempted this? A second question related to the first has to do with the time delay between the start of an epidemic (of infections) and the beginning of notification of new polio cases. Can you say something about this time delay?

There may be data available on acute polio cases that Eichner could use to compare with his model results. The oscillatory behaviour could be compared by looking for the time intervals during which no cases were reported although transmission was still occurring, as this is an indirect measure of the rate of transmission.

REPLY   If a polio virus infection is reintroduced into a vaccinated population that is free of wild polio virus infection, then the infection can spread unrecognised for an average time of three months to more than a year before the first paralytic case is observed. This duration depends on the vaccination coverage and the type of vaccine used.

Part 4
Consequences of treatment interventions

Conflicts between the Individual and Communities in Treatment and Control

G.F. Medley

1 Introduction

It is a central, if unspoken, tenet in medicine that interventions which alleviate disease only do good. For non-transmissible diseases this is certainly true. However, over the past decade, the quantitative study of transmissible diseases has shown several examples where the treatment of individuals has consequences on the untreated proportion of the population which may lead to overall disease being increased by the intervention. Whilst conflicts in resource allocation, between, for example, providing kidney machines or hip replacements, are discussed fairly widely, conflicts between treating an individual and increasing the risk of disease to those untreated receive very little attention. The purpose of this review is to raise these issues for discussion.

When evaluating the overall effect of a control policy on morbidity and mortality for any disease, the important considerations are the risks to individuals of infection and consequent disease, and the numbers exposed to those risks. Interventions against transmissible infections will reduce the risk of infection to some or all of the population, but may decrease or increase the risk of disease following infection and may decrease or increase the total number of people exposed to these altered risks. The risks of disease to individuals and groups within a population are, by design, always improved by interventions targetted at them, but the consequences to the remainder of the population who are not directly targetted are not guaranteed to be beneficial, and it is from this inequality that conflicts between population and individual benefits arise.

I begin by outlining the epidemiological differences between transmissible and non- transmissible diseases, for it is in these differences that the conflicts have their origins. In particular, careful consideration of the relationship between infection and disease is required. Specific examples of the effect of intervention on the non-treated population (some deleterious, some beneficial) are then presented.

2   Transmissible vs non-transmissible

There are two major differences between transmissible and non-transmissible disease. First, in the case of transmissible diseases, the exposure of an individual to a pathogen and the development of infection and infectiousness provides a source of pathogens for other individuals in the population, thus increasing population exposure. Likewise, the loss of infectiousness in an individual reduces exposure in the remaining population. By contrast, exposure to factors inducing non-transmissible diseases is not a direct consequence of the number of individuals previously exposed and diseased. However, it is possible that other, non-biological, mechanisms act to control exposure to factors, such as asbestos, in a manner dependent on the number of people suffering disease, through, for example, public awareness of the risk and the legislature.

Second, transmissible diseases are caused by biological agents which are using hosts as a resource to further their own reproduction and survival. As living organisms with genetically determined characteristics, infectious disease agents are open to the processes of selection and evolution such that they will adapt to changing environments. So that, for example, asbestos does not change its characteristics to circumvent control measures to reduce exposure, but infectious agents certainly do so. The development of genetic resistance to chemotherapeutic agents is well documented for parasites as diverse as malaria, veterinary helminths and bacteria. It is also likely that parasites' life cycle (e.g. age at sexual maturity, transmissibility and virulence), which is under genetic control, will adapt in accordance with changes to exposure as a result of public health interventions (Medley 1994).

These two differences between transmissible and non-transmissible diseases are central to understanding why these two types of disease behave differently, and have been, or should have been, treated separately when considering public health measures to control them. In particular, the consideration of infectious disease agents as biological entities is not widely appreciated by the medical community, which tends to consider the human host aspect alone, rather than regarding infectious disease as the interaction of two species, in the same way as an ecologist regards the interaction between predators and their prey.

A specific example of the difference between transmissible and non-transmissible disease is the concept of the threshold population density. For directly transmitted infections (i.e., those that are passed from person to person without the mediation of a vector or specific behaviours such as sex) there is a density of people below which the infection cannot invade and produce an epidemic. This notion arises because a transmissible epidemic requires that an infectious person passes the infection to more than one susceptible (i.e. infectable) person during the period of infectiousness. Thus, one can imagine chains of transmission stretching into time and space, with some chains dying out, and others burgeoning with many people becoming infected from one source. There is a level of infection and contact in the community below which transmission will be unsustainable, and the pathogen (= disease risk) will become extinct.

Although the idea of quarantining individuals with infectious disease is to prevent other individuals from acquiring infection, if it is practised diligently enough, the community-level effect can be the elimination of the pathogen from a population. The pattern of transmission dynamics depends quantitatively on the numbers (or some related quantity such as density) of both infected and susceptible individuals. Transmission increases the number of infected individuals and decreases the number of susceptibles, whereas the number of susceptible individuals is increased by immigration, birth and recovery from infection. Thus, population level processes of infection are inherently dynamic (changing with time) and non-linear. There is no such set of phenomena in non-transmissible disease epidemiology.

In attempting to draw a distinction between transmissible and non-transmissible disease, the overlaps must, of course, be acknowledged. In particular, non-transmissible diseases whose aetiology is wholly genetic (for example, muscular dystrophy), will behave epidemiologically as transmissible diseases whose route of transmission is solely from parent to offspring (vertical transmission).

3 Infection vs disease

Interventions against transmissible disease can be conveniently divided into two: those that are aimed at cure of disease or alleviation of symptoms within individuals already infected, and those that are aimed to reduce exposure of individuals to infection or to protect individuals against future infection and/or disease. Both have immediate consequences on the rate of transmission of infection between individuals in the whole population, and on the relationship between infection and disease. Generally, both of these types of intervention will reduce the overall rate of transmission within a population either by reducing the infectious period or by reducing the number of susceptible individuals available for infection and subsequent infectiousness. Exceptions to this rule are treatments to individuals which prevent disease but prolong the duration of infectiousness, as in the effect of AZT treatment on HIV infected patients.

However, the reduction in infection may not reduce the overall level of disease as the relationship between infection and disease is not usually simple. The development of clinical signs of infection and their severity is mediated by numerous factors such as age at infection, immunological status (e.g. previous exposure to the pathogen), genetic interaction of host and pathogen, nutritional status and gender. Making infection rarer always increases the average age at which individuals are exposed to infection. If the disease consequences of infection are increased by increased age, as in some childhood viral infections, then the protection of individuals in young age groups may actually increase the total number of disease cases as those individuals that did not receive treatment are more likely to suffer from the disease. However, the effect of the intervention may be enhanced if increased age at infection is associated with decreased risk of disease, as in the development of carriage on infection with hepatitis-B virus (Edmunds *et al.* 1993).

Many complications exist in determining the relationship between infection and disease, most of which are shared with non-transmissible diseases. Complications of reporting infection and disease are important given that it is not always easy to determine infection, and that most infections produce a wide spectrum of disease. Exposure to infection is very heterogeneous in terms of time, age and spatial patterns, and intervention will change these patterns, complicating diagnosis further. In addition for transmissible disease, both human hosts and the infectious agents themselves are heterogeneous in terms of genetics and behaviour, and these heterogeneities may change over time. For example, the definition of AIDS has changed over time creating discontinuities in data, and perhaps a change in the apparent incubation period distribution of AIDS (the distribution of times between infection and diagnosis) (Chaisson *et al.* 1993). New understanding may also change the way that data are interpreted, for example, Kaposi's Sarcoma, which was once the most common presenting conditions for AIDS diagnoses, has become much rarer and is now interpreted as a separate epidemic (Beral *et al.* 1990).

In many cases, morbidity develops in individuals as a consequence of the intensity of infection, i.e. the number of pathogens harboured by an individual. The measurement of the intensity of infection is usually not simple as most pathogens exist within their hosts, and measurements such as egg counts in faeces or density of parasites in the blood are relative rather than absolute. For example, it is common to measure intensity of parasitaemia in malaria as the number of parasites per white blood cell, but blood cell populations are dynamic entities in themselves and may change in consequence to infections other than malaria (Cox *et al.* 1994).

Almost without exception, the frequency distribution of intensities of infection is overdispersed within the host population, such that most individuals have little or no infection, but a minority of the host population have very high infection intensities (Anderson and May 1991). If disease occurrence and/or severity is correlated with intensity of infection then most individuals diagnosed with disease will have intermediate parasite intensities, even though those individuals with the highest parasite burdens have the greatest individual risk of disease (Medley and Bundy 1995, Medley 1994).

Furthermore, it is not uncommon for disease to be a consequence not of current infection or infection intensity, but to be a consequence of cumulative infection over an individual's total experience of infection. This effect is most likely in diseases in which intensity of infection is important, such as schistosomiasis and onchocerciasis, where disease is a result of the build up of eggs and microfilariae respectively. Severity and occurrence of disease is related to some function of the sum of all fecund female parasites that an individual has harboured over that individual's life rather than simply the number currently harboured (Medley and Bundy 1995). This may also be important in viral infections, where exposure to different genetic variants of the pathogen increases the effect of the pathogen. Such an effect has been implicated in dengue fever and dengue haemorrhagic fever (Halstead 1992).

4 Examples of conflicts

4.1 Childhood vaccination

The best understood examples of conflicts between community and individual benefits arise in consideration of vaccination to prevent childhood viral infections (especially rubella, pertussis and mumps). At least three conflicts have been documented. First, incidence of disease may not be reduced by vaccination. Vaccination reduces circulation of the infectious agent within the host population, thus increasing the age of infection of those unvaccinated. If the probability of severe complications increases with age (as with rubella), then there is the potential for increased disease in populations with vaccination compared to those without. This will occur when the product of the number of unvaccinated individuals and the increased risk of disease is greater than the product of the total population and a the lower risk of disease. Note that vaccinated people are essentially free of risk, but that the increased numbers of cases in the community comes from the increased risk in the unvaccinated fraction of the population. Whether the numbers with disease is increased by vaccination depends on the quantitative details of age-related transmission, vaccination and disease risk (Knox 1980, Dietz 1981, Anderson and May 1983, 1985, Anderson *et al.* 1987, Anderson and Nokes 1991, Nokes and Anderson, 1987, 1988). The best policy for an individual may be to be vaccinated, but if the remainder of the population do not follow the same policy, then vaccinated individuals may increase the numbers of disease cases in the community.

Rubella is the best example of this conflict, as the only risk of disease is to the foetus if the mother becomes infected during the first trimester of pregnancy. Ukkonen and Bonsdorff (1988) reported epidemiological data that clearly show that age at infection increases when vaccination begins, as the theory suggests. However, although it is theoretically possible that disease may be increased by vaccination, it has never been documented. This may be due the prevailing view within the medical community that prevention of infection of individuals is not harmful to the community.

The second conflict emanates from the fact that vaccines carry a risk of disease themselves. Vaccines can differ in efficacy (the proportion of vaccinations that confer protection to future infection) and complication rate (the proportion of vaccinations that produce harmful side- effects), and both these variables are usually positively associated through the vaccine's immunogenicity. Thus, the individuals' best interests are served if they are exposed to neither infection nor vaccination. This can be achieved for one individual if the whole community bar that individual is vaccinated. In the UK at present, over 90% of infants are vaccinated for measles, mumps and rubella, so that the risk to an individual of complications from vaccination may be greater than the risk of disease, and the individual's response may be to decline vaccination. If, however, a sufficient proportion of the population remain unvaccinated, then herd immunity will be reduced, and outbreaks and epidemics of infection may ensue. This situation is a variant of the 'tragedy of commons' model of conflict between individual and community benefits (Hardin 1968).

The third conflict is a subtle complication of the second. The optimum policy for eradication of the virus from the community may be, initially at least, the use of the more efficacious vaccine as the reduction in infection and consequent disease may be greater than the increased numbers of severe complications compared to a less efficacious vaccine. The community-level benefit can be maximised by reducing the numbers of disease cases from either source, which may involve switching the vaccines used depending on the proportion of the population vaccinated (Nokes and Anderson 1991). Again the best strategy for the individual who is vaccinated is for all others to receive the most efficacious vaccine, and reserve the safest for herself.

4.2   Vaccination against hepatitis-B

In not all cases does disease risk increase with age. Hepatitis-B virus (HBV) is an extremely common infection of man, acquired during childhood where it is highly endemic (in most of sub-Saharan Africa and south-east Asia), but confined to certain risk populations in the developed world. Although there is some morbidity and mortality associated with primary infection, the most important disease consequences arise if the infection is not cleared, and the person infected becomes a carrier. In this state, people remain infected and infectious for decades, and are at much greater risk of developing chronic liver disease including liver cancer and cirrhosis. The greater number of carriers than acutely infected people ensures that carriers provide most infections, even if they are less infectious individually. Edmunds *et al.* (1993) showed that the probability of developing the carrier state decreases dramatically with age. Consequently, the benefit of immunisation, which delays infection in those unimmunised, is greater than would be expected without age-related decay in carriage development (Edmunds *et al.* 1995a,b,c).

4.3 Prolonging the HIV infectious period

The management and treatment of people infected with HIV has improved continuously over the period of the epidemic as medical science has gained experience of the spectrum of disease in these patients. These developments have serious implications for the pattern of future AIDS diagnoses (Brookmeyer 1991). Generally, the effect has been to suppress the manifestations of disease that induce AIDS and consequently death, by prophylactic treatment against opportunistic infections and use of the anti-viral drug AZT. Consequently, people currently infected with HIV and under medical care are living longer, more healthy lives than those infected earlier in the epidemic. During this extended incubation period of AIDS (i.e., the distribution of times between infection and AIDS diagnosis), there is greater opportunity for transmission from the infected individual to susceptible people, therefore potentially increasing the total number of people infected with HIV (Anderson *et al.* 1991, Gupta *et al.* 1993). Thus, the overall benefit to the population (in terms of reduction in the total HIV-induced disease) is derived from the opposite effects of prolonging life in those infected versus increasing the total number infected. This relationship is complicated by changes in transmissibility (perhaps measured as the total amount of virus in an individual) bought about by the interventions. The conflict here is that treatment of an individual may result in infections of people who would otherwise not experience infection. Although this conflict is entirely in the mind of the theoretician as beneficial treatment will not be withheld on the chance of another infection resulting, it is important to recognise the possible community level impact of treatments to individuals so that public health planning and campaign design take place in an informed, quantitative setting.

It has been shown that HIV evolves resistance to AZT fairly rapidly following first administration (Erice and Balfour 1994). It may be that with wide-spread use of this anti-viral drug the frequency of the genetically resistant variant becomes fixed in the host population, thus showing that treatment of individuals now reduces the benefits to future infected individuals. Recently, the potential for transmission of AZT-resistant HIV has been highlighted (Erice *et al.* 1993). In this case, the conflict is between giving an effective treatment now and having one available in the future, as it would appear that the options are mutually exclusive. As with the previous example, this conflict is largely fictitious, but the processes that generate it should be uppermost when considering the future of HIV/AIDS.

4.4   Acquired immunity to parasitic infection

Unlike the childhood viral infections such as measles and rubella, most parasites (used in the broadest sense) do not elicit a fully protective immunity in their hosts. After repeat exposure, the host may be able to control infection, usually to prevent pathogenesis and disease, rather than to prevent infection. One can imagine that hosts have to allocate resources between fighting infections and other activities (such as growth and reproduction). Given that for many pathogens a significant component of pathogenesis is immune-related and that the host can be expected to be exposed to the pathogens many times, controlling the level of infection may be a more tenable option rather than ridding themselves of the pathogen at each exposure.

At the population level, partial, acquired immunity generates an age-related pattern with a peak of infections (and possibly disease) in younger ages, with increasing levels of immunity in the population with age reducing infection and disease. Malaria provides the archetypal example. Individuals that are exposed to parasite populations that they have previously not encountered suffer morbidity regardless of their age (whereas serious disease is largely confined to children in sympatric parasite and host populations).

Mass treatment of a community to reduce infection rates, will make the parasite population smaller. If the parasite population is controlled by an immune response that depends on the history of previous exposure to individuals, then reduction of that experience by treatment will cause an increase in the parasite population (and possibly disease) into older age classes. The same argument applies equally well to the relationship between infection and disease, in which the acquired response reduces the morbid consequences of infection as well as the infection intensity itself.

In this situation, the compromise that must be considered is between the individual now and at some point in the future. Infection now may prevent infection and disease at a later time. Will treatment now prevent more disease than will be generated in the future? If the intervention reduces the rate of infection significantly, then this question will have a positive answer, but if the intervention is intermittent or does not reduce infection rates, then the answer may well be negative. A complication exists in that the acquired immune response generated generally has a limited duration, so that lack of exposure to the parasite results in loss of immunity. This question has been specifically addressed generally for helminth parasites (Anderson and May 1985, 1991, Berding *et al.* 1986, Woolhouse 1992), and developed for two experimental situations (Crombie and Anderson 1985, Berding *et al.* 1987). Barnes and Dobson (1990) included a waning immune response in a model of helminth parasites of sheep, although it is difficult to see the separate effect of immunity in their results. The development of specific models to examine detailed, quantitative consequences of mass treatment in humans with respect to immunity is currently prevented by the lack of specific understanding of the immune response and its relation to infection and disease.

4.5 Reduction of transmission in parasite infections

In infections in which the intensity of infection is measurable and important, and in which intensity is related to the degree of exposure, then reducing the total parasite population by chemotherapy will reduce the infection rate in the remainder of the population. A model of helminth transmission (Medley *et al.* 1993, Chan *et al.* 1994), shows that the prevalence of heavy infections in the untreated portion of the community is reduced by reduction of the parasite population. This leads (*inter alia*) to a non-linear relationship between control effort (the number of people treated) and benefit of control. Essentially, the parasite population within an individual is kept at a high level by constant input of infective stages. If the level of transmission is reduced to the population (by killing the worms in a fraction of the population), then the parasite populations of even those untreated falls due to none replacement of parasite deaths. This effect may be small and difficult to detect in practice, but does deserve further field investigation. It is analogous to the situation of vaccination against viral and bacterial infections which reduces transmission to those who were unvaccinated.

5 Determinants of behaviour

The essential difference between transmissible and non-transmissible disease is the more non-linear and dynamic nature of the infection patterns in the former. Exposure to risks that induce non-transmissible disease are often implicitly considered to be relatively stable, and, although time dependent, not related to the number of people already exposed. However, the magnitude of an individual's behavioural risk factor, may be determined to some extent by the level of that risk behaviour within the population (Cavalli-Sforza and Feldman 1981, Boyd and Richardson 1985). Examples are mainly anecdotal, but there is evidence of 'epidemics' of injecting (rather than smoking) illicit drugs, and smoking tobacco, drinking alcohol, and aspects of diet and sun-bathing are all activities which are to some extent determined by the behaviour of other members of the population. The mechanisms responsible for the population modification of individual behaviour are social, but will also operate through the economic determinants of cost of these activities.

More obvious are those activities that depend on more than one individual, for example, penetrative sex or sharing drug injecting equipment, where the behaviour of an individual is directly constrained by the behaviour of the other members of the population. This particular activity has been of central interest in the study of sexually transmitted infections, but has not received full attention as a dynamic entity in itself (Blythe and Castillo-Chavez 1990). It is likely that mathematical models of behaviour would prove fruitful in understanding and predicting patterns of disease, although this area remains largely unexplored. It is also possible that such consideration of risk behaviour as a transmissible entity will reveal possible conflicts in terms of behaviour modification.

6 Conclusions

Conflicts between individuals and populations do not generally arise in non-transmissible disease epidemiology. These conflicts are, however, relatively common in infectious disease epidemiology because of the non-linear nature of transmission and its reduction that arises from intervention. They are not usually apparent when treating individuals without monitoring the whole population. Where such a conflict exists, the benefits of the individual are usually held to outweigh the detrimental effects to the whole population.

The other important area of conflict revolves around the capacity of the infectious pathogen to genetically adapt to changing circumstances – again a difference between transmissible and non-transmissible diseases. This has only been briefly touched upon here, but is central to many issues surrounding health policy. The general consequence is that current interventions become increasingly less useful at a rate depending on the manner in which they are currently used. Thus the conflict pivots on treating individuals now and having an effective treatment available for individuals in the future. Because of a combination of implicit discounting of benefits and lack of understanding of the biological and procedural relationships, the effects of current interventions on future success of interventions appear to be largely ignored.

Mathematical descriptions of infection transmission and disease development are becoming increasingly common in the design and implementation of public health policy. Two points are worth noting in this respect. First, interventions are not decided by their health consequences alone, but in conjunction with the economic consequences in terms of costs of implementation and benefits. The economic aspects can act either to enhance or to reduce the complications of individual versus population. This can be especially so if the future benefit/harm of a policy are discounted (i.e., by giving decreased weight to effects further in the future), in the same way that the costs are discounted. The choice of 'benefit measure' can also be crucially important, for example, the average reduction in disease cases over the next ten years, or the equilibrium difference in disease incidence with and without the control policy.

Second, much of the analysis presented is done with deterministic frameworks from which a single, hopefully mean, benefit measure is produced. However, a more accurate picture is generated if the benefit measure is a probability distribution. Public health policy should be 'risk-adverse', and should prefer a safer policy with lower expected benefit to one which may produce much greater benefit, but may fail disastrously.

The consequence of interventions in transmissible diseases are dynamic and non-linear, and therefore difficult to predict. It is a commonly held belief that no intervention that increases health of individuals will reduce the health of the whole population. There are no empirical examples of this tenet failing, but the belief that it will not occur is strong enough to ensure that it has not been sought. The theoretical work outlined here suggests that such a circumstance is perfectly possible.

Acknowledgements

I thank W. John Edmunds and an anonymous reviewer for comments on previous drafts. The author is a Royal Society University Research Fellow.

References

Anderson, R.M., Crombie, J.A. and Grenfell, B.T. (1987) 'The epidemiology of mumps in the UK: a preliminary study of virus transmission, herd immunity and potential impact of immunisation', *Epidemiol. Inf.* **99**, 65–84.

Anderson, R.M., Gupta, S. and May, R.M. (1991) 'Potential of community-wide chemotherapy or immunotherapy to control the spread of HIV-1', *Nature* **350**, 356–359.

Anderson, R.M. and May, R.M. (1983) 'Vaccination against rubella and measles: quantitative investigations of different policies', *J. Hyg. (Camb.)* **90**, 259–325.

Anderson, R.M. and May, R.M. (1985) 'Vaccination and herd immunity to infectious disease', *Nature* **318**, 323–329.

Anderson, R.M. and May, R.M. (1991) *Infectious Diseases of Humans: Dynamics and Control*, Oxford University Press, Oxford.

Anderson, R.M. and Nokes, D.J. (1991) 'Mathematical models of transmission and control'. In *Oxford Textbook of Public Health*, Volume 2, second edition, W.W. Holland, R. Detels, G. Knox, B. Fitzsimmons and L. Gardner (eds.), Oxford Medical Publications, Oxford, 225–252.

Barnes, E.H. and Dobson, R.J. (1990) 'Population dynamics of *Trichostrongylus colubriformis* in sheep: computer model to simulate grazing systems and evolution of anthelmintic resistance', *Int. J. Parasitol.* **20**, 823–831.

Berding, C., Keymer, A.E., Murray, J.D. and Slater, A.G.F. (1986) 'The population dynamics of acquired immunity to helminth infection', *J. Theor. Biol.* **122**, 459–471.

Berding, C., Keymer, A.E., Murray, J.D. and Slater, A.G.F. (1987) 'The population dynamics of acquired immunity to helminth infection – experimental and natural transmission', *J. Theor. Biol.* **126**, 167–182.

Beral, V., Peterman, T.A., Berkelman, R.L. and Jaffe, H.W. (1990) 'Kaposi's sarcoma among persons with AIDS – a sexually transmitted infection', *Lancet* **335**, 123–128.

Blythe, S.P. and Castillo-Chavez, C. (1990) 'Scaling of sexual activity', *Nature* **344**, 202.

Boyd, R. and Richarson, P.J. (1985) *Culture and the Evolutionary Process*, University of Chicago Press, Chicago.

Brookmeyer, R. (1991) 'Reconstruction and future – trends of the AIDS epidemic in the United States', *Science* **253**, 37–42.

Cavalli-Sforza, L.L. and Feldman, M.W. (1981) *Cultural Transmission and Evolution: A Quantitative Approach*, Princeton University Press, Princeton.

Chaisson, R.E., Stanton, D.L., Gallant, J.E., Rucker, S., Bartlett, J.G. and Moore, R.D. (1993) 'Impact of the 1993 revision of AIDS case definition on the prevalence of AIDS in a clinical setting', *AIDS* **7**, 857–862.

Chan, M.S., Guyatt, H.L., Bundy, D.A.P. and Medley, G.F. (1994) 'The development and validation of an age-structured model for the evaluation of disease control strategies for intestinal helminths', *Parasitology* **109**, 389–396.

Cox, M.J., Kum, D.E., Tavul, L., Narara, A., Raiko, A., Baisor, M., Alpers, M.P., Medley, G.F. and Day, K.P. (1994) 'Dynamics of malaria parasitaemia associated with febrile illness in children from a rural area of Madang, Papua New Guinea', *Trans. Roy. Soc. Trop. Med. Hyg.* **88**, 191–197.

Crombie, J.A. and Anderson, R.M. (1985) 'Population dynamics of *Schistosoma mansoni* in mice repeatedly exposed to infection', *Nature* **315**, 491–493.

Dietz, K. (1981) 'The evaluation of rubella vaccination strategies'. In *The Mathematical Theory of the Dynamics of Biological Populations*, R.W. Hiorns and D. Cooke (eds.), 81–97.

Edmunds, W.J., Medley, G.F., Nokes, D.J., Hall, A. and Whittle, H. (1993) 'The influence of age on the development of Hepatitis-B carrier state', *Proc. Roy. Soc. Lond. B* **253**, 197–201.

Edmunds, W.J., Medley, G.F. and Nokes, D.J. (1995a) 'The transmission dynamics and control of hepatitis B virus in a developing country', *Stat. Med.*, in press.

Edmunds, W.J., Medley, G.F., Nokes, D.J., Whittle, H.C. and Hall, A.J. (1995b) 'Epidemiological patterns of hepatitis-B virus (HBV) in highly endemic areas', *Epidemiol. Inf.*, in press.

Edmunds, W.J., Medley, G.F. and Nokes, D.J. (1995c) 'The design of immunisation programmes against hepatitis-B virus in developing countries', this volume.

Erice, A. and Balfour, H.H. (1994) 'Resistance of human immunodeficiency virus type 1 to antiretroviral agents – a review', *Clin. Inf. Dis.* **18**, 149–156.

Erice, A., Mayers, D.L., Strike, D.G., Sannerud, K.J., McCutchan, F.E., Henry, K. and Balfour, H.H. (1993) 'Brief report – primary infection with zidovudine-resistant human-immunodeficiency-virus type 1', *New Eng. J. Med.* **328**, 1163–1165.

Gupta, S., Anderson, R.M. and May, R.M. (1993) 'Mathematical models and the design of public health policy – HIV and antiviral therapy', *SIAM Review* **35**, 1–16.

Halstead, S.B. (1992) 'Dengure fever, viral hemorrhagic fevers and rabies', *Curr. Opin. Inf. Dis* **5**, 332–337.

Hardin, G. (1968) 'The Tragedy of the Commons', *Science* **162**, 1243–1248.

Knox, E.G. (1980) 'Strategy for rubella vaccination', *Int. J. Epidemiol.* **9**, 13–23.

Medley, G.F. (1994) 'Chemotherapy'. In *Parasitic and Infectious Diseases: Epidemiology and Ecology*, M.E. Scott and G. Smith (eds.), Academic Press, London, 141–155.

Medley, G.F., Guyatt, H.L. and Bundy, D.A.P. (1993) 'A quantitative framework for evaluating the effect of community treatment on the morbidity due to ascariasis', *Parasitology* **106**, 211–221.

Medley, G.F. and Bundy, D.A.P. (1995) 'Dynamic modelling of epidemiological patterns of schistosomiasis morbidity', *Am. J. Trop. Med. Hyg.*, in press.

Nokes, D.J. and Anderson, R.M. (1987) 'Rubella vaccination policy: a note of caution', *Lancet* **i**, 1441.

Nokes, D.J. and Anderson, R.M. (1988) 'The use of mathematical models in the epidemiological study of infectious diseases and in the design of mass immunisation programmes', *Epidemiol. Inf.* **101**, 1–20.

Nokes, D.J. and Anderson, R.M. (1991) 'Vaccine safety versus vaccine efficacy in mass immunisation programmes', *Lancet* **338**, 1309–1312.

Ukkonen, P. and Bonsdorff, C.H. (1988) ' Rubella immunity and morbidity: effects of vaccination in Finland', *Scand. J. Inf. Dis.* **20**, 255–29.

Woolhouse, M.E.J. (1992) 'A theoretical framework for the immuno-epidemiology of helminth infection', *Paras. Immunol.* **14**, 563–578.

The Design and Analysis of HIV Clinical Trials

T. Peto

1 Introduction

Clinical trials have been conducted in patients with AIDS or HIV for ten years. There is no obvious reason why the principles underlying good clinical trial design should be any different for trials on HIV than for any other disease. However, the social setting of the infection has demanded that some of these principles should be more clearly justified. Attempts have been made by some trialists to conduct trials that avoid the need for randomisation or placebos, or attempt to use early signs of disease progression or laboratory markers rather than death as an end-point. This paper will illustrate these issues by comparing the design and analysis of two large European studies, coordinated by the MRC at the Brompton Hospital (in collaboration with INSERM in Paris), with other trials studying the same questions.

2 Summary of some of the key trials

2.1 Trials on the early use of Zidovudine

Zidovudine is an anti-HIV drug which was shown in one study to reduce mortality in patients with advanced HIV disease over a median study time of four months. On the basis of this study, the drug has been licensed and widely used.

(i) Concorde (an MRC/INSERM study) is a study of immediate versus deferred use of zidovudine in asymptotic HIV+ patients. It is a double blind placebo-controlled trial of about 1800 patients followed for 3–4 years using death and objective disease progression as the end points. Patients were urged to stay on trial capsules until clinical progression occurred, but all patients were followed. The results are expected in Spring 1993 following unblinding of the trial as specified in the protocol. At least 150 deaths have occurred in the study.

(ii) ACT 019 is a similar double blind placebo-controlled study. Patients were expected to take trial capsules until a clinical end-point occurred. The trial was terminated early in 1989 after a median of one year follow up on the basis of a difference in the rates of disease progression. Only seven deaths occurred, so no difference in mortality could be inferred. Apart from Concorde, all other placebo-controlled trials on asymptotic patients were stopped in 1989 for 'ethical reasons'

2.2 Trials of didanosine (ddI)

Didanosine (ddI) is, like zidovudine, a nucleoside analogue. It has been licensed in the US and many European countries (not the UK), on the basis of small studies which demonstrate a change in laboratory markers of disease activity (and increase in the numbers of circulating CD4+ lymphocytes and a decrease in concentrations of HIV viral particles in the serum).

(i) Alpha, an MRC/INSERM coordinated European/Australian study, is a blinded randomised study of ddI in symptomatic HIV+ patients intolerant to zidovudine. Patients had the option of being entered into a placebo-controlled comparison of high and low dose ddI, or to be simply randomised between high and low dose ddI. All patients were to be followed for life, and the end-points were disease progression and death. The study was terminated in October 1992. Unfortunately, recruitment into the placebo-controlled option was too slow to provide any useful data. The dose comparison study recruited about 1800 patients with about 65% mortality: no difference in mortality between high and low dose was detected, although it did confirm the changes in laboratory markers which the earlier studies had described.

(ii) An open label study of ddI was conducted in a London hospital by the sponsoring company in the hope that historical controls could be used to provide sufficient clinical data to register the drug in the UK. The trial has been completed but the results have not been conclusive.

(ii) ACT 116a/116b/117 is a randomised blinded dose-comparison study of ddI compared to zidovudine in patients stratified according to previous zidovudine use. The trial showed a difference in the rates of new clinical events but not in overall survival. In some sub- groups low dose ddI was best while in other sub-groups zidovudine was best.

3 Issues of design and analysis

3.1 Historical controls and randomisation

The dangers of interpreting non-randomised controls were not appreciated by many HIV trialists. They argued that natural history studies showed such a high mortality that even modest treatment effects could be detected without the rigours of randomisation. However, the natural history of HIV infection is rapidly changing. The reasons for this are not entirely clear, but probably are a result of changing definitions of 'AIDS, HIV associated disease' and the decreasing incidence of 'AIDS defining infections', because of routine use of effective antimicrobial agents as prophylaxis.

Even allowing for these ascertainment biases, it is quite plausible that the observed natural history of HIV infection is attenuating. Obviously, patients presenting with symptomatic HIV infection in the early 1980s represented patients with fast incubation disease who are likely to have a high mortality. Patients infected at the same time but presenting 10 years later with symptoms, have a long incubation disease and therefore are likely to live longer. These changes are seen in the UK haemophiliac population, all of were infected at about the same time.

Finally, there is no reason that HIV, which is rapidly expanding in the human population, is not itself changing its virulence and pathogenicity. Such changes have not been measured, partly because epidemiological studies are likely to be confounded by the changing use of antiviral agents.

3.2   The need for placebo (no treatment) control groups

One of the paradoxes of the modern history of HIV trials is that the two most influential trials (the first zidovudine study and ACT 019) on the use of antiviral agents were placebo- controlled. These two studies have led to the widespread use of zidovudine. The evaluation of other drugs since then has been slowed by the feeling amongst clinicians that patients would not tolerate placebos. The MRC/INSERM/ALPHA trial represents an attempt to recruit patients into a placebo-controlled study in a manner which attempted to allow for the social pressure at the time. Great difficulties were faced from clinicians in launching the study; some ethical committees suggested that placebos were unethical. Some patients' advocate groups, more sceptical of the efficacy of antiviral agents, were supportive of the study. The role of the clinicians in the failure of recruitment into the placebo-controlled trial will be discussed. The publication of the dose comparison study of ddI, which failed to demonstrate a dose effect and therefore created doubt about the efficacy of ddI, has recreated a demand by many clinicians and patients for placebo-controlled trials in the future.

3.3   Choice of end-points

Although there is widespread agreement that mortality is the most important and valid end- point in clinical trials of anti-HIV drugs, there is a reluctance by trialists to include survival as an end-point in their trials. The reasons for this are both pragmatic and social.

Pragmatically, use of earlier end-points allows drugs to be evaluated more quickly and with fewer patients. Also, the large number of different early endpoints (both clinical and laboratory) increases the changes of finding some biological effect of the drug which may be related to efficacy. This was shown with ddI. Unfortunately, although ddI increased CD4 counts, this was not translated into a change in mortality.

Socially, trialists are under pressure by patient groups to design trials that allow the patients entering the trial to benefit from the results of that trial. Clearly, this contract between trialists and the participating patients is only possible if mortality during the trial is low.

The interpretation of the significance of early end-points is highly controversial. For example, the debate on the early use of zidovudine still lingers, 3.5 years after the end of ACT 019 (which had been terminated early on the basis of clinical progressions). It is clear that the decision to continue CONCORDE by its Data and Safety Monitoring Committee for at least two years beyond the duration of 019, has driven this debate. It is becoming increasingly clear that only long term survival data, which should be provided by the CONCORDE trial, will resolve the uncertainty.

4   Conclusion

The first two clinical trials conducted by the MRC/INSERM collaborative group have concentrated on using large scale double-blinded randomised trials using survival as a primary end-point and included placebo arms. Most other trials of anti-retroviral agents have attempted to avoid placebos, randomisation or death as an end-point in their trial design. It is becoming clear that attempts to design 'novel' trials that avoid the need for large-scale randomised studies using mortality as an end-point have so far failed to provide reliable evidence on the efficacy of new agents.

A Theory of Population Dynamics Used for Improving Control of Viral Diseases: AZT Chemotherapy and Measles Vaccination Policy

Z. Agur

1 Introduction

Virulence of pathogens, the origin and growth of neoplasias, and their treatment by chemotherapy or vaccination, are problems involving many complex processes on different organizational levels of the biological system. In recent years molecular biology has made an important step forward in identifying major elements in these processes. Yet, it becomes increasingly clear that in many cases prognosis is determined by the *dynamic interaction* between elements of the system, rather than by their presence or absence.

Today, thanks to the efforts of Anderson, Dietz, Hethcote, May and others, it is not a strange idea to employ population dynamics theory for identifying optimal vaccination strategies for human populations. In contrast, drug protocols for individual patients are still determined by *trial and error*.

The present paper attempts to show how a theory of population dynamics in perturbed environments proves useful for studying disease processes across several organizational levels of the biological system. A method for increasing selectivity of AZT treatment of HIV infected individuals, and a method for improving measles vaccination policy will be described, both being motivated by the same general theory.

2 The relation between the population and the environmental periodicities

Until recently, the approach to population dynamics was governed by the concept of equilibrium, and environmental disturbances, although much alluded to, were seldom incorporated in the analysis of life-history strategies. In contrast to the predominant view, my work investigates population dynamics over a wide spectrum of time-scales for the environmental perturbation. Using *non-Markovian* models it shows that, regardless of most details of intrinsic population growth, persistence is a non-monotonic function of the relation between the characteristic population and environmental periodicities and maximum persistence is obtained when the relation between the two periods has an integer value (Agur 1982, 1985a). These results are obtained under the assumptions that the organism's susceptibility to environmental disturbances varies during different stages of its life-cycle, and that environmental changes occur on the same time-scale as the average generation time in the population.

Now, if this mathematical description is indeed a good model of biological populations, then it is expected to be applicable to various biological systems: to molluscs in the marine intertidal that are subjected to the devastating effects of storms (Agur and Deneubourg 1985), to human populations suffering from periodic diseases, or to cell populations undergoing chemotherapy. Two such applications are briefly described below.

3 Improving selectivity of AZT

The inhibitors of HIV-1 reverse transcriptase, zidovudine (AZT), $2', 3'$-dideoxyinosine (DdI) and other antiviral agents, such as acyclovir and adenosine arabinoside, are cell-cycle-phase-specific, interrupting DNA synthesis while having no effect on cells that are not in the S-phase. These drugs typically have greater affinity for the viral polymerase than the host cell polymerase. Nonetheless their action on host cell polymerase results in the toxic side-effects associated with their use (Yarchoan and Broder 1987, Fischl *et al.* 1987). Recently it has been suggested that a daily dose of 500–600 mg AZT is as effective in eliminating the virus, but much less toxic to the host, than the original FDA approved daily dose of AZT (1200 mg) (Fauci 1990, Fischl *et al.* 1990). However, optimal dosing intervals have yet to be defined and individual practices vary from administering the drug five times a day to once a day.

Can cytotoxicity of AZT be decreased by altering the rationale of its application? Mathematical analysis suggests that the answer is positive and that factors, such as the large variability in the generation-time of HIV-1 (see below), can be exploited for increasing treatment selectivity. Based on the theory of population dynamics in perturbed environments (Agur 1982, 1985a) it was suggested that toxicity to the host of cell-cycle-phase-specific drugs can be reduced using high dose pulses, the dosing interval being an integer multiple of the generation-time in the susceptible host tissue (Agur 1985b, 1988a, Agur *et al.* 1988).

To test the above prediction, laboratory experiments were carried out in mice given varying doses of AZT at different intervals. This drug causes severe depletion to murine bone marrow pluripotent stem cells, committed cells and erythrocyte progenitors, whose generation-time is roughly 7h (Schofield *et al.* 1980, Nijhof *et al.* 1984). These experiments showed that mice, given short duration AZT protocols exactly every integer multiple of 7h, have significantly higher white blood cell counts and lower mean red blood cell volume than mice treated at other dosing intervals. In addition, a significantly lower proportion of cells arrested in early S-phase is detected in mice treated by AZT every 7h, or 14h, as compared to those treated every 10h, or its multiple (Agur *et al.* 1991).

These results suggest that bone marrow toxicity of AZT can be minimized by its administration at fixed intervals that are integer multiples of the average bone-marrow generation-time. The general implication is that mathematical models can be employed for predicting treatment outcomes. However, for achieving higher precision in such predictions for human patients the simple models had to be modified to take account of realistic assumptions about the drug's pharmacokinetics and pharmacodynamics, as well as of the exact distribution of cell division times. The resulting formal method for evaluating schedule efficacy is described elsewhere (Cojocaru and Agur 1992). Its use for evaluating current AZT protocols is brought forward below (recently, Webb (1992) has provided a very elegant analysis, supporting these results).

3.1   Selecting effective AZT protocols for human patients

Cell-cycle-phase-specific drug protocols that differ in the dosing interval, also differ in the rate of elimination of the target cells. In addition, the cellular intrinsic growth rate is expected to be patient-specific, as it reflects the effect of patient-specific cofactors, such as cytokines, on cell division. Clearly then, the same cell-cycle-phase-specific protocol will have different effects in different patients. These differences can be checked in conjunction with the Concorde trial.

In the same context, we are interested in predicting the *relative* toxicity of different interval AZT schedules for the host bone-marrow cells and for the HIV-1 virus, as a function of their different life-cycle parameters. Other differences between the two populations, such as the intrinsic growth rates, the initial population size and the drug's killing efficacy are ignored. For simplicity we also ignore the plausible emergence of drug-resistance, as well as the existence of latent viruses, or G_0 cells.

Our computations assume a conventional, first order kinetics of drug elimination

$$C(t) = C_0 e^{-kt}, \quad C_0 = C(0), \tag{1}$$

where k measures the drug's cellular half-life (about 3h in AZT (Yarchoan *et al.* 1989)). To account for a saturation effect of the drug, its killing efficacy $K(t)$, is defined as follows:

$$K(t) = 1 - e^{-k_1 C(t)}, \tag{2}$$

where k_1 is a measure of the drug's toxicity. As HIV-1 generation-time depends on availability of antigens or mitogens that stimulate the host T-cell replication (Haxie *et al.* 1986) we take it to be a random variable in the range of 10h–50h. The duration of the viral susceptible life-phase (reverse transcriptase activity) has not been measured directly, but appears to be less than 4h (Kim *et al.* 1989). In our computations this episode is assumed to be in the range of 1h–3h. The generation-time in human bone marrow cells is taken to be normally distributed with an average of 24h (Furukawa *et al.* 1987), and the duration of the susceptible cell-cycle phase (the S-phase) is taken to be constant in the range of 9h–11h. Lacking realistic evaluation of AZT killing efficacy, we examine two cases: (i) a very high killing efficacy, $k_1 = 0.0026$, for which 1500 mg drug eliminate 98% of the cells or viruses *that are in their drug-susceptible phase* and 370 mg eliminate 62% of these cells; (ii) a lower killing efficacy, $k_1 = 0.0013$, for which 1500 mg and 370 mg drug eliminate 85% and 38% of the susceptible cells or viruses, respectively.

The above parameters were implemented in the chemotherapy model (Cojocaru and Agur 1992), and the temporal changes of the virus and bone marrow populations were simulated.

In Figures 1 and 2, a schedule involving a single daily dosing is compared with a schedule in which the same daily dose is divided into four dosings. These results suggest that bone-marrow toxicity is very sensitive to the dosing interval. A schedule involving four daily dosings appears to exert extremely high bone-marrow toxicity, irrespective of the details of the pharmacokinetics or the variation in the bone-marrow generation-time (Figure 1). In contrast, the bone-marrow pool may be preserved under a single daily application of the same total dose (Figure 2a,b). Note, however, that if the drug's cellular half-life is 3h and the killing efficacy is extremely high, bone-marrow toxicity is expected to be significant even under a single daily dosing (Figure 2c). However, under a more realistic killing efficacy of the same drug, (case (ii) above) bone-marrow toxicity of this protocol will be relatively small (not shown). Results in Figure 2 also suggest that a large variability in the bone-marrow generation-time in a single host will result in a higher toxicity of the single daily dosing protocol. The same will be true for larger duration of bone marrow S-phase (not shown). Still, toxicity of this protocol will always be much smaller than that exerted by the same total dose, divided into several daily dosings. Above all, variation within the group of treated patients may be an extremely important factor when efficacy of AZT and its toxicity are concerned. This variation should be checked empirically to see its effect on AZT treatment success.

The prospects of virus elimination appear very sensitive to the duration of the viral drug-susceptible life-phase (reverse transcription): if this phase is completed within 1h or less, any intermittent drug schedule will fail to eliminate the virus. In contrast, if HIV-1 reverse transcription lasts 2h or

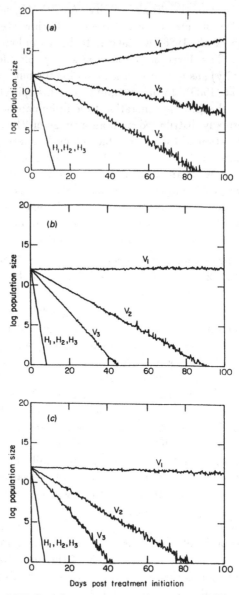

Days post treatment initiation

Figure 1. Effect of 100 days drug treatment, using a dose of 370 mg every 6h, on the number of bone-marrow cells and viruses. Bone marrow generation-time is 24h with standard deviation 0.0 (**H1**), 0.2 (**H2**), 0.5 (**H3**). Duration of susceptible life-phase (S-phase) is 10h. Virus generation-time is taken to be a uniformly distributed random variable in the range 10h–50h and the drug susceptible life phase (reverse transcriptase) is: 1h (**v1**), 2h (**v2**), 3h (**v3**); (a) half-life of the drug 1.5h, initial killing efficacy 62% ($k_1 = 0.0026$); (b) half-life of the drug 2.5h, initial killing efficacy 62%; (c) half-life of the drug 3h, killing 62%.

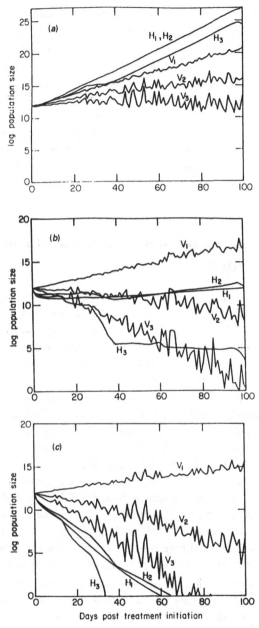

Figure 2. Effect of 100 days drug treatment, using a dose of 1500 mg every 24h, on the number of bone-marrow cells and viruses. Host and viral cycle parameters are as in Figure 1. (a) half-life of the drug 1.5h, initial killing 98% ($k_1 = 0.0026$); (b) half-life of the drug 2.5h, initial killing 98%; (c) half-life is 3h, initial killing 98%.

more, it will be effectively eliminated by AZT, whose cellular half-life is 3h. Under these conditions, elimination is expected to be effective even if the drug is applied only once daily, but a faster viral elimination is expected under a 6h dosing interval (Figures 1c, 2c). Viral elimination will require several daily dosings if drug's half-life is shorter than 2.5h (Figures 1a, 2a).

The above results suggest that if, indeed, the average bone marrow inter-mitotic interval is around 24h, then AZT selectivity (i.e. its efficacy in elim-inating the targeted cells vs. its damage to normal tissues) may be increased by relatively large doses, applied every 24h (Agur 1988b). However, increased selectivity of these protocols will be counterbalanced by a somewhat slower virus elimination. In addition, effectiveness of AZT can probably be enhanced if variation in responsiveness among patients early in the AZT treatment is monitored.

4   Pulse mass measles vaccination across age-cohorts

The successful containment of infectious diseases, such as poliomyelitis, led people to believe that most infections were curable one way or another. Thus, in the eighties, world health authorities were hoping that measles would be eradicated by standard vaccination measures. But this has not been the case: in spite of extensive vaccination efforts measles is still an active disease both in developing countries and in the industrialized world.

In the USA., Israel and other countries the current endeavor to prevent large-scale epidemics, involves new guidelines for vaccination. These are sim-ilar to the old guidelines in being based on the conventional concept of a time-constant immunization effort. One dose is still applied to all infants at about one year of age and a second dose is now given at the age of six years. In such strategies, vaccination affects the amplitude and the period of the epidemics, but it does not antagonize the natural dynamics of the disease. In contrast, the policy put forward here challenges the conventional concept of a constant vaccination effort. Admittedly, there may be some caveats in the new strategy, but our goal here is to convey the new idea, and only then to look at the corrections that ought to be made in the suggested approach.

The theory of population dynamics in harshly varying environments, which was discussed above, suggests that when the environmental pattern imposed on the population takes the form of discrete episodes of devastation, it is the spacing of these episodes that determines population persistence (Agur 1982, 1985a, Agur and Deneubourg 1985). Based on this theory it was hypothesized that measles epidemics can be more efficiently controlled when the natural temporal process of the epidemics is antagonized by another temporal process i.e., by a vaccination effort that varies significantly and abruptly in time (Agur *et al.* 1993, 1994). This policy was referred to as *pulse vaccination* and it was shown theoretically that pulse vaccination of children aged 1–7 years, once every five years, approximately, may suffice for preventing the epidemics.

4.1 Age-structure model with different vaccination strategies

Effects of the pulse strategy on the epidemics profile was studied using an age-structured compartmental model, which had been introduced by Anderson and May (1985) for analyzing the transmission dynamics of vaccine-preventable childhood infectious diseases. The model represents changes, with respect to age and time, in the population of (i) infants protected by maternal antibodies, (ii) susceptible individuals, (iii) infected, but as yet non-infectious individuals, (iv) infectious individuals, and (v) immune individuals. This model has been extensively studied under a large range of constraints and is widely employed in the investigation of epidemiological problems.

Simulations of the model with *no vaccination* yield a two-year-cycle epidemics, and most of the infected individuals are children under 10 years of age. Under no further perturbation the oscillations will decay and the system will slowly return to a steady-state level of infection. However, this will never be the case, since the total population size and epidemiological structure are frequently perturbed, due to immigration and other factors. Our simulations also support the known conclusion that the coverage levels in the industrialised world are too low for disease eradication, while a coverage level larger than 95%, required for herd immunity (May 1982) is difficult to obtain in practice.

To simulate *pulse vaccination*, the conventional policy, in which the level of vaccination is uniform over time, is replaced by a nonuniform *pulse* policy, i.e., periodic vaccination of several age groups at the same time. Some simulation results are shown in Figures 3 and 4. In Figure 3 a single pulse vaccination is applied to 85% of the children aged 1–7 years. The vaccination is timed to occur at about one year prior to the predicted onset of the next epidemic. These results show that a single pulse vaccination generates a 7 year epidemic-free interval. Continuing the simulations with a similar pulse vaccination one year prior to each prospective epidemic, we note that the inter-vaccination intervals become shorter until they stabilize at about 5 years. Under this strategy the epidemics are suppressed, and they continue to be suppressed as long as we continue to employ this strategy (Figure 4).

It should be noted that efficacy of the pulse vaccination depends on the vaccination level, p, and on the vaccinated cohorts. In the present simulations, with $p = 0.85$, efficacy is guaranteed only if 1–7 year age cohorts are immunized about every five years; lower levels of vaccination require smaller intervals between pulses to guarantee efficacy (see Agur *et al.* (1994) for

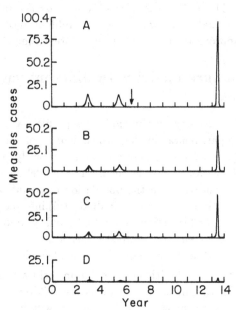

Figure 3. Temporal changes in the number of cases of measles infection with a single *pulse* vaccination (timing is denoted by arrow), $p = 0.85$, of children aged 1–7 years. Simulation results of the age-structure, 5 age classes, model. **A.** Total population; **B.** age class 0–4; **C.** age class 5–9; **D.** age class 10+. Simulations were carried out by perturbing the system from its equilibrium state (perturbation induced by reducing the fractions susceptible in each age class by a factor 0.8). Calculations were performed for 3.5 days intervals. Total population size is 3,717,000, for equations and other parameters see Anderson and May (1985).

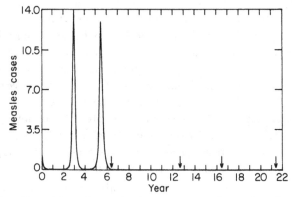

Figure 4. The effect of the *pulse* vaccination strategy on the number of cases of measles infection (timing is denoted by arrow), $p = 0.85$, of children aged 1–7 years. Simulation results of the age-structure, 5 age classes, model (see legend to Figure 3 for further detail).

analytic results).

The results of our analysis suggest that with the observed trend of age-specific infection rates (low in the very young, high in the child population and low in the adult age groups) a pulse vaccination of 85% of children aged 1–7, once every five years, may completely eliminate the epidemics. The cost of this strategy (measured by the total number of vaccinations) is lower than the current strategy of two doses, applied to all children at the age of one and six. An auxiliary advantage of the pulse strategy may be the higher compliance, due to the effect of "campaigning". Note, however, that due to stochastic effects, such as immigration waves, the national policy may be 'fool-proof' only if a constant vaccination at an early age is maintained.

5 Conclusions

This paper describes the use of population dynamics theory for optimizing control of viral or other pathogenic diseases on different organizational levels of the biological system. The general theory, suggesting that population persistence may be a highly non-monotonic function of the relation between the population and the environmental periodicities, implies that drug dosing can be manipulated for increasing treatment efficacy and tissue selectivity. Thus, a method for selecting AZT efficient treatments, and a method for reducing AZT cytotoxicity to the host is put forward, and it is suggested that side-effects are largely dependent on the choice of of specific dosing intervals. In particular, it is suggested that AZT toxicity to human patients can be reduced using high dose pulses, the dosing interval being an integer multiple of the generation-time in the susceptible host tissue (approx. 24h in humans).

The aim of this paper is to advocate a new general approach to protocol design. For this reason, detailed considerations are left out, e.g., the possible effects of AZT on cell-cycle progression or the effects of opportunistic infections. Such consideration will be discussed elsewhere (Agur *et al.* 1995).

This novel concept as applied to vaccination may be met with some scepticism. The possibility that, under the suggested policy, more infants may become infected certainly should not be neglected. Another concern may be the possible effect on the notoriously unstable measles dynamics, of the strong forcing implicated in the pulse strategy. These and other questions concerning the *pulse vaccination policy* will be dealt with separately. It should be noted, however, that simulations suggest a stabilizing effect of the pulse strategy on the system.

The approach suggested here is quite radical, and it is likely that many countries that have routine immunization programs will not easily yield to it. However, as current programs are experiencing extreme difficulties, equally extreme measures may be required. Clearly, more work is needed before the suggested policy can be implemented. Further work is warranted for exploring parameter sensitivity and programmatic vaccine uptake. However, the results we have already obtained provide encouraging indication that this option needs further consideration.

Acknowledgments

I am much obliged to L. Cojocaru and G. Mazor for useful discussion and for carrying out the simulations, to the reviewers for comments and to Jesus College, Oxford, for outstanding hospitality. The Rashi Foundation and the Sherman Foundation supported the work by grants.

References

Agur, Z. (1982) 'Persistence in uncertain environments'. In *Population Biology*, H.I. Freedman and C. Strobeck (eds.), Lecture Notes in Biomathematics, Springer-Verlag, 125–131.

Agur, Z. (1985a) 'Randomness, synchrony and population persistence', *J. Theor. Biol.* **112**, 677–693.

Agur, Z. (1985b) 'Increasing the half-life of cycle-specific drugs can increase elimination time'. In *2nd Cyprus Conference on New Methods in Drug Research, Limassol*, abstract 20.

Agur, Z. and Deneubourg, J.L. (1985) 'The effect of environmental disturbances on the dynamics of marine intertidal populations', *Theor. Pop. Biol.* **27**, 75–90.

Agur, Z. (1988a) 'A new method for reducing cytotoxicity of the anti-AIDS drug AZT'. In *Biomedical Modelling and Simulation*, J. Eisenfeld et al. (eds.), J.C. Baltzer AG, 59–61.

Agur, Z. (1988b) 'Clinical trials of zidovudine in HIV infection', *Lancet* **334** (ii), 734.

Agur, Z., Arnon, R. and Schechter, B. (1988) 'Reduction of cytotoxicity to normal tissues by new regimens of phase-specific drugs', *Math. Biosci.* **92**, 1–15.

Agur, Z., Arnon, R., Sandak, B. and Schechter, B. (1991) 'Zidovudine toxicity to murine bone marrow may be affected by the exact frequency of drug administration', *Exp. Hematol.* **19**, 364–368.

Agur, Z., Danon, Y.L., Anderson, R.M., Cojocaru, L., and May, R.M. (1993) 'Pulse mass measles vaccination across age cohorts', *Proc. Roy. Soc. Lond.* B **252**, 81–84.

Agur, Z., Cojocaru, L., Mazor, G., Anderson R.M. and Danon, Y.L. (1994) 'Measles immunization strategies for an epidemiologically heterogeneous population: the Israeli case study', *Proc. Nat. Acad. Sci. USA* **90**, 11698–11702.

Agur, Z., Tagliabue, G., Scechter, B., and Ubezio P. (1995) 'AZT effect on the bone marrow – a new perspective on the Concorde trials'. In *J. Biol. Sys.* **3**, 241–251.

Anderson, R.M. and May, R.M. (1985) 'Age-related changes in the rate of disease transmission: implications for the design of vaccination programmes', *J. Hyg. Camb.* **94**, 365–436.

Cojocaru, L. and Agur, Z. (1992) 'Theoretical analysis of interval drug dosing for cell-cycle-phase-specific drugs', *Math. Biosci.* **109**, 85–97.

Fauci, A.S. (1990) 'ddI – A good start, but still phase I', *N. Engl. J. Med.* **322**, 1386–1388.

Fischl, M.A. *et al.* (1987) 'The efficacy of azidothymidine (AZT) in the treatment of patients with AIDS and AIDS-related complex', *N. Engl. J. Med.* **317**(4), 185–191.

Fischl, M.A. *et al.* (1990) 'A randomized controlled trial of a reduced daily dose of zidovudine in patients with acquired immunodeficiency syndrome', *N. Engl. J. Med.* **323**, 1009–1014.

Furukawa, T., Ikeda, H. *et al.* (1987) 'Cinemicrography of human erythroblasts: direct measurement of generation time and delineation of their pedigree', *Blood Cells* **12**, 531–539.

Haxie, J.A., Haggarty, B.S., Rackowski, J.L., Pillsburg, N. and Levi, J.A. (1986) 'Persistent noncytopathic infection of normal human T lymphocytes with AIDS associated retrovirus', *Science* **229**, 1400–1402.

Kim, S. *et al.* (1989) 'Temporal aspects of DNA and RNA synthesis during Human Immunodeficiency Virus infection: evidence for differential gene expression', *J. Virol.* **63**, 3708–3713.

May, R.M. (1982) 'Vaccination programs and herd immunity', *Nature* **300**, 481–483.

Nijhof, W., Wierenga, P.K., Pietens, J. and Bloem, R. (1984) 'Cell kinetic behaviour of a synchronized population of erythroid precursor cells *in vitro*', *Cell. Tissue Kin.* **17**, 629–639.

Schofield, R., Lord, B.I., Kyffin, S. and Gilbert, C.W. (1980) 'Self maintenance capacity of CFU-S', *J. Cell. Physiol.* **103**, 355–362.

Webb, G. (1992) 'Resonances in periodic chemotherapy scheduling'. In *Proceedings of the World Congress of Nonlinear Analysis*, de Gruyter, Berlin, in press.

Yarchoan, R. and Broder, S. (1987) 'Development of antiretroviral therapy for the acquired immunodeficiency syndrome and related disorders', *N. Engl. J. Med.* **316**, 557–564.

Yarchoan, R. *et al.* (1989) 'Clinical pharmacology of 3'-azido-2', 3'-dideoxithymide (zidovudine) and related dideoxynucleosides', *N. Engl. J. Med.* **321**, 726–735.

The ONCHOSIM Model and its Use in Decision Support for River Blindness Control

J.D.F. Habbema, G.J. van Oortmarssen, and A.P. Plaisier

1 Introduction

The development and use of ONCHOSIM for studying epidemiology and control of onchocerciasis is a joint effort of the Onchocerciasis Control Programme (OCP) and the Department of Public Health of the Erasmus University, Rotterdam. ONCHOSIM uses the so-called microsimulation technique for modelling stochastic systems (Habbema *et al.* 1995). This technique is characterized by mimicking individual life histories of humans and – in the case of ONCHOSIM – parasites. Biological factors and characteristics of control measures can be modelled in detail. Output of microsimulation models can be detailed (age- and sex-specific tables for comparison with detailed data sets) and simple (trends in prevalence during control). New insights can readily be incorporated by redefining relationships in the model and adapting the computer program which is used to perform simulations with the model.

A model that is built and quantified using the ONCHOSIM computer program has two types of assumptions. One concerns the deep model of the transmission cycle and disease process of onchocerciasis. The other concerns the description of the relevant characteristics ('experimental setting') of the village or region under study and of the control measures. The degree of complexity of both the deep model and the descriptive part depends on the aims of the model use, the available data and other considerations. When compared to most other current epidemiological models, the most pronounced difference is probably the level of detail in which the descriptive part is modelled. This is a reflection of the primary reason for involvement of modelling in OCP: supporting evaluation and decision making in a particular control programme (Remme *et al.* 1995).

Elsewhere we have described the computer program (Plaisier *et al.* 1990), discussed model estimates from analysis of OCP data (Plaisier *et al.* 1991a), and demonstrated the use of ONCHOSIM in addressing control questions (Plaisier *et al.* 1991b). A review of questions addressed by OCP thus far is provided in Habbema *et al.* (1992) and in Remme *et al.* (1995). In the present paper we will first explain what basic transmission model can be thought of as underlying the more complex models that are specified within ONCHOSIM. Then, as an example of its application, the use of ONCHOSIM in analyzing the possibility of recrudescence of a serious endemic situation after a period of vector control will be discussed. In the annex we will give the structure and quantification of the model.

2 The basic model

The model consists of three parts: the transmission cycle, the development of blindness and subsequent excess mortality, and interventions (vector control and chemotherapy).

2.1 The transmission cycle

The basic transmission cycle is illustrated in Figure 1. Biting flies will transmit L3 larvae to humans at a rate that is expressed as the Annual Transmission Potential (ATP). Only a proportion sr of these infections will develop into mature worms, which have a life-expectancy of Tl years. Each worm will contribute cw microfilariae (mf) to the skin microfilarial density sl. In an equilibrium situation, the skin load in a person follows directly from the ATP:

$$sl = ATP.sr.Tl.cw. \qquad (2.1)$$

The main density-dependent step in the cycle occurs when microfilariae (mf) are engorged by a biting fly. The number of first stage (L1-) larvae resulting from a fly bite reaches a maximum at high skin mf densities. The functional relation $lu = F(sl)$ between the skin load of a human and the larval (L1 stage) uptake lu of a biting fly is directly based on experimental data.

The vectorial part of the basic model is summarized in two parameters: the annual biting rate ABR and the probability v for a L1 larvae to be released during one of the subsequent fly bites. Starting from the L1 uptake lu, the ATP equals:

$$ATP = ABR.v.lu. \qquad (2.2)$$

The shape of the uptake function will result in a threshold value for the biting rate (ABR) below which no stable infection occurs in the population.

For very low microfilarial densities, the uptake is approximately equal to $lu = F'(0).sl$, and the threshold level for the biting rate is:

$$ABR = \frac{1}{F'(0).cw.Tl.sr.v}. \qquad (2.3)$$

At present, the relation $lu = F(sl)$ is represented by:

$$lu = a(1 - e^{-b.sl})(1 + e^{-c.sl}), \qquad (2.4)$$

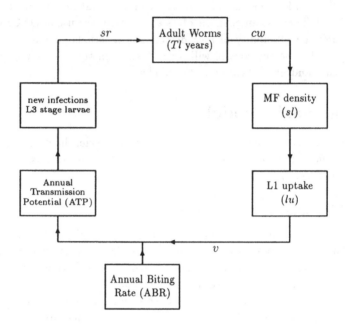

Figure 1. The transmission cycle of the basic onchocerciasis model

where the main parameters a, b and c are determined empirically. Parameter a denotes the maximum number of L1 larvae in a fly. Formula (2.4) results in the following ABR threshold level:

$$ABR = \frac{1}{2.a.b.cw.Tl.sr.v}. \qquad (2.5)$$

2.2 Blindness

In the model, blindness occurs when the cumulative past microfilarial load of a human exceeds a certain critical level. The remaining life-expectancy is lower for blind than for non-blind persons.

2.3 Intervention

Two types of interventions are included in the model. During the first decade, the OCP relied completely on vector control, which resulted in zero or very low biting rates (ABR levels) in large areas of the OCP. Alternatively, ivermectin treatment may considerably reduce the microfilarial load (sl) in humans and have an additional impact on the worm productivity (cw).

2.4 Refinements

A detailed description of the model is given in the annex.

In view of the questions that are being addressed by the model, which are directly related to the impact of interventions, the basic model has to be refined. For example, there will be low average worm loads after 10 or more years of vector control. When evaluating the possibility of recrudescence after so many years of control, it is important to take additional sources of variability and non-linearity into account. Microfilariae production requires regular mating of worms. Therefore a distinction is made between male and female worms and the process of mating is included in the model, resulting in a highly non-linear relation between worm loads and skin microfilarial loads at low numbers of worms.

Additional variability occurs because of exposure heterogeneity (partly related to age and sex of the human) and because of variation in the productive lifespan of worms. Earlier models assumed an exponential distribution for the lifespan (Dietz 1982, Anderson and May 1991). Analysis of OCP data shows that this is inappropriate, and that 95% of the worms have reached the end of reproductive life by the age of about 14 years, with an average lifespan of about 10 years (Plaisier et al. 1991a).

The human-parasite part of the model is truly stochastic: changes in the human population are modelled by adding (birth) or removing (death) individuals, and changes in worm load are recorded in individuals by adding or removing worms.

The vector-larvae part is represented in ONCHOSIM by distributions rather than by individual subjects. The probability v for an engorged L1 larva to be released as L3 at one of the subsequent bites is quantified through explicit modelling of the underlying mechanisms: duration of larval development and of the feeding cycle of the fly, daily fly survival, and the probability that an existing L3 larva is released during a bite. In the annex the expression for v is given for the case of variability in the durations of larval development and of feeding cycle, together with a simpler expression for v in the case of fixed durations.

3 Addressing control questions: possible recrudescence after vector control

Until recently the control strategy of OCP consisted exclusively of larviciding by aerial spraying of the breeding sites of the blackfly. This is an intensive and costly process, which is closely monitored in order to achieve (nearly) 100% effectiveness (Remme et al. 1986). Over the years, microfilarial loads became significantly reduced, and the question of the required duration of

vector control in view of possible recrudescence of the disease became increasingly opportune. Making a choice in this respect requires assessment of
chances of recrudescence in relation to duration of vector control. The OCP
modelling group was asked to use ONCHOSIM for analyzing the recrudescence problem and to support the decision making process by presenting
model based assessments of risk. We started by taking a closer look at the
concept of recrudescence in the context of disease control. It was agreed
that recrudescence is not completely described by the long-term chance of
occurrence alone. The time dynamics of the build up of recrudescence is also
important. Build up refers first to the fly population, then to the adult worm
population and finally, and most importantly from a public health point of
view, to the resulting blindness in the human population. These three aspects
have different time frames.

The recrudescence analysis has focussed on assessing the dependency of
the risk and dynamics of recrudescence on its most important determining
parameters. Although we have tried to arrive at valid estimates, based on
data analysis, scientific background knowledge and expert opinion, much uncertainty remains. The consequences of this uncertainty for the model predictions were assessed by a sensitivity analysis in which parameter values were
varied within their plausible range, with emphasis on parameter values that
favour the chances of recrudescence.

3.1   Determinants of recrudescence

An important determinant of the occurrence and dynamics of recrudescence
is the average microfilarial (mf) load at the end of a certain period of control, which mirrors the number of productive adults left (with a slight delay
reflecting the lifespan of mf). This remaining worm-load is proportional to
the number of worms at the start of control and depends on the reproductive
lifespan of the parasite and the variability in this lifespan. Since the pre-
control worm-load is highly dependent on the pre-control biting rate, we have
analyzed potential recrudescence for a highly endemic village in the OCP area
(Tiercoura, pre-control CMFL = 70 mf/s; here CMFL is the Community Microfilarial Load, i.e. the geometric mean skin snip mf count for adults) and
also for a medium endemic village (Folonzo, CMFL = 30 mf/s). By fitting
the model to the pre-control data in these villages we were able to estimate
the pre-control biting rates. On the basis of evaluation data collected during
vector control in the OCP area (in the same villages), we have estimated the
mean parasite lifespan at 9 to 11 years. The estimated lifespan variability
is such that 95% of the parasites will die before the age of 13 to 14 years
(Plaisier *et al.* 1991a). Apart from the standard model (mean = 10, 95th
percentile = 13.7), we also tested a 95th percentile of 15 years.

A second important factor for recrudescence is the potential of the *Simul-*

ium flies to attain a certain level of transmission once their population has built up after cessation of control. This depends on the relationship between the (remaining) human microfilarial load and the uptake by the fly of mf, followed by the subsequent development to the L1-stage and finally the infective L3-stage. A so called 'L1-uptake' curve as a function of human mf load could be estimated from experimental data (see (2.4) and (A10)). The data, however, also allowed for a curve with a higher ratio of initial slope to saturation level, which gives a stronger density regulation, but at the same time a relatively high uptake at low densities. Since this was presumed to favour recrudescence we also tested the impact of such an alternative curve. The transmission potential at low average densities also depends on the heterogeneity in exposure: if there is a lot of variation in exposure, then even at low mf-densities there will be a few frequently bitten persons who not only have a more than average (residual) worm load but also a more than average contribution to the infection of flies. Moreover, persons with higher worm-loads also have a higher probability that they harbour worms of both sexes, which is a condition for mf-production. We have, therefore, also analyzed the recrudescence risk and dynamics when there is more heterogeneity in exposure (variation coefficient of the biting rate 30–45% higher) in combination with a 5–10% higher biting rate than in the standard model.

Mating of worms and exposure heterogeneity are also important determinants for the reproductive potential of the newly generated worms. Combinations of male and female worms are most likely in persons with a relatively high exposure. Because Schulz-Key and Karam (1986) have demonstrated the necessity of regular insemination of female worms for mf production, we did not systematically analyze recrudescence for the hypothetical situation of hermaphroditic worms. A brief analysis, however, revealed that this would lead to a gross overestimation of the recrudescence probability or, conversely, of the estimated required duration of vector control.

3.2 Results

A summary of the results of the analysis is presented in Table 1 (see also Plaisier *et al.* (1991b)). The table indicates different model quantifications that have been tested. Vector control periods of 9–15 years have been tested (9, 9.5, 10, etc.; none of the simulations of 15 years of vector control showed recrudescence). Each combination of model quantification and vector control period is simulated 50 times. The risk of recrudescence is estimated by counting the number of simulations showing recrudescence divided by 50. A logistic curve was fitted through the simulated risks in order to be able to calculate a duration of vector control which leads to 50%, 5%, and 1% recrudescence. The required duration of vector control in Table 1 is defined as the estimated duration of vector control required to reduce the risk of recrudescence to be-

Level of endemicity[a]	Parameter quantification	Estimated required duration of control (years)	Estimated recrudescence time (years)[b]
High	standard	13.4	25.9 (23.8–27.9)[c]
High	increased biting rate and exposure heterogeneity	13.9	19.5 (18.9–20.0)
High	increased density regulation L1-uptake	13.8	20.8 (19.4–22.2)
High	increased *O. volvulus* lifespan variation	14.5	16.2 (15.7–16.8)
Medium	standard	11.6	N.a.[d]
Medium	increased biting rate and exposure heterogeneity	12.9	37.3 (30.7–43.9)

[a]High endemicity is modelled according to the village of Tiercoura and medium endemicity according to the village of Folonzo
[b]The estimated time to reach a post-control CMFL of 10 mf/s after 12 years of vector control when recrudescence occurs
[c]95% confidence interval
[d]After 12 years of vector control no recrudescence occurred

Table 1. Dependency of the estimated required duration of vector control on parameter quantification

low 1%. The recrudescence time is defined as the estimated time to reach a post-control CMFL of 10 mf/s when recrudescence occurs, after a period of 12 years of vector control.

From Table 1 we learn that the estimated required duration of control varies between 11.6 and 14.5 years depending on the quantification of the model. In a highly endemic village like Tiercoura increasing variability in *O. volvulus* lifespan prolongs the required duration of control by more than 1 year. The effects of other unfavourable scenarios are less pronounced, showing parasite lifespan to be the most important recrudescence determining factor. In a less highly endemic village like Folonzo, increasing the (pre- and post-control) biting rate and exposure heterogeneity has a more pronounced effect than in Tiercoura. Apparently in such villages the number of parasites (and the associated mating chances) is also an important limiting factor.

Another important finding of the recrudescence analysis is that, at least initially, recrudescence is a relatively slow process. Even after an apparently too short control period of 12 years in a hyper-endemic village like Tiercoura, it is estimated that it takes more than 25 years before infection levels are reached which are significantly associated with deterioration of ocular tissues and blindness (see Remme *et al.* 1989). The results further indicate that as the recrudescence risk falls below 5% (13–13.5 years of vector control) the recrudescence time exceeds 40 years.

4   Discussion

The duration of vector control which is sufficient to reduce the probability of recrudescence to very low levels depends on the assumptions made in the model. These assumptions concern both biological aspects and the specific circumstances in a village. If it is assumed that no immigration of infected persons or infected flies will occur, then according to the model a reasonable upper-bound for the duration of vector control seems to be 14 years. This value relates to a village with very high biting rates resulting in one of the highest endemicity levels encountered in the OCP area. The model estimates values for duration of control such that the probability of recrudescence will be less than 1%. Only the combination of extremely high biting rates and a (rather unlikely) assumption on the variability of *O. volvulus* lifespan resulted in slightly more than 1% risk after 14 years of control (see Table 1). These estimates should certainly not be taken as a final truth since the model is, despite its many parameters, still a tentative and simplified approximation of reality, and long-term prediction with or without models is always a hazardous enterprise. The OCP used results from the model as one of the many inputs in their decision making process and decided that in the central area, where larviciding has been completely effective and where the risk of infections imported by immigration is probably low, vector control can be stopped after 14 years (OCP 1990).

When recrudescence occurs, the projections made by the model give an indication of the duration until the emergence of serious visual impairment and blindness on a scale at which it becomes a public health problem. The prediction that it will take decades was regarded to be useful and encouraging, partly since it may well be that an effective and safe macrofilaricide will be developed in that time.

A policy question that arises naturally with regard to the possible build up of recrudescence is whether it can be detected early and be interrupted by mass ivermectin treatment. This question has been addressed using ONCHOSIM by investigating the use of epidemiological surveillance schemes, and subsequent treatment schedules. Questions studied thus far include: How often should surveillance be done? How sensitive and specific are different criteria for recrudescence detection? How well is recrudescence preventable subsequently by mass ivermectin treatment? See Habbema *et al.* (1992) for further discussion on the use and limitations of ivermectin in recrudescence control.

The example of the recrudescence analysis has been presented to discuss some of the reasons for using a microsimulation approach. In the simple deterministic basic model, recrudescence will always occur in villages where the biting rate is sufficiently high (i.e. all villages in the endemic region of the OCP) except when the worm load is zero. Some of the refinements in our model will increase the risk and speed of recrudescence, for example heterogeneity in exposure of humans to biting flies. Introduction of a finite (small) human population and keeping track of individual worms will lead to a high probability of a zero worm load after a sufficently long period of vector control. For shorter periods, the recrudescence risk will vary between zero and one. A refinement which has an important impact on the risk of recrudescence is the mating requirement, which causes a non-linearity at low worm loads, and considerably lowers the required duration of vector control compared to a no-mating model.

If it were only for the recrudescence analysis, one could argue that some of the refinements mentioned could also be achieved with an analytical approach, which has important advantages of its own, for example by giving the modeller a better understanding of the behaviour of his mathematical system. But there are additional considerations, and for example the following ones have played a role in the decision to use microsimulation within OCP.

First, microsimulation allows explicit modelling of all processes involved, enabling judgment by non-mathematical experts. This is important for the acceptance of the modelling work, and will enhance both intellectual commitment and appropriate use of model results in decision making and planning.

Second, microsimulation allows evaluation of realistic but complicated control options, including combinations of control options with incomplete coverage or compliance. This will of course require a considerable investment in programming an initial model. An additional advantage of a microsimulation program is its flexibility in implementing changes and extensions of the model.

Third, because experimental conditions can be described, data analysis can be done more rigorously with a microsimulation model than otherwise. For example, in a trial of yearly ivermectin administration in Asubende (Ghana), some additional irregular vector control took place in the area (Alley *et al.* 1994). This background phenomenon could be taken into account in ON-CHOSIM, and the age and sex specific ivermectin coverage could easily be modelled. Because individual life histories are simulated, output could be calculated and presented in exactly the same way as done in OCP field research, facilitating estimation and goodness-of-fit testing.

Taking the randomness into account is also instructive, as it shows the 'natural variation' in data (which is important in analysis of the large amount of data collected by the OCP) and in the impact of control activities.

In conclusion, we hope to have shown that the ONCHOSIM model can be seen as well-reasoned extension of a simple mathematical core model which can be placed in the tradition of analytical modelling of infectious diseases, and that there are compelling arguments for the use of micro-simulation, especially in an applied context where the goal of modelling is to evaluate control options in a complex real-world situation. We are aware that, despite its merits, ONCHOSIM has to be regarded as a first attempt to develop a modelling approach which is integrated in a control programme for a tropical disease. A lot of work has to be done, both on methodological issues and on improving the link between model and practice. Another important issue is to bridge the gap between theoretical analytical models and applied microsimulation modelling, which could enhance the value of modelling as a tool in decision making about control of infectious diseases.

Annex – description of ONCHOSIM model structure and quantification

This annex gives a complete description of the ONCHOSIM model structure and parameter quantification. Except for the quantification of the effect of ivermectin treatment, the version of the model presented is the same as used in Habbema *et al.* (1992). In other applications of the model, other quantifications may be used for situation specific parameter groups like demography, exposure, coverage of drug-treatment, etc. Since the model structure and quantification is regularly updated, in the future use of ONCHOSIM assumptions may differ from this description. Note that the ONCHOSIM computer program offers the opportunity to change parameter values, to choose other options regarding the type of probability distributions used, and to make structural changes in parts of the model.

Demography

The human population dynamics is governed by birth and death processes. We define $F(a)$ as the probability to survive to age a (apart from excess mortality due to onchocerciasis related blindness). The values used are as follows:

age (a)	0	5	10	15	20	30	50	90
$F(a)$	1.000	0.804	0.772	0.760	0.740	0.686	0.509	0.000

Survival at intermediate ages is obtained by interpolation.

The expected number of births (per year) at a given moment t is given by:

$$R_b(t) = \sum_{k=1}^{n_a} N_f(k,t) \times r_b(k) \qquad (A1)$$

with:

$N_f(k,t)$ number of women in age group k at time t.

$r_b(k)$ annual birth-giving rate of women in age-group k: 0.109 babies per year for women between 15 and 20 years; 0.300 between 20 and 30 years; 0.119 between 30 and 50 years; 0.0 for all other ages.

n_a number of age-groups considered.

Each month $R_b(t)$ is adapted according to the number of women and their age-distribution.

Exposure to blackflies

The number of bites $mbr_i(m)$ a person i gets in month m is given by:

$$mbr_i(m) = Mbr(m) \times Ex_i \qquad (A2)$$

with:

$Mbr(m)$ number of bites in month m (m = Jan., Feb., ...) for a person with relative exposure 1.

The relative exposure Ex_i is calculated as:

$$Ex_i = Exa(a_i, s_i) \times Exi_i \qquad (A3)$$

with:

$Exa(a,s)$ relative exposure of person with age a and sex s: Zero at birth, linear increase between age of 0 and 20 years to 1.0 for men and 0.7 for women, and constant from 20 years onwards.

$Exi_i \sim Weibull(1.0, \alpha_{Exi})$ exposure index of person i. The exposure index of a person remains constant throughout lifetime. For selected OCP villages, estimated α_{Exi} values vary between 1.3 (nearly exponential) and 4.5 .

The values of $Mbr(m)$ are obtained from six representative years of fly collections near the village of Asubende (Ghana). There, average monthly biting rates of 2570 bites per person, varying from 1500 in March to 3750 in November have been found. For the actual biting rates $(Mbr(m))$ inside this village we multiplied these figures by a factor (called the *relative biting rate*) of 0.95 (note: since we have no measurements of biting rates actually experienced by villagers, we have – arbitrarily – defined a relative biting rate of 1.0 – i.e. mean $Mbr = 2570$ – as the biting rate resulting in a geometric mean number of mf per skin-snip of 100 in a hypothetical village with all persons being permanently characterized with a relative exposure of 1.0). Assuming the same seasonal pattern, for other villages relative biting rates have been estimated to vary from 0.4 to 0.9.

Acquisition, development, longevity and productivity of parasites in the human host

If, during a bloodmeal of a fly in month m on average lr infective larvae are released, the force-of-infection $foi_i(m)$ — defined as the expected number of new adult parasites per year — acting upon person i in month m is calculated as:

$$foi_i(m) = 12 \times mbr_i(m) \times lr(m) \times sr \qquad (A4)$$

with:

> sr success ratio: fraction of injected L3-larvae succeeding in growing to adult male or female worms: $sr = 0.0031$. An average male:female sex ratio of $1 : 1$ is assumed.

The reproductive lifespan of male and female parasites is a random variable

$$Tl \sim Weibull(\overline{Tl}, \alpha_{Tl}), \quad \text{with } \overline{Tl} = 10 \text{ years and } \alpha_{Tl} = 3.8.$$

The mf-productivity $r(a, t)$ of a female worm of age a at time t is calculated as follows:

$$r(a, t) = R(a) \times m(t) \qquad (A5)$$

with:

> $R(a)$ potential mf-productivity of a female worm of age a (in years): $R(a) = 0$ for $0 \leq a < 1$ (immature period of one year); $R(a) = 1$ for $1 \leq a < 6$; $R(a) = 1 - ((a - 6)/15)$ for $6 \leq a < 21$; $R(a) = 0$ for $a \geq 21$.

> $m(t)$ mating factor at time t

To continue mf-production, a female worm must be inseminated each rc months (rc = reproductive cycle = 3). If insemination took place less than rc months ago, then $m(t) = 1$. Otherwise, the probability of (re-)insemination $P_{ins}(t)$ in month t is given by:

$$P_{ins}(t) = \begin{cases} W_m(t)/W_f(t) & \text{if } W_m < W_f \\ 1 & \text{otherwise} \end{cases} \tag{A6}$$

with:

> $W(t)$ number of male (W_m) or female (W_f) parasites in the human at time t.

If no insemination takes place then $m(t) = 0$ and the female worm has a new opportunity in month $t + 1$. If insemination occurs in month t_i then $m(t) = 1$ during $t_i \leq t < t_i + rc$.

The skin mf-density at time t ($sl(t)$) is calculated by accumulating the mf-production of all female parasites over the past Tm months:

$$sl(t) = cw \times el(t) \tag{A7}$$

$$el(t) = \frac{1}{Tm} \sum_{j=1}^{n_i} \sum_{x=1}^{Tm} r_j(a_j - x, t - x) \tag{A8}$$

with:

> $el(t)$ the *effective parasite load* at time t. This intermediate variable describes the female parasite load obtained by weighting each worm according to the mf-productivity during the past Tm months.

> cw average contribution of an inseminated worm at peak fecundity ($R = 1$) to the skin mf-density: $cw = 7.6$ mf/worm.

> Tm (fixed) microfilarial lifespan: $Tm = 0.75$ years.

> n_i number of parasites alive during at least one of the months $t - 1, \ldots, t - Tm$.

Skin-snip count

The expected number of mf in a skin-snip is given by:

$$\widehat{ss}(t) = \frac{cw}{Tm} \sum_{j=1}^{n_i} d_j \sum_{x=1}^{Tm} r_j(a_j - x, t - x) \tag{A9}$$

with:

d_j the *dispersal factor* of female parasite j. This is a random variable accounting for differences in the contribution of female worms to the mf-density at the site of the body where snips are taken. We assume an exponential distribution for describing these differences: $d_j \sim Expo(1.0)$.

The actual number of mf per skin-snip follows a Poisson distribution: $ss(t) \sim Poisson(\widehat{ss}(t))$. At each epidemiological survey 2 snips per person are taken.

Uptake, development and release of larvae in the vector

On the basis of fly-feeding experiments in OCP the following expression for the relation between L1-uptake (lu) and skin-microfilarial density (sl) has been derived (note: since most of the mf engorged during a bloodmeal are trapped in the fly, we consider L1-'uptake' rather than mf-uptake):

$$lu = a(1 - e^{-b.sl})(1 + e^{-c.sl}) \qquad (A10)$$

with: $a = 1.2$, $b = 0.0213$, and $c = 0.0861$ (the initial slope of this relationship equals $2ab$). The mean L1-uptake in the fly population in month m is now calculated as:

$$\overline{lu}(m) = \sum_{i=1}^{N(m)} (Ex_i \times lu_i) / \sum_{i=1}^{N(m)} Ex_i \qquad (A11)$$

with:

$N(m)$ number of persons in month m.

It is assumed that a fixed proportion of the L1-larvae develops to the L3-stage and will be released at one of the subsequent bites:

$$lr(m) = v \times \overline{lu}(m) \qquad (A12)$$

with:

$lr(m)$ mean L3-release per bite in month m.

v transmission probability: average probability that an L1-larva is released as an infective L3-larva.

The calculation of the transmission probability v is complicated. In calculating v we take into account the life-history of the fly starting from her first bloodmeal. We assume that bloodmeals are taken at fixed hours during daytime, so that we can use 1 day timesteps. Though we take into account differences in the length of the gonotrophic cycle between flies, in the model we assume that a particular fly has always the same cycle length (which equals the time between two successive bloodmeals). We further explicitly account for variation in the duration of development from L1 to L3. The basic assumption underlying the use of a fixed proportion v is that at any moment the fly-population has a stable age-distribution and that the number of bites per person is large enough to ensure that the flies biting a person always reflect this stable age-distribution.

Calculation of the transmission probability v

Assume that a fly engorges one L1-larva at her m^{th} bloodmeal, then the probability of releasing an L3-larva n bloodmeals later is given by:

$$P_{rel}(n|i,j,m) = P_{L1 \to L3} \times (1 - P_{L3 \to})^i \times P_{L3 \to L3}^i \times P_{L3 \to} \times S(m, n \times j) \quad (\text{A}13)$$

with:

$P_{rel}(n|i,j,m)$ The probability to release one L3 larva at the $(m+n)^{\text{th}}$ bloodmeal if one L1 larva has been engorged at the mth bloodmeal, given that:

   • a gonotrophic cycle takes j days

   • between bloodmeal m and $m + n$ there have been i potentially infective bloodmeals (i.e. bloodmeals at which the L1-larva had already developed to the L3-stage)

$P_{L1 \to L3}$ The probability that an L1-larva develops to the L3-stage, given survival of the fly: $P_{L1 \to L3} = 0.85$.

$P_{L3 \to L3}$ The probability that an L3-larva which is not released at a given bloodmeal survives to a next bloodmeal, given survival of the fly: $P_{L3 \to L3} = 0.90$.

$P_{L3 \to}$ The probability that an L3-larva is released at a bloodmeal: $P_{L3 \to} = 0.65$.

$S(m, t)$ The probability that a fly survives for t days since bloodmeal m.

In order to arrive at a general solution for all possible values of i, we use the probability distribution of the number of potentially infective bloodmeals since the intake-meal and before the release meal:

$$P_{rel}(n|j,m) = \sum_{i=0}^{n-1} [P_{rel}(n|i,j,m) \times P_{ib}(i|n,j)] \qquad (A14)$$

$$P_{ib}(i|n,j) = F_{dL1 \to L3}(j(n-i)) - F_{dL1 \to L3}(j(n-i-1)) \qquad (A15)$$

with:

$P_{ib}(i|n,j)$ The probability that before the nth bloodmeal since intake, i bloodmeals have been potentially infective (L1 has become L3), given a cycle length of j days.

$F_{dL1 \to L3}(t)$ The probability that the duration of development of L1 to L3 is equal to or less than t days ($F_{dL1 \to L3}(t) = 0.0$ for $t \leq 5$; 0.07 for $t = 6$; 0.86 for $t = 7$; 1.0 for $t \geq 8$ days).

A general solution for all possible values of m can be obtained by incorporating the probability that a fly takes her m^{th} bloodmeal:

$$P_{rel}(n|j) = \sum_{m=1}^{m_{max}} [P_{rel}(n|j,m) \times P_b(m|j)] \qquad (A16)$$

$$P_b(m|j) = L(j(m-1))/ \sum_{m=1}^{m_{max}} L(j(m-1)) \qquad (A17)$$

with:

$P_b(m|j)$ The probability that a feeding fly takes her m^{th} bloodmeal at a cycle length of j days.

$L(t)$ The probability that a fly lives for at least t days. At present we assume an age-independent daily survival of 0.78.

Generalizing for j can be achieved by summation, weighted for the probability distribution of the duration of the gonotrophic cycle:

$$P_{rel}(n) = \sum_{j=j_{min}}^{j_{max}} [P_{rel}(n|j) \times P_{gc}(j)] \qquad (A18)$$

with:

$P_{gc}(j)$ Probability that a gonotrophic cycle takes j days
(i.e. j days between successive bloodmeals;
$P_{gc}(j) = 0.0$ for $j \leq 2$; 0.2 for $j = 3$; 0.6 for $j = 4$;
0.2 for $j = 5$; 0.0 for $j \geq 6$ days).

Using the following equality

$$S(m, n \times j) = L(j(m + n + 1))/L(j(m - 1)) \qquad (A19)$$

the average probability that an L1-larva taken from a human will develop to
the L3-stage and be released to another human is given by:

$$
P_{rel} = P_{L1 \to L3} \times P_{L3 \to} \times \sum_{j=j_{min}}^{j_{max}} \left\{ P_{gc}(j) \times \sum_{m=1}^{m_{max}} \left[\frac{1}{\sum_{m=1}^{m_{max}} L(j(m - 1))} \right] \right.
$$

$$
\times \sum_{n=1}^{n_{max}} \left\{ L(j(m + n + 1)) \times \sum_{i=0}^{n-1} [(1 - P_{L3 \to}) \times P_{L3 \to L3}]^i \right. \qquad (A20)
$$

$$
\left. \left. \times [F_{dL1 \to L3}(j(n - i)) - F_{dL1 \to L3}(j(n - i - 1))] \right\} \right\}
$$

In equations (A16), (A17) and (A18):

$$
m_{max} = \left\lfloor \frac{a_{max}}{j} + 1 \right\rfloor \quad n_{max} = \left\lfloor \frac{a_{max} - (m \times j)}{j} \right\rfloor \qquad (A21)
$$

with:

a_{max} Maximum attainable age of the fly (i.e. age at
which $L(t)$ approaches zero). ($\lfloor \cdot \rfloor$ denotes
truncation to integer).

The transmission probability v is now given by:

$$v = P_{rel} \times (1 - z) \qquad (A22)$$

with:

z Fraction of fly-bites on non-human objects
(zoophily; $z = 0.04$).

Using the indicated quantifications, we have calculated the value of v as
0.073 released larvae per L1-larva resulting from a given mf-uptake. Note
that formula (A20) reduces to a much simpler form if we assume that each
day a fraction S of the flies survive, that the gonotrophic cycle has a fixed
duration of dgc days, and that the number of bloodmeals needed to complete
the development of L1 to L3 is fixed at $n1 \to 3$:

$$
P_{rel} = P_{L1 \to L3} \times P_{L3 \to} \times \frac{S^{n1 \to 3 \times dgc}}{1 - S^{dgc} \times (1 - P_{L3 \to}) \times P_{L3 \to L3}} \qquad (A23)
$$

Blindness and excess mortality

The probability of a person going blind at age a (months) depends on the *accumulated parasite load* (elc) of a person:

$$elc(a) = \sum_{x=0}^{a} el(x) \qquad (A24)$$

Each person has a threshold level of elc (denoted as Elc) at which a person goes blind. Elc follows a probability distribution: $Elc \sim Weibull(\overline{Elc}, \alpha_{Elc})$, with $\overline{Elc} = 10,000$ and $\alpha_{Elc} = 2.0$. Person i goes blind at age a when:

$$elc_i(a) \geq Elc_i > elc_i(a-1) \qquad (A25)$$

At that moment the remaining life-span at age a is reduced by a factor rl which follows a uniform distribution on $[0,1]$ (hence, on average, $rl = 0.5$).

Ivermectin: mass treatment coverage and compliance

The primary characteristic of a certain ivermectin mass treatment w is the coverage C_w (fraction of the population treated; typically 0.65). However, a difficulty in calculating individual chances of participation is that there are several exclusion criteria for the drug. Moreover, compliance to treatment differs from person to person. Exclusion criteria can be either permanent (chronic illness) or transient (children below 5 and pregnant or breast-feeding women). We define the eligible population as the total population *minus* a fraction fc ($= 0.05$) which is permanently excluded from treatment (in the model from birth to death). The coverage among the eligible population is now given by:

$$C'_w = C_w/(1 - fc) \qquad (A26)$$

The transient contra-indications and other age- and sex-related factors are taken into account in the age- and sex-specific relative compliance $c_r(k, s)$ for each age-group k and sex s. Based on OCP data we use:

age-group (k)	0–4	5–9	10–14	15–19	20–29	30–49	50+
$c_r(k, \text{male})$	0.00	0.75	0.80	0.80	0.70	0.75	0.80
$c_r(k, \text{female})$	0.00	0.75	0.70	0.74	0.65	0.70	0.75

Note that in $c_r(k, s)$ only the ratio between the values for the different groups is relevant. The coverage $c(k, s, w)$ in each of the age- and sex-groups at treatment round w is calculated as:

$$c(k, s, w) = \frac{c_r(k, s) \times N(w)}{\sum_{s=1}^{2} \sum_{k=1}^{n_a} c_r(k, s) \times N(k, s, w)} \times C'_w \qquad (A27)$$

with:

$N(k, s, w)$ Number of individuals eligible to treatment
              in age-group k and sex s at treatment
              round w.

$N(w)$ Total number of eligible individuals at
        treatment round w.

Finally, the probability of participating in treatment round w for an eligible person i of age-group k and sex s is given by:

$$Ptr_{i,w} = co_i^{(1-c(k,s,w))/c(k,s,w)}$$ (A28)

with:

co_i Personal compliance index. This is considered as
        a lifelong property and is generated from a
        uniform distribution on $[0, 1]$.

Note that for all k and s the average value of $Ptr_{i,w}$ equals $c(k, s, w)$.

Ivermectin: the parasitological effect of treatment

In the model we assume that an effective treatment with the drug causes elimination of 100% of the microfilariae from the skin-tissues. The impact of the drug on the subsequent productivity r of a female parasite j in person i is given by:

$$r_{j,i}(t) = \begin{cases} r_{j,i}^0(t) \times (1 - v_i d) \times \left(\frac{t}{v_i Tr}\right)^s & \text{if } u_j > v_i m \text{ and } v_i d < 1 \\ 0 & \text{otherwise} \end{cases}$$ (A29)

with:

t Time (months) since treatment. Note: the last
     term of the equation is truncated to 1 if $t \geq Tr$.

$r_{j,i}(t)$ mf-productivity of female worm j at t months
             after treatment with ivermectin of person i (see
             (A5))

$r_{j,i}^0(t)$ The mf-productivity of this worm j had person i
              not been treated at the last round.

v_i Relative effectivity of treatment in person i.

d Average permanent (unrecoverable) reduction in
     mf-productivity resulting from treatment
     ($d = 0.35$).

Tr Average duration of the period of recovery, i.e. the period during which the mf-productivity of the female worm increases from 0 to the new equilibrium ($Tr = 11$ months).

s Shape parameter of the recovery function ($s = 1.5$).

u_j Random number on $[0,1]$ generated for each female worm j.

m Average fraction of female worms killed as a result of treatment (at present: $m = 0$).

The relative effectivity v_i is a random variable generated from a probability distribution: $v_i \sim Weibull(1.0, \alpha_v)$, with $\alpha_v = 2.0$. In the model we explicitly allow for persons (5% of the treated population) on whom the drug has no effect on a particular round (malabsorption, e.g. due to vomiting).

Vector control

Vector control is modelled as a percentage reduction r of the monthly biting rates during a given period of time. A period of vector control is specified as the year + month + day of the beginning of the strategy and the year + month + day of the end of a strategy. If in a certain month during a period of d days larvicides have been applied, then the reduction in $Mbr(m)$ in that month equals $d/30 \times r$.

References

Alley, E.S., Plaisier, A.P., Boatin, B., Dadzie, K.Y., Remme, J., Zerbo, G. and Samba, E.M. (1994) 'The impact of five years of annual ivermectin treatment on skin microfilarial loads in the onchocerciasis focus of Asubende, Ghana', *Trans. Roy. Soc. Trop. Med. Hyg.* **88**, 581–584.

Anderson, R.M. and May, R.M. (1991) *Infectious Diseases of Humans*, Oxford University Press, Oxford.

Dietz, K. (1982) 'The population dynamics of onchocerciasis'. In *Population dynamics of infectious diseases*, R.M.Anderson (ed.), Chapman and Hall, London, 209–241.

Habbema, J.D.F., Alley, E.S., Plaisier, A.P., Van Oortmarssen, G.J. and Remme, J.H.F. (1992) 'Epidemiological modelling for onchocerciasis control', *Parasitol. Today* **8**, 99–103.

Habbema, J.D.F., De Vlas, S.J., Plaisier, A.P. and Van Oortmarssen, G.J. (1995) 'The microsimulation approach to epidemiological modeling of helminth infections, with special reference to schistosomiasis', *Am. J. Trop. Med. Hyg.*, in press.

OCP (1990) *Report of the Eleventh Session of the Expert Advisory Committee of the Onchocerciasis Control Programme in West Africa*, OCP/EAC/90.1

Plaisier, A.P., Van Oortmarssen, G.J., Habbema, J.D.F., Remme, J. and Alley, E.S. (1990) 'ONCHOSIM: a model and computer simulation program for the transmission and control of onchocerciasis', *Comp. Meth. Programs in Biomed.* **31**, 43–56.

Plaisier, A.P., Van Oortmarssen, G.J., Remme, J. and Habbema, J.D.F. (1991a) 'The reproductive lifespan of *Onchocerca volvulus* in West African savanna', *Acta Trop.* **48**, 271–284.

Plaisier, A.P., Van Oortmarssen, G.J., Remme, J., Alley, E.S. and Habbema, J.D.F. (1991b) 'The risk and dynamics of onchocerciasis recrudescence after cessation of vector control', *Bull. WHO* **69**, 169–178.

Remme, J.H.F., Ba, O., Dadzie, K.Y. and Karam, M. (1986) 'A force-of-infection model for onchocerciasis and its application in the epidemiological evaluation of the Onchocerciasis Control Programme in the Volta River basin area', *Bull. WHO* **37**, 195–212.

Remme, J.H.F., Dadzie, K.Y., Rolland, A. and Thylefors, B. (1989) 'Ocular onchocerciasis and intensity of infection in the community. I: West African savanna', *Trop. Med. Parasit.* **40**, 340–347.

Remme, J.H.F., Alley, E.S. and Plaisier, A.P. (1995) 'Estimation and prediction in tropical disease control: the example of onchocerciasis'. In *Models for Human Infectious Diseases: Their Structure and Relation to Data*, D. Mollison (ed.), Cambridge University Press, Cambridge, 372–393.

Schulz-Key, H. and Karam, M. (1986) 'Periodic reproduction of *Onchocerca volvulus*', *Parasitol. Today* **2**, 284–286.

Invited Discussion

A.K. Shahani

1. General comments

One connecting theme for these papers is modelling. A standard terminology for modelling work could ease the communication between various disciplines and perhaps it may be helpful to classify the nature of the models and their solutions along the following lines:

Model	Solution
Deterministic	Analytical
Stochastic	Numerical
Other	Simulation/Monte Carlo
	Other

For example, a semi-Markov process is a useful general stochastic model for disease processes and it is often solved for particular numerical values through simulation.

It is instructive to trace the development of statistical data analysis and the current modelling work. Before about 1900 medical and biological knowledge about humans was insufficient for the development of models for disease and attention was focused on mortality statistics. This early work could be classified as Death Modelling. The medical, microbiological, epidemiological, statistical, mathematical, and computing advances have resulted in many Disease Models where attempts are made to describe the development of a disease over time in a community. In Disease Models important events, additional to Death, could be clinical or microbiological events. There is a good spectrum of disease models at this workshop. A Disease Model opens up the possibility of more efficient trials and data analysis in comparison with the use of mortality statistics only. Perhaps with a greater understanding of the control processes in a human body we can look forward to Health Models in which particular diseases will be symptoms of particular kinds of microbiological, genetic, electro/chemical events in the body. Perhaps a useful class of models will turn out to be Integrated Survival and Health Augmenting Models (ISHAM).

The four high quality papers in this session have been thought provoking and instructive.

2. Paper by Dr. Peto

Dr. Peto, in a very lucid and interesting talk, reminded us about the importance of properly designed clinical trials: Death as the well established end
point of a trial is a 'gold standard'; randomisation and blindness are essential
for avoiding bias.

Whilst acknowledging the vital importance of survival, I feel that perhaps
we should encourage a few 'novel' trials for dealing with the threat of HIV
infection. There seems to be a good agreement about the use of some clinical
events, for example listed in the CDC (1987) classification, in judgements
about treatments, and the seriousness of decreased life span. These early
events, compared with Death in a data set will mean less noisy data. In
other words trials based on early clinical events would be quicker and cheaper.
Disease models for the progression of infection in a cohort of HIV+ patients
could point to the design of some 'novel' trials. The opposition by clinicians
to the use of gold standards in the design of trials for evaluating treatments
for HIV patients is a good stimulus for a discussion about other possible, and
desirable, standards.

Randomisation and blindness are excellent for guarding against bias in
judgements about the general goodness of a treatment. Is there a role for novel
trials that test whether clinicians, or HIV patients, can 'spot the winner'?
The starting point for discussion of this issue is the idea that a treatment
will be beneficial for some but not all patients. Maybe some clinicians can
spot the people for whom the treatment is more likely to be beneficial. Is it
possible to design trials that test these differential effects without the danger
of a total waste of effort?

One particular point of detail on which I would welcome Dr. Peto's comments is the evaluation of the two survival curves for the data from one of
the HIV trials. The strong graphical impact was that between years 1 and
2 there seemed a difference and that the overall difference was influenced by
the sharp drop in the top curve towards the end of the trial. Some of the
questions raised by this graphical evidence are: Is the large drop due to an
outlier? What would be the conclusion from the statistical analysis if the
large drop is treated as an outlier? Is it a good idea to discuss confidence
limits, rather p values, in the consideration of conclusions from statistical
analysis?

3. Paper by Dr. Medley

Dr. Medley has drawn attention to the conflicts between public good and
individual good that can result from public health policies.

Perhaps a sharper focus for discussions about this important issue could
be provided by a simple dichotomous classification of 'good result' and 'poor

result' for a community and for an individual. This classification results in four possible outcomes, two of which have conflicts.

In the absence of a Health Model, public policy for dealing with diseases has to be evolved through the consideration of a particular group of diseases. Complexity, uncertainty, variability and use of scarce resources are the typical challenges that have to be met. Use of appropriate models is likely to be a growth area and Dr. Medley draws attention to the importance of probability distributions, rather than mean values obtained commonly from deterministic models. It is perhaps a good idea to use a standard result to remind ourselves about the dangers of a bias in the mean value calculated from a deterministic model.

Consider $Y = f(X)$, where Y is an outcome measure. The mean value of X is μ and the use of a deterministic model corresponds to the use of the approximation

$$E(Y) \simeq f(\mu).$$

Taylor series expansion of Y, yields

$$E(Y) \simeq f(\mu) + f'(\mu)E(X - \mu)2/2! + f''(\mu)E(X - \mu)3/3! \ldots$$

Thus if Y is a non-linear function of X and there is variation in X, then the use of results from deterministic models as the mean value for the community could be incorrect. The bias will depend on the degree of variability in X and on the nature of the function f. In comparison of two policies, for example, it may be that the deterministic models would yield good answers. With Y_1 and Y_2 as two outcome measures we have

$$E(Y_1) = f_1(\mu) + \text{Bias}_1$$
$$E(Y_2) = f_2(\mu) + \text{Bias}_2$$

so that

$$E(Y_1) - E(Y_2) \simeq f_1(\mu) - f_2(\mu) \quad \text{if Bias}_1 \simeq \text{Bias}_2.$$

Experience in the development and use of models that take conflicts into account is needed. The pressures against such explicit considerations in a discussion of public policy are easy to understand. For example, vaccine damage is an illustration of individual loss for public good; however there would be an anxiety that public debate fuelled perhaps by headlines about vaccine damage would simply result in unnecessary refusals for vaccination. A false HIV+ result is another example of individual damage. It may be that explicit modelling of such conflicts may result in policy about looking after damaged individuals without assigning specific blame to particular doctors or health organisations.

Dr. Medley feels that non-transmissible diseases do not give rise to conflicts between individuals and populations. This would be so if the definition of conflict is conditional on achieved health benefits. However the development of public policy requires decisions about allocation of resources and these decisions do give rise to conflicts. Diverting resources from, for example, a disease which is not very common will benefit a community as a whole at the expense of the individuals with the disease.

4. Paper by Dr. Agur

There is a growing literature on the development of models that can help to design improved treatments, and the use of population dynamics for AZT chemotherapy is an important contribution to this work. Practical models for evaluating treatments should take different types of side effects explicitly into account. Another important issue is that of variability in responses to treatment from individual to individual. It is likely that side effects and variability are major challenges to analytical work and in the absence of general solutions, simulation models could give valuable insights.

5. Paper by Professor Habbema

Professor Habbema's paper is concerned with the development of practical models that can help to control disease in a community. Necessary conditions for developing good models are:

Joint work by a number of appropriate experts and dedicated work over a period of time for evolving the models.

Data for validating such models is a major problem. Internal verification of large simulation models, that is checking that the model does what it is supposed to do, is also a challenging task. I would welcome Professor Habbema's comments on validation and verification. Comments on the use of the model by OCP and other users would be welcomed.

Are there some well defined clinical/biological events, in addition to microfilarial load and blindness, that can be used to extend the model? Such additional states, if feasible, could provide further measures of the effects of interventions. Is it a good idea to extend the model with explicit calculations of the resources needed and, perhaps, the resulting costs?

Professor Habbema asked whether this modelling approach has been used for other diseases. At the University of Southampton, our experiences of modelling through the Operational Research approach of joint work has been used for work on a number of diseases. Recent examples are: Resource planning and patient care for HIV infection; Control and treatment of trachoma, Detection and treatment of genital chlamydial infection; Surveillance of patients with Barrett's oesophagus; Care of asthma patients, Maternity care in community and hospital; Community, GP and hospital consultant interactions on patient care through outpatient clinics. Given the willingness for joint work, adequate data for developing and validating models is a major challenge. In the absence of data, models that provide an easy access of expert opinion can yield valuable insights for dealing with disease and for highlighting the need for particular kind of data. There are a number of other examples of this sort of modelling work. In the UK it may be that one of the effects of the national documents on health targets and health policy will be an increased modelling activity involving community care, General Practitioner's work, and hospital care.

Invited Discussion

C. Dye

The preceding papers have been sufficiently diverse to expose (at least) two apparent dichotomies in quantitative epidemiology. These concern the kinds of models needed to solve epidemiological problems: simple versus complex models, and dynamics versus statistical models. A minimum of three papers is needed to highlight the issues: this session has done it with just four.

Those who prefer to begin with complex (Habbema) or simple (Agur, Medley) dynamic models take different views of how many parameters and variables are needed to make these models useful. Crudely, the former hold that model utility is a monotonically increasing function of the number of parameters and variables, whilst the later believe that the slope of this graph will usually be negative. The two schools have different approaches because they have different aims. The view of the complex modellers is epitomized by the statement (Habbema *et al.* 1992):

> *Ideally, epidemiological modelling should serve as a scientific framework for studying many aspects of disease control: choice of control policy, prediction, planning, operational decision making, data analysis, evaluation and surveillance.*

The effort to deal with 'many aspects' is characteristic, but so too is the attempt to construct a model which is sufficiently detailed to predict the absolute (Habbema *et al.* 1992):

> *14 years of full-scale vector control will be sufficient to reduce the risk of [onchocerciasis] recrudescence to less that 1% even in the most afflicted areas.*

It is clear, however, that the more robust policy statements will emerge when detailed models of this kind are used in a comparative way – to choose the best among available options.

The Onchocerciasis Control Programme (OCP), of which ONCHOSIM is a product, has been a multi-million dollar effort, an unusually large investment in parameter estimation. Two questions emerge: To what extent is the complexity of ONCHOSIM devoted to answering the most unanswerable absolute questions: how, for example, do we act on the statement that 14 years of control will reduce the risk of recrudescence to less than 1%? Could much simpler models which are less data-hungry lead to a robust choice of the best among available control options?

Accepting that even very complex simulation models are crude represen-
tations of reality, pupils of the second, minimalist school (Agur, Medley)
generally believe that making detailed predictions is the most demanding
task given to modellers. They question the view that complex models do indeed provide a useful 'scientific framework': the behaviour of big simulation
models often remains inexplicably counter-intuitive, even after investigative
numerical experiments. Their emphasis is on using models to lay bare the
fundamental processes, looking at one phenomenon at a time. Understanding
in each case will, it is thought, be most easily gained by working from the
bottom upwards.

Advocates of big models may ask for evidence that the bottom-up approach
does not overlook important interaction effects when trying to understand basic epidemiological processes. It is worth noting that the function of simple
models sometimes slips unnoticed from qualitative explanation to absolute
prediction. For example, published estimates of the proportions to be vaccinated for eradication come from calculations of R_0 based on very simple
models (Anderson and May 1991). How should these estimates be treated by
policy makers?

From the two poles of dynamic and statistical epidemiology have been
heard cries of 'sterile' (the former on the latter) and 'simply unbelievable'
(the latter on the former). The more temperate view is, of course, that the
best epidemiology will exploit both. Here, Agur's discussion of drug treatment regimes in terms of perturbations to systems with natural resonance
or periodicity raises a general question for drug trialists (Peto). Could dynamic models of the human immune response to HIV infection be used to
identify surrogate markers, bringing forward the end-points of clinical trials?
At present, the answer is that they certainly could not. But would medical
statisticians ever accept arguments of this kind?

The conflict between individuals and communities in the treatment of
AIDS patients, made plain by viewing infectious disease epidemiology on
both levels (Medley), raises an additional, obvious question for those concerned with the introduction of new drugs (Peto): do longer-lived HIV cases
which are more durably infectious constitute (yet) another serious ethical
issue for clinicians? Conceivably, the dilemma here would be dismissed by
simultaneous appeal to the individual responsibility of infected patients, and
to the Hippocratic Oath.

References

Habbema, J.D.F., Alley, E.S., Plaisier, A.P., van Oortmarssen, G.J. and Remme,
J.H.F. (1992) 'Epidemiological modelling for onchocerciasis control', *Parasitol.
Today* **8**, 99–103.

Anderson, R.M. and May, R.M. (1991) *Infectious Diseases of Humans: Dynamics
and Control*, Oxford University Press, Oxford.

Hydatid Disease

M.G. Roberts

Introduction

Hydatid disease is caused by accidental infection with the intermediate stages of tapeworms of *Echinococcus* species, principally *Echinococcus granulosus* and *E.multilocularis*. The adult worm parasitises the small intestine of carnivores, usually Canidae, and sheds proglottids containing eggs which pass with the host's faeces. If the eggs are then ingested by a herbivore they develop into a larval stage (cyst) within the liver or other viscera. The cycle is completed when the carnivore consumes the herbivore, ingesting a mature cyst. *Echinococcus granulosus* originated in a wolf-deer life-cycle, and has evolved in dogs and sheep and other domesticated and wild animals. The definitive hosts of *E.multilocularis* are foxes, and the intermediate hosts small rodents such as voles and lemmings. *Echinococcus granulosus* is ubiquitous but *E.multilocularis* is confined to the Northern Hemisphere. Cystic hydatid disease in man is caused by the larval form of *E.granulosus*. Surgery provides a cure in 50–90% of cases, but recurrence is common. Alveolar hydatid disease caused by *E.multilocularis* results in metastases throughout the soft organs. Until recently it was invariably fatal, but chemotherapy may retard the proliferation of cysts. For further information on the epidemiology of echinococcosis and hydatid disease see Roberts and Gemmell (1994). This paper presents two examples where models of the dynamics of *Echinococcus* species have been used to investigate control policies.

Echinococcus granulosus in farmed animals in New Zealand.

The first case of cystic hydatid disease in New Zealand was recorded in 1862. The annual number of cases peaked at 7.2 per 100,000 in 1946, and then declined to 0.37 per 100,000 in 1987, largely due to the control programme that was initiated in 1959. From that time all dogs were subjected to regular chemotherapy to remove tapeworms. The prevalence of *E.granulosus* in dogs and sheep had been 37% and 89% respectively in 1958, but by 1990 no dogs were found to be infected, and infected sheep were confined to a few farms. Prior to the control programme a related parasite *Taenia ovis*, which does not infect humans, was rare, but by 1968 it was being detected in 5% of lambs and ewes at meat inspection.

388

A model for the population dynamics of cestodes in domestic life-cycles was described by Roberts *et al.* (1986, 1987). Define h as the mean rate at which an intermediate host animal (sheep) would acquire larvae in the absence of density-dependent constraints. As acquired immunity in the intermediate host is the only such constraint in this system, h is proportional to the mean number of worms in dogs, and also the mean density of eggs on the pasture. The dynamics of h are described by

$$h'(t) = -\mu h + \lambda \int_0^t f(t - \tau)h(\tau)S(\tau)d\tau \qquad (1)$$

where $S(t)$ is the proportion of sheep that are susceptible to infection, μ is the rate at which parasites are lost by processes such as the desiccation of eggs or the mortality of adult parasites, and λ is an overall transmission rate. The function $f(t)$ is the probability density of the time from the establishment of a cyst to it being mature and ingested by a dog, conditional on this occurring.

The proportion of sheep that are susceptible to infection decreases as the infection pressure increases, and increases as immunity wanes. As acquired immunity is boosted by re-exposure the rate of decrease (γ) is a function of h and

$$S'(t) = -ahS + \gamma(h)(1 - S) \qquad (2)$$

Equations (1, 2) have two steady states: $h = 0$, $S = 1$ where the parasite is extinct and all sheep are susceptible to infection; and a second where $S = \mu/\lambda$ and h is the solution of $ah = \gamma(h)(\lambda/\mu - 1)$. As $\gamma'(h) \leq 0$ the second steady state exists and is uniquely determined if the basic reproduction ratio $R_0 = \lambda/\mu > 1$. The extinction state ($h = 0$) is globally asymptotically stable for $R_0 < 1$ and unstable for $R_0 > 1$. The stability of the non-zero steady state depends on the function $\gamma(h)$, and insufficient data are available to determine this.

Roberts *et al.* (1987) estimated the values of R_0 for *E.granulosus* in male and female sheep in New Zealand in 1958 to be not greater than 1.3 and 1.6 respectively. Similar estimates for *T.ovis* were 2.5 and 4.3. In addition Roberts *et al.* (1986) estimated that the dog-dosing programme reduced R_0 for these parasites by 69%. Hence the control programme was able to eradicate *E.granulosus*, but was largely ineffectual against *T.ovis*.

Echinococcus multilocularis in wild animals in France.

Echinococcus multilocularis is found in wildlife in mountainous regions of France. Its major definitive host is the red fox, and intermediate hosts are rodents (especially voles). Approximately twenty human cases per year are reported (Delattre *et al.* 1991). In Eastern France foxes also serve as a reservoir for rabies, and a programme of distributing baits containing oral vaccine by helicopters is in progress. If a helminthicide were added to the baits a mass chemotherapy of foxes would be achieved, but at a level dictated by the policy governing the control of rabies. The possibility of such a campaign being successful was investigated by Roberts and Aubert (1995).

The proportions of foxes and voles that are susceptible, infected but not yet infectious, or infectious are denoted by F, H, J or U, V, W respectively, $F + H + J = U + V + W = 1$. The dynamics of the adult *E.multilocularis* population in the fox are described by

$$H'(t) = \lambda FW - (\nu + s + c)H, \qquad (1)$$
$$J'(t) = \nu H - (\mu + s + c)J, \qquad (2)$$

where s is the death rate of foxes, parasites mature at a rate ν, adult parasites have a mean life-expectancy of $1/\mu$ years and c is the control effort, defined as the increase in the rate of mortality of adult parasites due to control.

Similarly the dynamics of the larval population in the vole are described by

$$V'(t) = \gamma NUJ - (\eta + b)V, \qquad (3)$$
$$W'(t) = \eta V - bW, \qquad (4)$$

where b is the death rate of voles and parasites mature at a rate η in the intermediate host. The parameters λ and γ in equations (1) and (3) respectively are transmission rates, and the fox population density N has been explicitly incorporated to emphasise the dependence of transmission on this parameter.

Equations (1–4) have two steady states: the trivial one $F = U = 1$, $H = J = V = W = 0$; and an endemic equilibrium which exists if and only if $R_0 > 1$, where

$$R_0 = \frac{\lambda \nu \eta \gamma N}{b(b + \eta)(\nu + s + c)(\mu + s + c)}$$

is the basic reproduction ratio. The trivial steady state is globally asymptotically stable when $R_0 < 1$, and unstable for $R_0 > 1$. The prevalence of infection is low in the intermediate host ($\ll 1\%$), hence R_0 may be approximated by $1/(1 - P_{fox})$, where P_{fox} is the prevalence of infection in foxes. The control effort required to eradicate *E.multilocularis* can then be calculated as a function of P_{fox}.

This model assumes that superinfection does not occur. As yet no data are available to support or refute this assumption. If this were not valid, the model would have be modified to incorporate an intensity framework. Also, the results are sensitive to the life expectancy of *E.multilocularis* in the definitive host, but in the absence of data Roberts and Aubert (1995) assumed this to be the same as that of *E.granulosus*. The model demonstrates that if the prevalence of *E.multilocularis* in foxes is low in a particular region, incorporating chemotherapy into the existing antirabies treatment could eliminate the parasite from that region. More importantly it highlights deficiencies in the available data. If an experiment could determine the longevity of the parasite in the definitive host, or a trial could establish the distribution of parasites in that host population, then confidence in the results would be much greater.

References

Delattre, P., Giraudoux, P. and Pascal, M. (1991) 'L'échinococcose alvéolaire', *La Recherche* **22**, 295–303.

Roberts, M.G. and Aubert, M.F.A. (1995) 'A model for the control of *Echinococcus multilocularis* in France', *Vet. Parasitol.* **56**, 67–74.

Roberts, M.G. and Gemmell, M.A. (1994) 'Echinococcosis'. In *Parasitic and Infectious Diseases*, M.E. Scott and G. Smith (eds.), Academic Press, 249–262.

Roberts, M.G., Lawson, J.R. and Gemmell, M.A. (1986) 'Population dynamics in echinococcosis and cysticercosis: mathematical model of the life cycle of *Echinococcus granulosus*', *Parasitology* **92**, 621–41.

Roberts, M.G., Lawson, J.R. and Gemmell, M.A. (1987) 'Population dynamics in echinococcosis and cysticercosis: mathematical model of the life cycles of *Taenia hydatigena* and *T.ovis*', *Parasitology* **94**, 181–97.

Vaccines and Herd Immunity: Consequences for Vaccine Evaluation

Mart C.M. de Jong

Introduction

Vaccines activate the immune system so that it is hoped that the response of the host to subsequent infections will be less harmful for the host. Leaving aside the mechanisms by which vaccination works, one can observe three changes in the host-pathogen interaction, i.e. compared to a non-vaccinated individual, a vaccinated individual has: (1) A lower probability of becoming infected when exposed (reduced susceptibility), (2) fewer clinical signs when it is infected (clinical protection), and (3) less infectivity when it is infected (reduced infectivity).

For a first vaccine evaluation, reduced infectivity would not be considered as a positive effect of the vaccine, because it is not of direct benefit to the individual receiving the vaccine. It is important to take reduced infectivity into account, when estimating the combined effect of reduced susceptibility and clinical protection, i.e. vaccine efficacy, because reduced infectivity lessens the exposure of the other individuals in the population. Thus for the estimation of vaccine efficacy one should compensate for differential exposure, and reduced infectivity is a nuisance parameter.

It is especially important to consider how vaccines differ in their effect on infectivity whenever several vaccines are available, that all have similar efficacy. It is known for some vaccines, for example those against measles and polio, that although in vaccinated individuals clinical signs are either absent or very mild, vaccinated individuals are susceptible and they can replicate and excrete virus (infectivity). This implies that virus could circulate in vaccinated populations and therefore it is important to quantify and compare the amount of virus circulation in groups of individuals vaccinated with various vaccines.

Results and Discussion

The extent to which virus circulates is measured by the number of secondary cases per infectious individual, the reproduction ratio of the infection. Maximally, this reproduction ratio equals the basic reproduction ratio R_0 which is the (theoretical) number of secondary cases per infectious individual in

'experiment'	incidence among vaccinated individuals average(s.d.)	incidence among unvaccinated individuals average(s.d.)	correlation coefficient
community level randomisation	0.62(1.21)	8.56(1.93)	–
individual level randomisation: vaccine effect is 100% due to change in susceptibility	2.47(1.67)	8.91(0.86)	0.15
vaccine effect is 50/50 due to change in infectivity and susceptibility	7.17(1.95)	8.67(1.64)	0.71
vaccine effect is 100% due to change in infectivity	8.39(2.22)	8.46(2.03)	0.99

Table 1. Simple numerical example of numbers of individuals infected (incidence) among vaccinated and unvaccinated individuals in various trials.

a wholly susceptible population. Let R_{vac} be the reproduction ratio in the vaccinated population, when $R_{vac} < 1$ the infection will disappear from the population. It is possible that in spite of residual infectivity and susceptibility after vaccination, R_{vac} is below one and thus the infection will never spread. In other words there can be sufficient herd immunity even when individual immunity is not complete.

It follows from the definition of reproduction ratios that these ratios are the product of contact rate, infectivity and susceptibility. Thus, assuming that the contact rate does not change because of vaccination, the effect of vaccination on the reproduction ratio depends on changes in the product of infectivity and susceptibility. In vaccine trials that have as unit of randomisation the community, the incidence in the vaccinated population as compared to that in the unvaccinated population is a measure of the change in the reproduction ratio after vaccination (see Table 1). Note, however, that a decrease in the reproduction ratio due to vaccination cannot be detected in trials based on randomisation on the individual level whenever this decrease is the due to the decrease in infectivity after vaccination (see Table 1).

Consider the simple example where the two types of trials are compared: (1) a trial with two populations each of 10 individuals (9 'susceptible' individuals and one infectious individual) where in one of these populations all individuals are vaccinated and in the other population no individuals are vaccinated, and (2) a trial in a population of 20 individuals with 10 vaccinated individuals (18 'susceptible' individuals and two infectious individuals). In the latter case the outcome critically depends on how the vaccine works: how much of the vaccine effect is due to a change in infectivity after vaccination and how much is due to a change in susceptibility?

Conclusion

Vaccine trials with randomisation at the individual level are unsuitable to quantify the herd immunity after vaccination.

An Epidemiological Approach to the Evaluation of Disease Control Strategies for Intestinal Helminth Infections: an Age Structured Model

M.S. Chan, G.F. Medley and D.A.P. Bundy

Introduction

It is estimated that one quarter of the world population is infected with one or more of the intestinal helminth species *Ascaris lumbricoides*, *Trichuris trichiura* and hookworms (*Ancyclostoma duodenale* and *Necator americanus*) (WHO 1987, Bundy 1990). Approximately one hundred million people worldwide may suffer morbidity as a result of each of these infections (Chan *et al.* 1994b). A relatively cost-effective method of controlling the more serious consequences of all these infections is the use of mass or age-targetted chemotherapy.

When designing community based chemotherapy programs, the cost-effectiveness of different treatment strategies must be taken into account. In the absence of adequate field data, the likely benefit of treatment in terms of infections and morbidity prevented can be assessed by epidemiological modelling. An epidemiological model has been developed which incorporates observed patterns of infection in the community and can be used to estimate the rate of reinfection following treatment interventions (Medley *et al.* 1992). The output from the epidemiological model can be combined with actual cost data from chemotherapy operations to provide a cost-effectiveness analysis of different control options (Guyatt *et al.* 1993).

The aim of this study is to develop an age structured version of the Medley *et al.* (1992) model. The rationale for this approach comes from the well known age differences in prevalence and intensity of infection. For *Ascaris lumbricoides* and *Trichuris trichiura*, highest prevalence and intensity is found in school age children, whereas with the hookworms, highest prevalence and intensity is found in adults. The model also allows treatment to be targetted at one age group only. This means that the effect of treatment in the most highly affected age group on transmission in the whole community can be investigated.

The Model

The Medley *et al.* (1992) model simulates the dynamics of infection and disease in a community of constant population size after one or more cycles of treatment by mass chemotherapy. The main features of this model are:

1. The model is formulated as a set of coupled differential equations (Anderson and May 1985,1991)

2. Heterogeneity between hosts in susceptibility to infection is included.

3. Disease is assumed to be a function of current worm burden. A threshold worm burden is defined above which morbidity is assumed to be observed.

4. The changing worm burden distribution over time is simulated explicitly as opposed to using a fixed theoretical distribution.

5. Random mass chemotherapy treatment can be carried out once or several times during the simulation at given coverages (proportion of people treated) and drug efficacies (proportion of worms in treated individuals killed by the treatment).

In the present model (Chan *et al.* 1994a), the community is divided into two constant sized groups, adults and children. The following assumptions are made:

1. The contact rate represents the combined effect of exposure and establishment of adult worms in the host and will generally be higher in children compared with adults (except for hookworms).

2. It is assumed that there is only one pool of infective stages. This means that the pattern of mixing is random.

3. At equilibrium, the worm burden distribution within each group is assumed to be negative binomial with separate mean worm burdens and aggregation parameter (k) for adults and children.

4. Fecundity and mortality of worms and the effect density dependence are assumed to be the same for both groups.

Results

The age structured model enables the assessment of age targetted treatment. The simulation results show that the treatment of children only can result in the reduction of prevalence, mean worm burden and disease in adults through the reduction in transmission. The per capita benefit is lower in adults as compared to children but the total community benefit may be similar due to the generally larger number of adults.

The presence of untreated adults also reduces the effectiveness of treatment in the children as compared to a hypothetical population of children isolated from transmission from adults. This reduction is of the order of 50% which suggests that the modelling of children as a single population will give misleading results.

The treatment of children six-monthly instead of yearly leads only to a marginal increase in benefit which is unlikely to be justified due to the increased cost of control. The treatment of both adults and children at the first treatment time followed by subsequent yearly treatment of children leads to only a marginal increase in benefit for children but benefits the adults significantly. The justification for use of this strategy will depend on the extra cost involved for the initial mass treatment.

The model results were compared to data from Thein Hlaing et al. (1991). In this study children were treated at three month intervals and in one sample there was also a mass treatment initially. The model was able to reproduce the results for mean worm burden accurately.

References

Anderson, R.M. and May, R.M. (1985) 'Helminth infections of humans: mathematical models, population dynamics and control', *Adv. Parasitol.* **24**, 1-101.

Anderson, R.M. and May, R.M. (1991) *Infectious Diseases of Humans: Dynamics and Control*, Oxford University Press, Oxford.

Bundy, D.A.P. (1990) 'Is the hookworm just another geohelminth?' In *Hookworm Disease, Current Status and New Directions*, G.A. Schad and K.S. Warren (eds.), Taylor and Francis, London, 147-164.

Chan, M.S., Guyatt, H.L., Bundy, D.A.P. and Medley, G.F. (1994a) 'The development and validation of an age-structured model for the evaluation of disease control strategies for intestinal helminths', *Parasitology* **109**, 389-396.

Chan, M.S., Medley, G.F., Jamison, D. and Bundy, D.A.P. (1994b) 'The evaluation of global morbidity attributable to intestinal helminth infections', *Parasitology* **109**, 373-387.

Guyatt, H.L., Bundy, D.A.P. and Evans, D. (1993) 'A population dynamic approach to the cost-effectiveness analysis of mass anthelmintic treatment: effects of treatment frequency on *Ascari lumbricoides* infection', *Trans. Roy. Soc. Trop. Med. Hyg.* **87**, 570-575.

Medley, G.F., Guyatt, H.L. and Bundy, D.A.P. (1992) 'A quantitative framework for evaluating the effect of community treatment on the morbidity due to ascariasis', *Parasitology* **106**, 211-221.

Thein Hlaing, Than-Saw and Myat-Lay-Kyin (1991) 'The impact of three monthly age-targetted chemotherapy on *Ascaris lumbricoides* infection', *Trans. Roy. Soc. Trop. Med. Hyg.* **85**, 519–522.

WHO (1987) *Prevention and Control of Intestinal Parasitic Infections*, WHO Technical Report Series **749**, World Health Organisation, Geneva.

The Control of Directly Transmitted Infections by Pulse Vaccination: Concepts and Preliminary Studies

D. J. Nokes

The vaccination of a range of age cohorts on a periodic basis – termed pulse vaccination – for the control of common childhood infections, may, under some circumstances, be an attractive alternative or addition to routine infant immunization schedules (Quadros *et al.* 1991, Agur *et al.* 1993). Following from the recent work of Agur *et al.* (1993), studies are in progress in an attempt to gain a better understanding of the mechanism by which pulse vaccination influences the infection dynamics of directly transmitted 'close contact' infections and to explore the merits of such immunization programmes when compared with routine continuous cohort immunization. The preliminary work presented here outlines a conceptual framework for understanding how pulse vaccination programmes effect control on infection transmission, and for establishing rough criteria for the necessary interval between pulses, T_v, for a defined age range vaccinated, and analyses some of the temporal changes induced by pulse strategies.

The basic criterion for control of an infection transmitted by close contact, such as measles, is to keep susceptible numbers, X, below that required to establish an epidemic, i.e. the equilibrium or threshold number of susceptibles, X_T (or proportion $x^* = 1/R_0$). Assume a closed homogeneously mixing stationary population, exhibiting Type I survival (step function mortality), with an infection at stable endemic equilibrium. Further assume that all individuals are born susceptible, remaining so until of age A, the average age at infection, whence they become infected (for a negligible period of time), and rapidly move into the immune class in which they remain until death at age L (Anderson and May 1991). Under these simple conditions where, additionally, vaccination is assumed to suppress infection rates to negligible levels, the interval between pulses T_v, required to maintain $X \leq X_T$ ($x \leq x^*$), will be related to the reduction in the susceptible pool from its equilibrium, $x^* - x$, i.e. dependent upon the proportion of the population vaccinated, p, and the time taken for births to replenish the susceptible deficit, which depends upon L. It follows that

$$T_v = (x^* - x).L$$

and if $x^* = A/L$, and $p = 1 - x/x^*$ then

$$T_v = pA.$$

This was previously defined more formally by Agur *et al.* (1993). Relaxing the implicit assumption that individuals of any age may be vaccinated, then the interval between pulses T_v can be calculated numerically by a minimization procedure, for a variety of values of V_a, the age range from birth over which vaccination is applied, p, the level of coverage, A and L.

From this conceptual approach some general trends emerge. First, the interval between pulses, T_v, never exceeds a value equivalent in years to the average age at infection, for the common sense reason that a period $T_v > A$ will inevitably allow susceptible numbers to exceed the equilibrium proportion (defined as $x^* = A/L$). Second, that most benefit will be gained, in terms of maximising the interval between pulses by vaccinating a range of ages at least equivalent in years to the average age at infection, A, particularly for high values of p, and that the benefits of increasing the age range vaccinated still further progressively diminish (particularly for infections with low ages at infection) as the pulse interval asymptotes at $T_v = pA$. Third, whilst the eradication criteria $(x < x^*; \, p > 1 - x^*)$ are the same for pulse as for routine immunization, it is possible for a pulse coverage, p, over age range V_a, to be less than the critical value p_c, and yet achieve an average coverage across all ages which is in excess of p_c, because individuals have more than one opportunity to be vaccinated whist in the vaccinated age range V_a. Fourth, it is clear that by reducing the effective reproductive ratio well below unity, pulse vaccination effects far more rapid control of transmission than can routine/continuous vaccination.

Moving on from this conceptual framework, age-structured deterministic models have been used to explore the dynamical aspects of the impact of pulse immunization programmes on infection transmission. A deterministic SEIR model, with age-structure, but an age-independent mixing pattern, is used. Pulses of vaccine across age range V_a are administered whenever the fraction susceptible equals x^*. It is noted that (i) incidence rapidly declines to negligible proportions as R is continually maintained below unity, (ii) the pulse interval, T_v, oscillates over a time period L, life expectancy, as susceptibles are redistributed over the age classes, and (iii) nevertheless, in the long term T_v settles out to an equilibrium value equal to that estimated by the conceptual model given above. The rate at which the system approaches this stable result depends upon the age-range vaccinated and proportion covered, but is at least of the order of life expectancy in years.

The influence of a variety of factors on these initial findings are now being explored. They include, (i) incorporation of a convex age-dependent pattern for the force of infection, typical of childhood viral infections, (ii) seasonality in contact rates, forcing longer-term oscillatory fluctuations in incidence, (iii) age-dependence in the severity of infection and (iv) a growing population.

References

Quadros, C.A., Andrus, J.K., Olive, J-M., Silveira, C.M., Eikhof, R.M., Carrasco, P., Fitzsimmons, J.W. and Pinheiro, F.P. (1991) 'Eradication of poliomyelitis: progress in the Americas', *Pediatr. Infect. Dis. J.* **10**, 222–229.

Agur, Z., Cojocaru, L., Mazor, G., Anderson, R.M. and Danon, Y.L. (1993) 'Pulse mass measles vaccination across age cohorts', *Proc. Nat. Acad. Sci. USA* **90**, 11698–702.

Anderson, R.M. and May, R.M. (1991) *Infectious Diseases of Humans: Dynamics and Control*, Oxford Science Publications, Oxford.

Discussion

DIETZ In reference to Nokes' presentation, eradication and elimination of virus are best thought of as different. Eradication is best defined as the total extinction of the infectious agent, as in the case of smallpox, whereas elimination is best used to describe the local extinction of the infectious agent within a local population. In the case of elimination, the population remains at risk of infection by introduction, and this state can only be maintained by continued vaccination to make the population impervious to immigrating virus. As regards the use of pulse vaccination versus continuous vaccination, it would be informative to know the distribution of size of outbreaks under both strategies, as outbreaks will occur, and one of the aims of a vaccination policy is to limit their size.

REPLY I agree with the first point: it is useful to make a distinction between 'eradication' and 'elimination'. Let us hope this phrasiology is generally adopted.

The second point is of importance in assessing the merits of pulse vaccination as a method of control. Pulse vaccination has the potential to induce marked changes in the age-distribution of susceptibles in a population. The method of repeated application across a wide age range, which characterises pulse vaccination, is likely to (a) induce such changes over a far shorter time scale than those resulting from continuous infant immunization and (b) develop cycles of change in the susceptible age distribution, such that the prediction of age groups most at risk of outbreaks will be difficult without continuous surveillance (e.g. serosurveys). The importance of dynamical changes set up by pulse vaccination will need to be investigated under conditions of age-dependence in mixing and in the risk of severe disease following infection.

Operational Models for the Prevention of Blindness

D.J. Gove, A. K. Shahani, S.E. Meacock, H.H.J. van der Hoorn, R. Bailey, M.E. Ward and D.C.W. Mabey

Trachoma is the world's largest cause of preventable blindness. About 500 million people suffer from trachoma and about 7 million people are blind (Dawson *et al.* 1981). The aetiological agent is a bacterium, *Chlamydia trachomatis*, which causes progressive damage that can lead to blindness.

The prevalence and intensity of trachoma in a community is strongly associated with the degree of poverty and the resulting environmental conditions. The infection can be treated with antibiotics, but reinfection is common in heavily infected communities. At present, a vaccine is not available, although it is acknowledged that a suitable vaccine would be important for the control of trachoma, and research is actively pursuing such a vaccine. Trachoma could, like most other infectious diseases, be eradicated by a dramatic improvement in environmental conditions (especially clean water supply) , public health and nutrition, but these are long-term goals. In the shorter term, control of trachoma can be acheived in varying degrees by combinations of strategies involving chemotherapy and other targeted medical interventions. Operational modelling work provides a practical tool for evaluating various strategies for the treatment and control of trachoma.

The main data used for developing and testing the models is from a series of longitudinal surveys carried out in the village of Jali, Gambia, West Africa, from 1984. In these surveys the villagers were examined clinically and microbiological samples were also obtained. Suitable demographic data was also used. The data collection, analysis, and the development of the models involves team work by medical doctors, microbiologists, statisticians, and operational researchers (Bailey *et al.* 1989, Ward *et al.* 1990, Shahani *et al.* 1992).

The transmission dynamics of trachoma are not well understood. There is a great deal of uncertainty and variability in the natural history of the disease leading up to blindness. A simulation model was chosen as being appropriate at the necessary operational level, in order to obtain detailed information over time. An analytical approach was not attempted. A simulation model has a further advantage of easier acceptability by non-mathematicians in a team of workers.

In the simulation model the force of infection is defined as the probability of a new infection in a chosen time period in a defined community. The model takes an individual through time and this structure enables us to evaluate proposed treatment and control strategies at detailed operational levels. The individuals are given relevant attributes such as age, sex, membership of a family. This means that the effects of interventions at the whole community level or at selected group levels can be studied.

An individual can be in one of three basic states: Susceptible, Infected, and Immune. A susceptible individual has a risk of contracting the infection. The probability of becoming infected depends on individual characteristics, such as age, and global characteristics, such as the prevalence of the infection in the population. An infection can be of three types: severe, moderate, or inapparent. Severe and moderate infections are determined by the clinical signs of infection, graded by the WHO scheme (Dawson *et al.* 1981). Inapparent infection is only detectable microbiologically.

At the end of a particular infection, an individual may have a short period of resistance to another infection and this resistance can, again, be measured microbiologically. Resistance wanes over time so that the individual becomes susceptible again, and consequently, individuals suffer from repeated infections. The clinical signs of infection can persist longer than the microbiological infection, i.e. disease is not synonymous with infection. Thus the number of people exhibiting clinical signs need not correlate to the level of infection.

Two types of model are being produced: a clinical model that requires clinical data only, and a microbiological model that requires data from laboratory investigation. The clinical model is designed to be used by those who do not have access to the necessary detailed microbiological information — clinical signs only show that an individual has had the infection recently. The microbiological model can be used by those who require a more accurate model of the infection and who have access to microbiological data, which can be used to determine infection (including inapparent) and resistance. There are a number of other differences between the models: for example, the mean duration of active disease is about 15 weeks and that of inapparent infection is 5 weeks.

New-born babies are assumed to be susceptible for there is little evidence of derived maternal resistance. Repeated infection causes Conjunctival Scarring and ultimately Severe Visual Loss or Blindness. Demographic data is used to define birth and death rates. Trachoma alone is not a fatal disease, but resulting blindness may have some effect on life expectancy.

The effects of chemotherapy (use of antibiotics) and socio-economic actions are modelled through changes to the force of infection. The calculations from the model provide guidance for effective strategies involving both chemotherapy and socio-economic interventions. The effect of vaccination is modelled by extending the period of immunity. The inclusion of vaccination provides quantitative guidance about both the necessary quality of a vaccine and the design of an appropriate vaccination strategy.

The model has many parameters. Easy methods of providing the model with the necessary inputs have been a major consideration in this work. We have provided default files that can be edited by the user. The simulation models have been implemented on a standard microcomputer.

Results from the models show that the best solution to the problem is socio-economic change, however this may not be a readily achievable aim. Chemotherapy is an alternative but its effects are short term. Vaccination would provide a longer term alternative but as yet no vaccines are available.

Acknowledgement

This work is supported by a grant from the Edna McConnell Clark Foundation, New York.

References

Bailey, R., Osmond, C., Mabey, D.C.W., Whittle, H.C. and Ward, M.E. (1989) 'Analysis of the household distribution of trachoma in a Gambian village using a Monte Carlo simulation procedure', *Int. J. Epidemiol.* **18**, 944–951.

Dawson, C.R., Jones, B.R. and Tarizzo M.L. (1981) *A Guide to Trachoma Control*, World Health Organization, Geneva.

Shahani, A.K. Ward, M.E., Gove, D.J. and Meacock, S.E. (1992) 'Prevention of Blindness'. In *Proceedings of the International Conference on Operational Research for Development, 1992, Ahmedabad*, to appear.

Ward, M.E., Hawkins, J.D. and Shahani, A.K. (1990) 'Evaluation of trachoma control strategies'. In *Human Chlamydial Infections*, Bowie *et al.* (eds.), 591–594.

Part 5
Prediction

AIDS: Modelling and Predicting

P. J. Solomon

1 Introduction

AIDS continues to place enormous demands on health-care resources and it is essential for public health planning that useful estimates are available of current and future numbers of individuals at different stages of HIV disease. People with HIV infection are eligible to receive treatments at ever earlier stages of the disease, and accurate estimates are required to ensure adequate resources are available. People sick with advanced HIV disease may be in need of special care. Estimates are also crucial for developing policy on awareness campaigns and intervention programs, as well as for investigating the value of needle exchange and other prevention, including vaccination, programs.

Many unanswered questions about the epidemic are essentially statistical in nature, for despite efforts over the past decade to improve both the collection and quality of data on HIV and AIDS, the data are still often incomplete, and there remain large gaps in our knowledge on many key epidemiological parameters.

In particular, the *infectivity* of HIV is a fundamental unknown and there is uncertainty about the *incubation period* and its space-time trends. The available data are therefore an incomplete description of phenomena which are, on the whole, relatively poorly understood, and predictions of the epidemic based on the available data are subject to considerable uncertainty. This uncertainty makes AIDS grimly interesting to statisticians, but the prediction problems have been forced upon us because of their practical urgency, regardless of whether or not we can solve them. The role of markers such as CD4 cell counts, IgA and other markers in HIV disease is currently receiving considerable attention by AIDS researchers and statisticians. A further major uncertainty is that of treatment efficacy.

It is essential to bring to bear on the prediction problem as much external information as possible on HIV prevalence and treatment effects. This has led to increasing interest in empirical Bayes and fully Bayesian approaches where prior knowledge, external information, and major sources of uncertainty are combined in a single, and more realistic, model. The fully Bayesian approach is made feasible by the increased availability of computational power, which makes practical the application of Monte Carlo Markov chain methods (Gibbs sampling, for example, is a very special case).

Predictions must be done separately for important groups, and in particular, by geographical region and transmission categories within regions, and possibly also by disease presentation at diagnosis.

The literature on AIDS has grown enormously ever since the late-1980's. This paper overviews current statistical approaches to estimating and predicting future numbers of people with HIV disease, and AIDS deaths. I will begin with some general remarks on the major sources of statistical uncertainty and the notation used in the paper. I will then describe the different statistical techniques and outline the advantages and disadvantages of each. The uncertainty about the epidemic and the incompleteness of the data affect the results of the different methods, each of which has its specific set of assumptions, in different ways, and these are discussed.

Many points concerning my own work in this area are based on collaborative work with Dr S.R. Wilson at the Australian National University.

2   The major sources of uncertainty

The focus in this overview is on countries like Australia, the US and most of Europe, where HIV-1 is prevalent, and where infection is predominantly seen amongst men who have sex with men, injecting drug users, people with haemophilia and recipients of transfused blood, and their sexual partners.

The nature of the uncertainties can be classified as statistical or epidemiological. The lengthy, variable, and nonstationary incubation period is a fundamental epidemiological unknown, and moreover, the spread of infection of the virus and behavioural changes are effectively unobservable. There is also considerable uncertainty about the efficacy of available prophylactic and antiviral treatments.

The incompleteness of the available information leads to the following major statistical errors in prediction:

- By far the major source of error is from 'model errors', which means that the use of a single model or technique for prediction can be very misleading. Models which fit the observed data equally well can lead to quite different predictions over a period of just a few years (Report of a Working Group 1988, Solomon *et al.* 1990b) and it is therefore important in prediction to consider as broad a range of plausible models as feasible. A crucial point here is that model errors arise from two, nested, sources: firstly, from the choice of technique for prediction (e.g., curve fitting, backcalculation or epidemic models); and secondly from various specific choices that may be made for a particular technique (e.g., several different mathematical forms can be used for curve fitting, parametric versus nonparametric approaches to backcalculation, and so on).

- Errors of estimating the unknown parameters in a chosen model are less important in this context, although effort has been devoted to obtaining confidence intervals by both bootstrapping and more conventional methods.

- Poisson-distributed variations in the data contribute additional uncertainty to the resulting estimates, even if the model parameters are known exactly, and there is evidence of over-Poisson variation.

- Data errors resulting from artefacts in the reporting process, including delays in reporting HIV and AIDS to national surveillance registers, underreporting, and trends in reporting practices and procedures, for instance, due to early cases of AIDS not being recognised.

Sensitivity to the assumed model and to other choices and assumptions must be investigated using *sensitivity analyses* and supplemented by external information wherever possible, particularly on HIV prevalence, and especially regarding the recent past. It is not possible to remove all the uncertainty surrounding the epidemic, but statisticians can help provide *plausible* ranges of estimates as a quantitative basis for planning.

3 Notation

The rate of new infections at time t is denoted by $h(t)$. Infection is followed by the incubation period, which is currently thought to have a median duration of about 10 or 11 years. The incubation distribution is denoted by $f()$ and is now usually taken to be a function of both calendar time of infection s and time elapsed since infection u i.e., $f(u|s)$. This reflects attempts to capture temporal changes in the incubation period associated with treatment and other therapeutic advances, as well as possible changes in the evolution of the virus, and the etiology of HIV disease. $\rho()$ denotes the hazard of progression to AIDS, and $F()$ is the corresponding distribution function. The incidence of new cases of AIDS at time t is denoted by $a(t)$.

4 Empirical models

4.1 Extrapolation forecasting

The simplest technique for predicting AIDS is to extrapolate from empirical curves fitted to observed AIDS (or other well-defined endpoint) incidence data. In some ways, curve-fitting is the most natural way to proceed for quite short-term forecasting for one or two years ahead. The simplicity of the approach stems from the fact that it depends only on data of the type usually collected under routine surveillance and maintained on state or national data registries. Usually Poisson errors are assumed and the 'goodness of fit' measured by the deviance and degrees of freedom.

Early on in the epidemic (or sub-epidemic) the growth rate is approximately exponential i.e., the number $a(t)$ of new diagnoses at time t is $e^{\alpha+\beta t}$ with constant doubling time $\log 2/\beta$. This curve has the advantage of being the simplest mathematically and corresponds approximately to the solution of several simple theoretical models which incorporate characteristics of the population at risk. Exponential growth is also often useful as a very local approximation to the growth rate when the epidemic is a little more advanced, although not when the peak is reached, and is therefore broadly useful in practice.

As the growth rate slows according to epidemic theory, mathematical forms incorporating subexponential growth become appropriate. In the mid to late 1980's observed AIDS diagnosis rates were fitted using a number of curves based on the exponential, such as the quadratic exponential model

$$a(t) = e^{\alpha+\beta t-\gamma t^2}.$$

Here, the rate of new diagnoses of cases rises to a maximum then falls away symmetrically to zero. The model is a statistically convenient way of representing early and small departures from exponential growth. Although it is not very plausible for AIDS diagnoses for most transmission groups, the model is a reasonable approximation to the pattern of new diagnoses of AIDS amongst recipients of blood or blood products (Solomon and Wilson 1993b), amongst whom nearly all new infections stopped in Australia (and elsewhere) when widespread screening of donated blood was introduced in 1985. The power curve model with $a(t) = e^{\alpha+\beta \log t}$ can be regarded as one of exponential type, and is more appropriate for the early phase of an epidemic.

The linear logistic model has provided the best fits to observed AIDS incidence data in Australia and in England and Wales. The rate of new cases of AIDS is assumed to pass from exponential to linear growth according to the expression

$$a(t) = \frac{\alpha + \beta t}{1 + e^{\gamma - \delta t}}.$$

This is appropriate in the second phase of the epidemic, but not as the stationary point is approached and subsequently.

Differences between geographical regions, transmission groups and other categorical effects can be easily evaluated by comparing the relevant parameter estimates. Temporal changes such as those due to changes in the definition of AIDS and the introduction and availability of treatments, can be incorporated in a number of ways, for example, by change-point models (Solomon et al. 1990b) but explicit modelling will depend on the actual processes involved. For further details see for example the Report of a Working Group (1988), Solomon et al. (1990b), Taylor (1989).

These curves, among others such as the logistic, are also used for estimating the size and shape of the past HIV epidemic in the parametric backcalculation method (see section 5).

Nonparametric curves have also been fitted where the observed numbers are sufficiently large. Lowess (locally weighted scatterplot smoother, Cleveland (1979) has been used to smooth observed AIDS counts for the purpose of describing trends in incidence (see, for instance, Rosenberg, Levy, *et al.* (1992)). Zeger *et al.* (1989) used splines to model the US AIDS data, and others have proposed semiparametric curves which combine parametric and nonparametric components (De Angelis *et al.* 1993) or fit piecewise constant, linear or nonlinear models.

An advantage of fitting parametric curves is that the parameter estimates can provide a concise summary of observed trends, ideally have some meaningful interpretation, can be applied to relatively small sets of data, and be a basis for cross-counts conferring, which is very important. The major disadvantage is that medium-term predictions depend crucially on the choice of model, whereas in numerically smoothing the observed counts, no model need be assumed. However, nonparametric procedures which numerically smooth the counts provide no apparent basis for inference or prediction, require reasonably large numbers, and are sensitive to the amount of smoothing or choice of smoothing parameter. The question arises here as to whether the use of splines is at all enlightening.

It is crucial that the data are of high quality. Predictions based on fitted curves are very sensitive to reporting delays, artefacts of the reporting process, and to under-reporting. Predictions are also influenced by the level of aggregation of the data (monthly, quarterly, yearly, etc; see Wilson *et al.* (1992)), and the errors do not usually look Poisson.

Regardless of what type of curve is fitted, knowledge of important features of the epidemic cannot be directly incorporated in this approach. This is in contrast both to epidemic models which attempt to simulate the actual pattern of HIV infection, and to the backcalculation method which can incorporate 'external' information observed from survey, cohort and other studies.

4.2 Reporting delays and underreporting

There have been numerous statistical methods, both formal and informal, proposed for dealing with reporting delays, which can be substantial. It is often simplest to adjust the observed counts for reporting delays before analysis and then treat these as the observations, although this will tend to underestimate the variance of the resulting estimates (Lawless and Sun 1992).

A general approach to forecasting AIDS in the presence of reporting delays is to correct simultaneously for delays when fitting a composite model. If diagnosis time and delay time pairs (t_i, x_i) are observed over a period $(-\infty, t_0)$ (or $(0, t_0)$) the likelihood assuming a continuous time Poisson process of rate $\lambda(t; \rho)$ and reporting delays X with probability density function $f_X(x; \theta)$, where ρ and θ are unknown parameters, is

$$\prod_{i=1}^{n} \lambda(t_i; \rho) f_X(x_i; \theta) \exp\{\int_{-\infty}^{t_0} \lambda(u; \rho) F_X(t_0 - u; \theta) du\}.$$

Cox and Medley (1989) describe this parametric approach, and consider a variety of models for λ, including the quadratic exponential, logistic and linear logistic, and some interesting mixture distributions for f e.g., a mixture of two gamma distributions of index one. Heisterkamp et al. (1989) also explicitly model the reporting delay distribution to adjust observed AIDS incidence in Europe.

A useful overview of recent work is given by Lawless and Sun (1992), who use an estimating equation approach. The reporting delay distribution in the US has been changing, and various suggestions have been made to deal with this. Harris (1990) divides calendar time into stationary intervals, whereas Lawless and Sun (1992) estimate the distribution using the most recently reported cases (their resultant predictions are of cases that will ultimately be reported). They report that more than 15% of cases that will ultimately be reported in the US have reporting delays longer than three years.

Right-truncated data in this context have been analysed by both parametric and nonparametric methods (see Pagano et al. (1995) for an overview), including survival analysis techniques. The main problem with the conditional approach is that if t_{max} say, is the longest observed incubation time, one can only estimate the conditional distribution given that the incubation period is less than or equal to t_{max}. This is fine only if t_{max} is in the upper tail of the distribution, and otherwise virtually useless. The parametric approach is the optimal way to proceed, in which case the full distribution is estimated.

Other authors have proposed handling reporting delays via Poisson regression models (Zeger et al. 1989, Brookmeyer and Liao 1990b). Brookmeyer and Liao's method is useful and popular (see, for instance, Rosenberg et al. (1992)). Rosenberg (1990) suggests a simple approach which can be done on a pocket calculator.

Bacchetti et al. (1993) estimate the delay distribution nonparametrically and jointly with the infection curve and incubation distribution. Their approach uses a computationally expensive EM algorithm based on a penalized likelihood and incorporates an adjustment for grouping of early diagnoses. Two approaches to adjusting for reporting delays are considered in the latest prediction work by the Cambridge MRC group. Firstly, they obtain 95% confidence intervals for the delay probabilities and adjusted AIDS incidence by generating bootstrap estimates based on a product multinomial model. Secondly, they propose a Bayesian approach which combines the different sources of uncertainty into a single model. The true number of diagnoses N_i in an interval $(i - 1, i)$ is assumed to be Poisson with rate η_i, where the η_i define a (smoothed) autoregressive process, and the probability of reporting is assumed to depend on the length of the reporting delay interval, as well as exhibiting extra-binomial variation. Gibbs sampling is used to estimate both models simultaneously and to produce a posterior distribution with confidence intervals for the N_i.

In Australia, new diagnoses of HIV infection and AIDS are routinely notified from all States and Territories, and the data have been more homogeneous and complete that those from the US and England, where the datasets are larger and more complex. At present, under-reporting of Australian AIDS cases is thought to be between 10% and 20% depending on region and transmission category. This is similar to the US situation, where it is estimated that 15% of cases are never reported. Reporting is thought to be virtually complete in Australia within 18 months (a figure based on empirical observation and analysis), although date of report has only recently been routinely included on the national surveillance register. It may be that the under-reporting rate is decreasing as treatment becomes more readily available to those in earlier stages of HIV disease and people with HIV are more actively seeking treatment both at an earlier stage and because it is more effective. It is also possible that reporting delays are shortening because these individuals will be monitored fairly closely.

4.3 Predicting trends in small groups and empirical Bayes

For health planning, a common requirement is to predict future numbers of a disease or infection for which just a few cases have been observed so far. Sparse data arise in a number of contexts, and particularly in the early phases of an epidemic. A simple and useful method for obtaining prediction limits in such situations was proposed by Cox and Davison (1989) in which the basis for the prediction is the total number of events observed in the past in the local area under study, together with the assumption that the overall pattern of growth can be determined from a larger body of data. They argue that for short-term predictions for one or two years ahead, Poisson variations in the data are the major source of uncertainty.

Suppose that in the area or subgroup in question n_{12} cases have been diagnosed in the time period t_1 to t_2, and that it is required to predict the number n_{34} of new cases to be diagnosed in a future time period (t_3, t_4). Suppose further that in the region or subgroup under study and in the time period t_1 to t_4 being considered (retrospectively and prospectively) diagnoses occur in a Poisson process of rate $\lambda v(\theta, t)$, where v is a known function with known parameters θ, but λ is unknown. Let

$$g(t_i, t_j) = \int_{t_i}^{t_j} v(\theta, t)dt.$$

Then the value n_{34} to be predicted is such that the split (n_{12}, n_{34}) is consistent with a binomial distribution with known probability

$$p = \frac{g(t_3, t_4)}{g(t_1, t_2) + g(t_3, t_4)}$$

of a case. p depends only on the future time interval, the functional form for the rate of incidence of new cases of AIDS, and the 'window' of observation i.e. whether $t_1 = -\infty$, or whether a finite interval is considered for observation. Ideally the 'window' of observation will represent the part of the process that is homogeneous and continuing. Cox and Davison (1989) consider the special case $t_1 = -\infty$ and $v(t) = e^{\theta t}$ and Solomon and Wilson (1993b) extend the methodology to accommodate the fact that the process is known to not be homogeneous over time, but is known to be relatively homogeneous over a recent, known, time interval in which observations are made (it is assumed that only the total number of cases in that interval, or 'window', of time is known); and that the preferred model for the growth of incident cases over the recent past is not necessarily a simple exponentially growing epidemic. Solomon and Wilson also provide a table which considerably simplifies the application of the method. The advantage of the first of these extensions is that, in practice, it is not always possible or desirable to use all the available data for a local area or subgroup, for instance, when early cases are likely to have been missed (perhaps because a new disease or infection was not recognised) or when the data are of poor quality. Model choice is useful when the incidence of cases is known to follow some path which is not exponential e.g., for transfusion-caused cases of AIDS.

The small group method is broadly applicable for short-term predictions for infectious disease data. Obviously the best approach would be one based on careful analysis of the spatial and temporal features of the epidemic, giving formulae based on local characteristics and experience, but relevant information for implementation of this approach is not, in general, available for HIV disease.

Zeger et al. (1989) describe a variety of statistical methods for monitoring the AIDS epidemic in the US, and one of these methods applies empirical Bayes shrinkage to separate model-based estimates of AIDS prevalence in different geographical regions and transmission groups. Essentially, the aim is to constrain the current estimates to conform to an overall model of the variation between groups. Diggle et al. (1990) apply Zeger et al.'s approach to the Australian data, where there is significant regional variability in the course of the epidemic and where very small numbers have been observed for some subgroups. They considered three regional groups (New South Wales, Victoria and the rest of the country) and three transmission categories (men who have sex with men, injecting drug users, and recipients of blood or blood products). c_{ij} is the ratio of rates of incidence of new cases over yearly intervals in the ith region and jth transmission group i.e. $\log\{\mu_{ij}(t_1)/\mu_{ij}(t_2)\}$, where $\mu_{ij}(t) = \exp(\beta_0 + \beta_1 t + \theta_2 t^2 + \theta_3 t^3)$, or the quadratic exponential model with $\theta_3 = 0$. $\hat{c}_{ij}$ is the estimate based only from the local information, and has standard error $\sqrt{v_{ij}}$ and $\hat{p}_{ij}$ is an estimate of c_{ij} based on fitting the model

$$p_{ij} = \alpha_i + \beta_j$$

for variation in the c_{ij}s amongst the different regions and transmission categories. p is fitted using weighted least squares with weights v_{ij}^{-1}, and the estimated residual variance is $\Sigma_{i=1}^3 \Sigma_{j=1}^3 (\hat{c}_{ij} - \hat{p}_{ij})^2/4$. The empirical Bayes estimate of c_{ij} is then the weighted average $w_{ij}\hat{p}_{ij} + (1 - w_{ij})\hat{c}_{ij}$, where $w_{ij} = v_{ij}/(v_{ij} + \sigma^2)$.

The basic idea is that separate estimates $\hat{c}_{ij}$ with relatively large standard errors are unreliable, and should be shrunk more towards the overall estimates $\hat{p}_{ij}$, than should estimates $\hat{c}_{ij}$ with small standard errors. Diggle *et al.* (1990) illustrate that shrinkage can guard against relying on estimates with relatively large standard errors.

Mariotto (1989) compared observed growth rates of AIDS in different European countries, and also calculated empirical Bayes estimates of the rates and their standard errors. There was little gain in using the empirical Bayes approach to improve the estimates from the UK, where the number of incident cases was large, but the approach did induce an appreciable gain for countries where the observed numbers of cases were small.

5   Backcalculation

Backcalculation is widely used by statisticians both for estimating the past HIV infection curve and for predicting future AIDS incidence. It is the predominant method of choice for prediction in the US, Australia (see Solomon *et al.* 1991, Becker *et al.* 1991) and the UK (De Angelis *et al.* 1993, Raab *et al.* 1993). Several authors have reviewed backcalculation in the context of the US epidemic, where the emphasis is on computationally intensive methods designed specifically to deal with the complexities of US databases which are typically large, incomplete and inhomogeneous (Jewell 1990, Gail and Rosenberg 1992, Bacchetti *et al.* 1993, among others).

In terms of mathematical complexity, backcalculation lies between empirical curve-fitting and epidemic models for the transmission dynamics of HIV infection. In backcalculation, the incubation distribution is incorporated directly into the model, and a big advantage over simpler models is that 'external' information, such as recent observed trends in HIV prevalence can be included. This is important since most AIDS cases observed now are from infections that occurred up to 10 years ago, or earlier, and current trends in AIDS incidence contain little information about recent trends in HIV incidence. It is well known that HIV estimates reconstructed via backcalculation are quite reliable up to the mid-1980's or thereabouts. Estimates beyond then must be based on, or at the very least supplemented by, external information or other knowledge.

The basis of backcalculation is that a process of infection has occurred, and is possibly still occurring, in the population under study, and that infection with the virus is followed by the lengthy and variable incubation period until (at least in a majority of cases) an AIDS-defining illness is diagnosed. It is still too early to determine whether a proportion of people will remain infected indefinitely without ever developing an AIDS-defining illness.

The relationship is represented mathematically by

$$a(t) = \int_0^t h(s)f(t-s)ds, \tag{1}$$

where $s = 0$ denotes the start of the epidemic, which is usually taken to be 1981 in Australia. Knowledge of any two of the distributions determines the third. For instance, if $f(t-s)$ and $h(s)$ for $s \leq t$ are known, then the rate of new diagnoses of AIDS $a(t)$ can be calculated. Alternatively, if a and f are assumed known, then h can be determined, and this is known as 'backcalculation'. Once the past infection curve has been reconstructed, (1) is used again to project the estimates forward in time to predict future AIDS incidence, usually for periods up to five years. New infections are usually assumed to arise according to a Poisson process, so that AIDS incidence also arises according to a point process with intensity $a(t)$ given by (1).

For application, it is often convenient to use a discrete form of the convolution (1), or to focus on the number of events occurring in equally spaced intervals e.g., per month, quarter or year. If y_c represents the number of AIDS cases diagnosed in the calendar time interval $[t_{c-1}, t_c)$ and $F(x)$ is the probability that an individual will develop AIDS in the interval $(s, s + x)$ following infection at calendar time s, then the expected value of y_c is

$$\mu_c = \int_{t_{c-1}}^{t_c} h(s)\{F(t_c - s) - F(t_{c-1} - s)\}ds.$$

Extra-Poisson variation can be allowed for by taking $\text{var}(y_c) = \sigma^2 \mu_c$, where σ^2 is an overdispersion parameter. This model defines a quasilikelihood (McCullagh and Nelder 1989). However, since the extra-Poisson variation is largely an artefact of the reporting process, it is better not to adjust for it.

The method of backcalculation was demonstrated by Brookmeyer and colleagues and Isham (Brookmeyer and Gail 1988, Brookmeyer and Damiano 1989, Isham 1989). Taylor (1989), Solomon and Wilson (1990) and others also used backcalculation early on to both reconstruct the size and shape of the past HIV infection curve, and to predict future AIDS incidence.

It is helpful at the outset to distinguish the different ways these two things have been done. a can be treated parametrically by fitting appropriate curves to the observed AIDS incidence and estimating the parameters to give $\hat{a}$ (Isham 1989, Solomon and Wilson 1990). Estimates of HIV infection incidence $\hat{h}$ are then obtained by iteratively solving the resulting equations, although the fitted values for AIDS incidence are used only up to the current time point. Implausible negative estimates and oscillations have been observed in successive values. Strategies for dealing with these include imposing ad hoc constraints, for example, by replacing negative estimates with zero. Isham (1989) gives further comments on the various problems that arose in the context of the epidemic in England and Wales. Alternatively, h can be treated parametrically, where the parameters are estimated by comparing the (usually delay-adjusted) observed and estimated AIDS incidence. Brookmeyer and Damiano (1989) consider the log logistic, Day *et al.* (1989), De Angelis *et al.* (1993) and Raab (1993), investigate a quadratic exponential form, which has also been investigated by Wilson *et al.* (1992), Lawless and Sun (1992), among others. Several authors (including those just mentioned) consider a number of different parametric forms for h. The resulting HIV estimates are extremely sensitive to the choice of parametric form for h, the different choices often being virtually indistinguishable statistically, owing to the lack of information about recent HIV infections in observed AIDS counts.

Sensitivity analyses are essential: Wilson *et al.* (1992) have evaluated the sensitivity of estimates of HIV and AIDS predictions to major uncertainties in the backcalculation method, including the quadratic exponential, linear logistic and power models for h, as well as Weibull and gamma incubation distributions and the level of aggregation of the data. Goodness of fit was based on the χ^2 statistic, and parameter estimates were obtained using a subroutine for unconstrained nonlinear least squares. We found that the least sensitive estimates were short term predictions of AIDS.

It is also important to consider different forms for h according to transmission category. In Australia, the rate of new infections is consistent with slow but exponential spread amongst injecting drug users and heterosexuals (Solomon *et al.* 1991), and the rate of new infections amongst men who have sex with men has been modelled as quadratic exponential up to the recent past, followed by linear decreasing or a constant rate, to allow for the known (nonsymmetric) HIV incidence. De Angelis *et al.* (1993) assume quadratic expontial growth amongst heterosexuals and injecting drug users,

and a 'quadratic exponential-linear spline' for homosexual and bisexual men
i.e.,

$$\alpha \exp \left(\beta(t - \eta(t)) - \gamma(2T_0\eta(t) - t^2 + \eta(t)^2) \right),$$

where

$$\eta(t) = \left\{ \begin{array}{ll} t - T_0 & \text{if } t > T_0 \\ 0 & \text{if } t \le T_0. \end{array} \right\}$$

Other variations include fitting a piecewise constant infection intensity (see
Lawless and Sun 1992). De Angelis *et al.* backcalculate their bootstrapped N_i
to eventually provide 'bootstrap' estimates of past HIV infection rates, and
corresponding estimates and predictions of AIDS incidence, and pointwise
95% confidence intervals. Bootstraps which give implausible infection curves
are excluded.

An advantage of assuming a parametric form for h is that plausible infection intensities may be summarized and interpreted in terms of one or more
estimable parameters. They are easy to fit, and give reliable short-term predictions. A single curve is too restrictive and does not represent the major
source of uncertainty associated with the technique, namely, model errors. It
is therefore important to consider a range of plausible models and to obtain
corresponding ranges of plausible estimates.

Weakly parametric or nonparametric estimates for h are popular in applications of backcalculation in the US, where the emphasis is on computer
intensive methods based on the EM algorithm. A general framework for analysis was suggested by Rosenberg and Gail (1991), who fit families of infection
curves of simple regression structure

$$h(s) = \sum g_i(s)\beta_i \tag{2}$$

for real, unknown β_i's, and known and well-behaved g_i's, such as spline functions and step functions (see Brookmeyer and Liao (1990a) for the latter).
Parameter estimates can be obtained by iteratively reweighted least squares.
These families of models provide flexible, weakly parametric models for the
size and shape of the HIV epidemic. There are difficulties, however. In the
step function models, the HIV estimates are sensitive to the choice of knots,
or jump points, and implausible oscillations and negative estimates may be
observed. Brookmeyer (1991) smooths the step estimates by minimising a
Poisson-weighted residual SS, plus a penalty function. The smoothed estimates are more appealing and give a better idea of trend, but they are very
sensitive to the amount of smoothing, and too much can lead to increased
bias. Brookmeyer and Liao (1992) discuss the trade-off between bias and
variance and suggest a strategy for choosing the smoothing parameter, which
should perhaps vary over parts of the infection curve (also see Rosenberg,
Gail and Pee (1991)).

Becker, Watson and Carlin (1991) smooth estimates of the Australian HIV epidemic by taking 'running' weighted averages over a 'window' of adjacent steps at each step of the EM algorithm. Their computer-intensive nonparametric approach with various modifications are reviewed by Becker (1992), where he also uses bootstrapping to assess the precision of the estimated infection curve (other authors have bootstrapped too e.g., Gail and Rosenberg (1992), and De Angelis *et al.* (1993)). A time transformation for reducing bias is proposed by Becker and Watson (1992), and a discrete time multiplicative model in which the infection intensity is allowed to depend on age is described in Becker and Marschner (1993). This enables smoothed, nonparametric estimates of age-specific susceptibility to infection to be found, even though age at infection is not generally observable. The expected number of individuals aged a who are infected with HIV at time t is

$$\pi_a \beta_a \lambda_t,$$

where π_a is the known proportion of individuals in the population under study of age a and β_a attempts to capture the relative susceptibility to infection with HIV. For identifiability, the authors suggest imposing the constraint $\sum_{a=1}^{\text{max. obs. age}} \pi\beta = 1$, in which case λ_t can then be interpreted as the baseline infection intensity ignoring age.

It is interesting that Becker *et al.*'s projections for AIDS in Australia give similar estimates to those of Solomon and Wilson's parametric approach (National Working Group 1992).

Spline and step function models suffer from the disadvantage of yielding much larger variances of the estimated infection rates than the parametric models. Second moment properties of the various estimation procedures have been investigated (See e.g., Rosenberg and Gail, (1991), and Jewell (1990) for an overview), although these remain secondary to model errors. Ultimately, it is crucial to undertake considerable sensitivity analyses, and the precise strategy for analysis will depend mainly on the data under study.

Uncertainty about trends in recent infection rates is reflected in increasingly large standard errors of the estimates. For the purpose of predicting AIDS, a number of suggestions to account for recent infections, both formal and informal, have been made. Brookmeyer and Liao (1990a) incorporate directly external epidemiological information on the epidemic. Some authors assume that infections have effectively stopped with the observed data and estimate a minimum size for the epidemic, others assume the infection rate will remain constant for the forseeable future, or they extrapolate from a certain point, such as the average of recent values, or assume a linear decline in incidence. In recent predictions for Australia, Solomon *et al.* (1991) constrain the number of new infections to not fall below 150 in each quarter. The best assumption is probably the one which appears to be the most plausible in the light of observed cohort or survey data on past and present HIV prevalence, and any other external information.

There is currently a move away from the traditional approaches to backcalculation towards more flexible models and methods for analysis which incorporate evolving levels of knowledge and uncertainty about the key features of the epidemic. De Angelis *et al.* (1993) refer to a fully Bayesian approach using Gibbs sampling that they are developing. Raab *et al.* (1993) also describe a fully Bayesian approach in which posterior confidence sets are obtained for the parameters of the incubation distribution and the infection curve. A nonparametric approach based on external estimates of the incubation period and reporting factors is proposed in Bacchetti *et al.* (1993), and Farewell *et al.* (1994) incorporate a model for HIV infection diagnosis into backcalculation.

5.1   The nonstationary incubation period

There is uncertainty about this key epidemiological quantity, and estimates of HIV and predictions of AIDS are well known to be sensitive to the assumed incubation distribution. The upper tail of the distribution has yet to be observed, and the situation is further confounded by the recent change in the definition of AIDS in the US. Excellent reviews of data sources and methods for estimating the incubation period are to be found in Jewell (1990) and Bacchetti *et al.* (1993).

There is considerable heterogeneity between individuals concerning the incubation distribution, and in the availability and effects of a variety of treatment regimes which have been evolving continuously over the recent past. Temporal trends in the incubation period need to be taken into account in predicting AIDS, otherwise the extent of the past epidemic may be underestimated. More generally, assumptions about treatment availability, efficacy and use have a strong influence on HIV estimates and projections – the stronger the treatment effect in delaying the onset of an AIDS defining illness, the higher the estimates of the number of people infected.

Treatment advances for HIV disease are believed to have lengthened the duration of the incubation period, but the effect is difficult to measure quantitatively. Recent evidence from clinical trials and population-based studies indicate that antiretroviral therapies such as zidovudine and/or prophylaxis for PCP are prolonging the incubation period and improving quality of life. However, the issue of treatment efficacy remains wide open following the release of the preliminary results of the European Concorde trial during the present Workshop (Aboulker and Swart 1993). The results show no additional benefit for disease progression or survival of using zidovudine in symptom-free HIV-infected individuals over deferring its use.

A great deal of effort has been expended on sensitivity analyses for the incubation period. Wilson *et al.* (1992) compare two incubation distributions for the Australian data commonly used in this context, namely the Weibull with shape parameter 2 and mean 10 years before mid-1987 and 11 years after (assumed to be the effect of treatment), with the two-parameter gamma distribution of index 2 and corresponding means 14.3 and 15.3 years. As expected, the gamma distribution gave higher estimates of the number of people infected with HIV, but short-term predictions of AIDS were not greatly affected by the choice of distribution. We also considered a Weibull with shape 2.55, but the goodness of fit was not much changed. Allowing a three-year lengthening of the incubation period (Solomon *et al.* 1991) gave estimates that were too high to agree with surveillance data on HIV and AIDS in Australia.

Bacchetti, Segal and Jewell (1992) recently compared several different estimated incubation distributions which represent a variety of shapes and sizes of the epidemic in subgroups in the US. The authors reach the rather pessimistic conclusion that uncertainty in the true form for the incubation distribution renders backcalculation too unreliable for quantitative estimates of infection incidence. They found, among other things, that estimated incubation distributions can differ substantially between cohorts, and that a single-stage Weibull distribution may be inappropriate. However, a more optimistic interpretation of the available data and knowledge about the incubation period is possible. Not all distributions will give plausible scenarios in all situations, and analyses should be done separately for regions and transmission categories within regions. It is also important to distinguish the blood transfusion-related data, which are quite different. Incubation distributions are clearly important, but other factors appear to alter independently HIV estimates and AIDS projections, particularly treatment effects and surveillance definition changes. For example, Rosenberg and Gail (1992) use comparable incubation distributions to Brookmeyer (1991), but obtain lower ranges of forecasts for AIDS in the US.

Solomon and Wilson (1993a) compare Bacchetti *et al.*'s (1992) incubation distributions Random Sample, Hepatitis B Vaccine Trial, the Hemophiliac Cohort and their own, comparable, treatment model on the Australian data. Based on information from studies of HIV incidence in clinic and cohort populations in Australia, the Hemophiliac Cohort and the Random Sample incubation models are unrealistic, but yielded the lowest deviances. The first predicts slowly decreasing numbers of new infections that are too high, and the second predicts a dramatic peak in infections in the second half of 1980, whereas it seems fairly clear that infections amongst men who have sex with men peaked in Australia around 1984/85.

5.2   Accommodating treatment effects in backcalculation

A number of approaches have been suggested to accommodate observed temporal changes in the incubation period and in AIDS incidence.

If infection occurs at calendar time s and u denotes time since infection, we can take the hazard of progression to AIDS as a function of s, and rewrite (1) as

$$a(t) = \int_0^t h(s)\rho(t - s|s) \exp\left(- \int_0^{t-s} \rho(u|s)du\right) ds. \qquad (3)$$

Suppose treatment becomes available at some (known) calendar time T and that its effect on the hazard of progression to AIDS is

$$\rho(u|s) = \begin{cases} \rho_0(u) & \text{if } s + u \leq T \\ \rho_1(u) & \text{if } s + u > T. \end{cases}$$

A simple adjustment for treatment which captures the overall 'average' effect on the population under study is, for infection times up to T, to take $a(t)$ as in (3) above with $\rho = \rho_0$, and for $t > T$, to take $a(t)$ equal to

$$\int_T^t h(s)\rho_1(t - s) \exp\left\{- \int_0^{t-s} \rho_1(u)du\right\}ds$$

$$+ \int_0^T h(s)\rho_1(t - s) \exp\left(- \int_0^{T-s} \rho_0(u)du - \int_{T-s}^{t-s} \rho_1(u)du\right) ds. \quad (4)$$

(4) is the contribution from an individual infected before T, for whom the survivor function is the product of the probability of survival after spending time $(t - T)$ with hazard ρ_1 with the probability of surviving time $(T - s)$ with hazard ρ_0. Solomon and Wilson (1990) proposed this adjustment for predicting AIDS in Australia using single-stage gamma and Weibull incubation distributions. Information available in Australia at the time suggested that zidovudine was widely introduced into clinical practice in mid-1987 and anecdotal evidence suggested that its effect was to prolong the incubation period by about a year. So we took T to be 30 June 1987 and assumed the mean incubation increased to 9 years for the Weibull and to 14.3 years for the gamma, but that the distributional shape remained the same. No adjustment was made for the proportion actually receiving treatment, or for the stage at which treatment commenced.

Raab et al. (1993) make this adjustment for the effects of pre-AIDS treatment from 1989 onwards, which improves the goodness of fit between observed and expected AIDS incidence to the Scottish data. Moreover, Raab et al. constrained the total size of the epidemic to match other knowledge of the likely number of people infected with HIV in Scotland, which determined the shape of the Weibull incubation distribution, which was found to be implausibly high. This is an interesting attempt to incorporate increasing knowledge of seroprevalence in Scotland and increasing uncertainty about the incubation period. Raab *et al.* also consider gamma incubation distributions. McNeil (1993) reports using a Weibull distribution with shape 4.1 in a Scottish injecting drug user cohort. De Angelis *et al.* (1993) assume a 'fixed' Weibull distribution with shape 2 and mean 11 years, and comment that the mean incubation time is thought to be longer for younger patients.

The simple adjustment for treatment in (3) and (4) is essentially equivalent to taking $\rho_1(s) = \theta\rho_0(s)$ for known, constant θ, which is the proportional effect of treatment on the baseline hazard. Solomon and Wilson's assumptions give $\theta \approx 0.8$ for the Weibull distribution. Brookmeyer and Liao (1990a) consider $\theta = 0.35$ based on clinical trial data and make the more realistic assumption that treatment was available only to those with CD4 cell counts of less than 200, which they define as the second stage of a two stage model for the incubation period. Stage one is from infection to 200 which is modelled according to a Weibull distribution. They assume only a proportion are in treatment and compare this fixed-time model with a random-time model where treatment is phased in over calendar time according to a Weibull distribution, whence the probability survival in their stage two is

$$\int_s^{s+t} \exp\left(-\int_0^{w-s} \rho_0(u)du - \int_{w-s}^t \rho_1(u)du\right) v(w|s)\exp\left(-\int_s^w v(u|s)du\right) dw$$

$$+ \exp\left(-\int_0^t \rho_0(u)du - \int_s^{s+t} v(u|s)du\right),$$

where ρ_0 and ρ_1 are the pre-and post-treatment hazards for stage two and $v(w|s)$ is the known hazard function for the treatment initiation at calendar time w for an individual who enters stage two at calendar time s. Once started, individuals are assumed to stay on treatment. In addition, some information needs to be available on the hazard of treatment initiation.

Brookmeyer (1991) models the early stage of the incubation period as a Weibull distribution of median 6.5 years, shape parameter 2.08, and the later stage as an exponential distribution of median 1.5, 2.5 or 3.5 years, and treatment phased in from mid-1987 according to an exponential distribution with rate 0.2 per year (in the second stage). The model provides vital ranges of estimates of the numbers of infected individuals with early or advanced HIV disease in the US. Solomon *et al.* (1991) have applied Brookmeyer's algorithms to the Australian data, and in addition consider $\theta = 0.65$, since it is reasonable to assume that treatment efficacy may be less for the population as a whole than for the effect observed under controlled conditions. Based on information about treatment coverage from cohort and clinic data in Australia, we assumed that treatment was phased in according to an exponential distribution of rate 0.5 per year i.e. of those eligible for treatment in mid-1987, 40% were in treatment by mid-1988, 63% by mid-1989, and so on. There was little to guide the choice of smoothing parameter, so we used those estimates which gave 1,000 new infections in 1990 for the 'high' bound (in retrospect this is too high, so the resulting predictions are a high upper bound), and compared the results assuming no new infections from 1990 ('low' bound). All estimates and predictions were sensitive to the uncertainty about the effects and coverage of pre-AIDS treatment.

De Angelis *et al.* also propose a model that adjusts for treatment and the proportion in treatment, although not for when treatment is received. For homosexual men and injecting drug users, they take the proportions treated in 1988, 1989 and from 1990 onwards as 5, 10 and 25%, and halve all proportions for heterosexuals as a basis for 'low treatment' effect estimates. All the proportions are doubled for 'high treatment' effect estimates. They compare one year to four year lengthenings of the incubation period, although the one year increase gave the best fits to the data from England and Wales, as we also observed for the Australian data (see also Becker and Motika (1992) who describe a compartmental model which attempts to reflect the efficacy and use of treatment).

A more realistic, although more complex, formulation of the treatment effect is to take θ as a function of time, for example, by modelling the 'transient' effect of treatment as

$$\theta(t) = \exp\left(\beta_1 + \beta_2 e^{-\beta_3 t}\right),$$

(Cox and Oakes 1984). If $\beta_2 = 0$ this reduces to the simple proportional treatment effect described above; if $\beta_1 = 0$ and $\beta_3 > 0$ then the post-treatment hazard eventually reverts to the pre-treatment hazard; if $\beta_3 > 0$ then the post-treatment hazard eventually becomes proportional to the pre-treatment hazard and so on. This would apply to individuals in different stages of HIV disease who are eligible for treatment, and different effects may hold in the different disease stages, which would need to be modelled in detail. Of course such detailed modelling of the effects of treatment would depend largely on the available data and information.

A related hazard model has been proposed by Rosenberg *et al.* (1991). Called a 'time since infection model', it also accommodates the effects of treatment and broadenings in the surveillance definition of AIDS. The hazard for AIDS u years after infection at calendar time s, where first access to effective treatment is at calendar time τ is

$$\rho(u|s,\tau) \;=\; \rho_0(u)\left(\theta(u)I(u+s \geq \tau) + I(u+s < \tau)\right) \times$$
$$(\delta I(u+s \geq T) + I(u+s < T)).$$

Here, $I()$ is the indicator function, ρ_0 is the hazard in the absence of treatment intervention under the old US surveillance definition (i.e $T = 1$ October 1987 in the US), δ captures the increase in the hazard for AIDS resulting from broadening the definition, and $\theta(u)$ reflects the effects of treatment, defined to be one for u near zero, but decreasing to an asymptote at $\theta = 0.5$ by about year seven. The model is designed to reflect official treatment policies in the US to late 1990, which restricted the availability of zidovudine and equivalents to people with advanced HIV disease. The model specifies the relative hazard for AIDS in treated individuals as a function of time since infection, where 'in treatment' refers to the fact that the individual is being monitored, and not necessarily receiving active treatment. The authors consider transmission categories separately, although not regional groups. For a useful and robust approach to estimating and predicting AIDS, see Rosenberg *et al.* (1992) in which they use backcalculation and the time-since-infection model to predict trends in HIV and AIDS in the district of Columbia, and obtain similar (disturbingly high) estimates to those collected from seroprevalence surveys.

Bacchetti *et al.* (1993) suggest modelling nonstationarity in the incubation period directly. They consider models where the probability of being diagnosed at time j and reported at time k, given that infection was at time s, is the product of independent terms, for example,

$$D_{ij} R_j e^{\beta_j + S(j)},$$

where $S(1) = 0$ and $S(j) = S(j+12)$ for all j capture seasonal effects fitted to monthly data, the β_js represent smooth secular trends, D_{ij} is the probability of diagnosis at j given infection at i, and R_j is a reporting 'completeness' factor incorporating underreporting and reporting delays. The authors fit their overall model by maximizing a penalized likelihood with the progression probabilitites and reporting factors estimated in advance. The model involves a large number of parameters which may not be directly interpretable, and lengthening incubation times and temporal changes in reporting delays cannot be separately estimated. An alternative way of modelling periodicity is to fit the first few terms in a Fourier series (Solomon and Wilson 1993a).

5.3 A general multistage incubation distribution

It is helpful for the purpose of estimating the numbers of individuals at different stages of disease to consider a quite general multistage model from initial infection with HIV to death.

A progressive disease semi-Markov model which describes multiple stages of HIV disease assumes M stages and that stage m is less severe than stage $m+k$ (for $k = 1, \ldots, M-m$). Assuming the times spent in the different stages are independent random variables with densities $f_i(u|s)$ (the independence assumption may not be reasonable for HIV disease, but the assumption could be modified), the incubation period is a random variable defined to be the sum of the times spent in the earlier stages, and the general form for the incubation period distribution is simply

$$F_{1+2+...+m}(t|s) = \int_0^t f_1(u_1|s)F_{2+...+m}(t - u_1|s + u_1)du_1$$

and so on recursively, to equal

$$\int_0^t f_1(u_1|s) \int_0^{t_1} f_2(u_2|s_1) \ldots$$

$$\int_0^{t_{m-1}} f_{m-1}(u_{m-1}|s_{m-2})F_m(t_{m-1}|s_{m-1})du_{m-1} \ldots du_1$$

(Wilson and Solomon 1994), where $t_k = t - u_1 - \ldots - u_k$ and $s_k = s + u_1 + \ldots + u_k$.

We assume that all infected individuals pass through all stages of the disease, and that they cannot 'improve' i.e., cannot move back to an earlier stage. These conditions may be relaxed if the relevant data are available. The advantage of this model is that changes in treatment regimes at different stages of disease as well as other temporal effects, such as the proposed broadening in the surveillance definition of AIDS to CD4+ $\leq$ 200 in the US, can be readily accommodated by appropriately defining the later disease stages, especially if the data are still collected with the old definition before the change-point. Expansions in the surveillance definition of AIDS have served to increase the observed incidence and therefore to decrease the length of the incubation period, partially counteracting the effects of treatment in prolonging incubation, and these effects should be modelled explicitly.

Example

Since treatment is now available to people with CD4 cell counts of $\leq$ 500, a natural extension of Brookmeyer and Liao's (1990a) model is to split their first stage into two i.e., to define a new stage-1 as CD4 counts of 500 or more, and a new stage-2 as counts in the range 499 to 200. The third stage is from < 200 to AIDS, and the fourth stage is from AIDS to death. Solomon and Wilson (1994) consider a stage-wise Weibull incubation distribution, where the hazard of progressing from stage j to $j + 1$ in the absence of treatment or other individual effects is $\rho_j(t) = \kappa_j \gamma_j t^{\kappa_j - 1}$.

Estimates of the probability of progression to first drop in CD4 cell count below 500 was based on data from subjects in the NCI Multicenter Hemophilia Cohort Study, enrolled at the Pennsylvania State University Medical Center. At months 12, 25 (correct), 36, 48, 60, 72, Kaplan-Meier estimates of the proportions with CD4 counts never below 500 were 0.904, 0.723, 0.566, 0.422, 0.299 and 0.113 respectively (personal communication, Goedert J.J.,

Years since infection	1	3	5	7	9	11	13	15
Treatment effect								
None	0.001	0.03	0.14	0.30	0.48	0.63	0.75	0.83
One year	0.0007	0.03	0.11	0.25	0.41	0.56	0.68	0.78
Three years	0.0004	0.02	0.07	0.18	0.31	0.44	0.56	0.67

Table 1. Cumulative probabilities of progression from the initial
HIV infection to AIDS for the multistage incubation distribution.

Eyster M.E. and Gail M.H., 1991). We approximated these probabilities using a Weibull distribution with shape parameter 1.62, rate 0.0962/year and
a median stage-1 duration of 3.38 years, which was in good agreement with
Longini's (1990) estimate of the mean time for CD4 count to fall from > 899
to the 200–499 range.

Longini (1990) estimated the mean time from infection to < 200 CD4 as
8.3 years, on which we based taking the stage-2 duration to be exponentially
distributed with mean 4.5 years (hazard 0.222/year), and the duration of the
advanced stage (< 200 to AIDS) to be exponentially distributed with mean
2 years (i.e. hazard 0.5/year), without treatment. The estimated mean of
the overall incubation distribution from infection to AIDS is 10.3 years, and
the cumulative probabilities of progression from initial infection to AIDS are
given in the first row of Table 1.

Assuming treatment was available from mid-1987 only to those infected individuals whose CD4 counts dropped below 200, as was the treatment policy
in Australia until the latter part of 1990, its effect was assumed to decrease
the hazard of progressing to AIDS to 0.33/year and 0.2/year. These rates
correspond to assuming that the effect of treatment is to prolong the mean
incubation period of stage-3 by one year or three years. The overall progression probabilities according to the treatment model (3) and (4) are given in
the second and third rows of Table 1. At the time, we were analysing observed AIDS incidence data in Australia to the end of 1990, when the change
in treatment policy would have had only minimal impact on the observed
AIDS incidence. Future analyses should, however, adjust for any emerging
effects and these could be incorporated by extensions of the model just described. In applications, choice of model will be driven at least in part by the
available data and information on the disease process.

5.4 A Markov model for the incubation distribution

An important recent paper by Longini *et al.* (1992) introduces the method
now being used by the Centers for Disease Control (CDC) for predicting AIDS

in the US. They base their staged Markov model for the incubation period on interval CD4 counts, so backcalculation based on the time-dependent Markov model can yield estimated numbers of individuals at different stages of HIV disease, as measured by CD4 count. There are seven irreversible states from initial infection to AIDS with transition intensities (i.e. progression rates) $\lambda_1, \ldots, \lambda_6$ for those not receiving treatment, and $\lambda_k^* = \theta_k \lambda_k$, $0 < \theta_k \leq 1$ for those receiving treatment.

The mixture probability density function for the incubation period for infection taking place at time $\tau \in [t_m, t_{m+1})$, and subsequent AIDS diagnosis at time $t \in [t_n, t_{n+1})$, where $n > m$, is

$$(1 - p_n)p_{16}(\tau, t; \lambda_1, \ldots, \lambda_6)\lambda_6 + p_m p_{16}(\tau, t; \lambda_1^*, \ldots, \lambda_6^*)\lambda_6^*$$
$$+ \sum_{j=m+1} \left((p_j - p_{j-1}) \sum_{r=1}^{6} p_{1r}(\tau, t_j; \lambda_1, \ldots, \lambda_r)p_{r6}(t_j, t; \lambda_1^*, \ldots, \lambda_6^*)\lambda_6^* \right),$$

where $p_{ik}(\tau, t; \lambda_i, \ldots, \lambda_k)$ is the probability that an individual in stage i at time τ will be in stage k at time t, and the pairs $\{t_j, p_j\}$ denote the proportions receiving treatment in the population. For instance, at time t_1, a proportion p_1 of the HIV population is receiving treatment. The first term in the density function is the incubation period for individuals with HIV who do not receive treatment by time t_n; the second term is the incubation period for those who receive treatment on or after time t_m; and the third term is for those receiving treatment in increasing numbers between times t_{m+1} and t. Treatment is assumed available from March 1987, and the overall hazard reductions due to treatment are broadly comparable to those discussed above.

Backcalculation based on this approach will easily accommodate the new US definition of AIDS, which includes all individuals with CD4 counts below 200, as Longini *et al.*'s last CD4 count interval is from 0 to 200.

6   Epidemic models and other methods of prediction

Epidemic models for the transmission dynamics of HIV infection provide a mathematical representation of patterns of spread of the virus by systems of equations in which the rates of transition between defined states are specified quantitatively. This approach to forecasting AIDS is the most analytically and computationally complex.

It is well known that transmission dynamic modelling of HIV is not the technique of first choice for short- to medium-term quantitative predictions. The limitations again result from a lack of accurate quantitative information on key epidemiological parameters. The socially sensitive nature of HIV infection and the variable, lengthy incubation period means that fifteen years after the start of the epidemic, there is still insufficient information available to produce a realistic model capable of giving reliable forecasts. We know which parameters are important, but not their quantitative values with any degree of accuracy. Early on in the epidemic however, transmission models were recognised as the best available means of identifying important future health policy considerations. Epidemic models are the way to study the dynamics of the spread of the virus, for evaluating the impact of prevention and intervention strategies, for understanding the epidemic and the tool for forecasting long-term demographic impact. They are also the tool for mathematical study of the underlying disease process i.e., how the virus interacts with the immune system to cause disease and death (Anderson 1989).

I am in less familiar territory with this topic, and will restrict my contribution to a brief outline of articles and reviews that I have found useful reading. Excellent entry points to the literature in this field are the overviews by Isham (1988), Anderson *et al.* (1989), Anderson and May (1991) and Dietz (1992) and references contained therein. Anderson and May (1991) overview how models can be used to clarify thinking about the kinds of information needed to anticipate the future course of the epidemic, and how incomplete information can be combined with mathematical models to gain realistic insight and predictions of the epidemic's future path; mathematical details are avoided, but can be found in Isham (1988) or Anderson *et al.* (1989). The latter study in detail a general model for HIV transmission dynamics in a one-sex population with heterogeneity of sexual behaviour. The authors refer to over 100 recent articles and include tabulations of estimates of key epidemiological parameters, such as proportions developing AIDS, the incubation period, probability of heterosexual transmission, and the numbers of sexual partners amongst men who have sex with men. Dietz (1992) describes models for heterosexual and injecting drug user populations. Most models studied are deterministic, but a simple stochastic model for epidemic spread is described by Isham (1993). Jewell, Dietz and Farewell (1992) contains a number of relevant articles on epidemic models for AIDS.

Studies of heterosexual activity are relatively uncommon. Studies that have been done suggest that the rate of acquisition of sexual partners amongst heterosexuals in developed countries is much slower than amongst men who have sex with men. Consequently, the spread of HIV amongst heterosexuals will be much slower, and this is certainly true in Australia, although sensitivity analyses for the infection curves show that slow, exponential spread cannot be excluded amongst heterosexuals and injecting drug users (Solomon *et al.* 1991). This is in contrast to some developing nations with naturally high birthrates, where HIV is spreading substantially through heterosexual contact. Some predictions suggest this is leading to severe effects on population growth (see Dietz 1992).

Actuarial projections need to be very long-term and age-specific, no matter how speculative or variable. So the purpose of prediction differs slightly, and certain parameters have to be incorporated at the exclusion of others. For instance, extra sickness and mortality from AIDS must be included, whereas assumptions about sexual behaviour need not be as elaborate. The purpose is also to follow cohorts of individuals. See for example, Wilkie (1989) in which he gives sets of differential equations that define the transitions between different states in populations of homosexual men. Solomon, Doust and Wilson (1989, Appendix 7) describe the results of Wilkie's model applied to the Australian data.

The ideal starting point for predicting future AIDS incidence, or other stage of HIV disease, would be accurate knowledge of the size and shape of the HIV infection curve, coupled with accurate knowledge of the incubation distribution. Such data would be ideally obtained by anonymous, randomized seroprevalence surveys coupled with close monitoring of large cohorts of susceptible groups. In the absence of the ideal data, we have already seen how the main techniques attempt to answer the prediction problem. Other, less common, approaches have been applied as well, some of which are useful in the early phases of an epidemic when there is little survey and other data available.

An approach which has been widely used by government departments is the so-called direct method, which essentially attempts to simulate the results of a random survey by piecing together various estimates of seroprevalence in subgroups of the population rather like a crude jigsaw (see, for instance, Hillier, Appendix 3 in Report of a Working Group (1988)). This approach can be fraught with difficulties, and as the epidemic progresses, the plausible bounds become so wide as to be virtually useless. Specific problems are: the comparability of studies, defining the subgroups, multiple counting estimating the size of the populations at risk, biased samples of seroprevalence, and more. There are various ways of trying to overcome some of these difficulties, such as basing the risk populations on known prevalence of risk behaviours over a limited period. Such studies can, however, provide useful evidence of the size of the epidemic if the results are broadly in agreement with those obtained from other approaches, and can help identify at an early stage where further information is needed. Moreover, Hillier's results were remarkably good in retrospect. Researchers have also attempted to reconstruct the HIV epidemic using mortality data (McCormick, 1989, for example).

A recent and interesting suggestion has been to reconstruct the past HIV infection curve using serial cross-sectional measurements of a marker of disease progression, namely CD4 cell counts (Satten and Longini 1994). If samples from the start of the epidemic are not available, then under a Markov assumption, one can calculate the conditional distribution of infection times.

In other recent work, Frydman (1992) describes a nonparametric procedure for estimating the incubation distribution in a cohort of hemophiliacs using a three-stage Markov process, where the probability of developing AIDS following infection depends on chronological time (see also related models in Keiding (1991)).

7 Predicting AIDS deaths and prevalence

The discussion so far has focused on methods for reconstructing the past HIV epidemic and projecting HIV estimates forward in time to predict future incidence and prevalence at difference stages of HIV disease. It is essential for health-care planning to have available predictions of AIDS prevalence i.e., the number of people sick with advanced HIV disease or AIDS, for which we need accurate forecasts of the numbers of AIDS deaths. Few surveillance systems are able to distinguish AIDS deaths which we define to be deaths from any cause amongst patients diagnosed with AIDS.

Changes in the definition of AIDS and consequent changes in the survival distribution will alter the magnitude of the estimates in a way dependent on the changes. The purpose and various approaches to estimation and prediction are essentially unchanged, but are made more difficult when the revelant data on emerging effects are not available.

Several of the prediction methods already discussed can be modified or extended to include estimating AIDS deaths and prevalence. For instance the staged models and the backcalculation method can define 'death' to be the endpoint of interest. Other modelling approaches, such as transmission models, produce qualitative rather than quantitative results, at least from a health planning perspective. Exceptions are actuarial models for AIDS which encompass rather pessimistic scenarios i.e., high death rates and AIDS prevalence, as these are required for advising insurance companies and pension funds (see Wilkie 1989).

For very short-term forecasting, say for one year ahead, simple extrapolation of curves fitted to recent observed death incidence data could, in principle, be used. The usefulness of this direct approach depends largely on the quality of the AIDS death data. Cox (Appendix 11 in Report of a Working Group (1988)) suggests simply adding together the expected contributions from deaths from AIDS cases diagnosed and reported, cases diagnosed but not yet reported, and those not yet diagnosed. The rationale for this is that the majority of deaths in the near future will be from cases already diagnosed and reported, and possibly from cases diagnosed and not yet reported where reporting delays are known to be substantial (e.g. Report of a Working Group, Scotland (1993)). In Australia, the AIDS incidence data are thoughtto be relatively complete with few serious reporting delays, as discussed previously.

There are problems however with the reporting of deaths, including delays and under-reporting.

For longer-term predictions, most deaths will be from cases of AIDS not yet diagnosed. A more sophisticated approach which uses more of the available information is to combine predictions of AIDS incidence with the 'known' survival distribution from diagnosis to death. This is essentially the approach used by compartmental and epidemic models, and the so-called staged models.

The rate of occurrence of deaths at time t is the convolution

$$\lambda_F(t) = \int_0^t a(u)f_S(t-u)du, \tag{5}$$

where $a()$ is the rate of new diagnoses of AIDS cases, and $f_S()$ is the probability density function of survival time. The prevalence of AIDS at time t is then simply the difference of diagnoses and deaths

$$\int_0^t \{a(u) - \lambda_F(u)\}du.$$

Detailed analysis depends on assuming particular functional forms or numerical quantities for a and f_S.

Early on in the epidemic, some countries reported a significant proportion of AIDS cases detected only after death, which was probably aggravated by a lack of familiarity with diagnosing AIDS and other artefacts of the reporting process. For survival data from England and Wales, Reeves (1989) proposed an adjustment for a proportion θ of 'zero' survivors i.e., the survival probability density function is $\theta = 0$ for $t = 0$ and $(1-\theta)f_S$ for $t > 0$. Reeves estimated θ to be 0.08 and found an exponential distribution provided an excellent fit to the positive times. Survival data from a study of New York City patients gave virtually the same answer (Rothenberg et al. 1987).

Changes in survival associated with treatment availability, other temporal trends, and definitional changes can be accommodated in (5) in ways directly analogous to modelling changes in the incubation distribution. Solomon and Wilson (1992) have incorporated changes in survival in Australia associated with the widespread availability of zidovudine in mid-1987, as well as Reeves's zero survivor proportion. Substantial improvements in survival were observed in cases diagnosed with AIDS in Australia after June 1987 over those who were diagnosed and reported up to that time (Solomon et al. 1990a). We took

$$\lambda_F(t) = \begin{cases} \theta a(t) + (1-\theta)\int_0^t a(u)\rho e^{-\rho(t-u)}\,du & t \leq T \\ (1-\theta)\int_0^T a(u)\rho e^{-\rho(t-u)}\,du + \theta'a(t) \\ \quad +(1-\theta')\int_T^t a(u)\rho' e^{-\rho'(t-u)}\,du & t > T \end{cases}$$

where θ, ρ and θ', ρ' are the parameters from the exponential survival models for diagnoses made before and after $T = $ mid-1987. The first two terms give the contribution to the death rate up to time T, the next term gives the contribution from cases of AIDS diagnosed before T and surviving beyond T, and the final two terms give the contribution from diagnoses made after T.

Similar, simpler approaches have been taken by the Working Group in England and Wales (1990), the Scottish Working Group (1993), and others.

In recent work Professor B.D. Ripley and I modelled the effect of the availability of treatment on Australian AIDS survival using time-dependent covariates. The analysis was based on a proportional hazards model which allowed a proportional change in the hazard from 1 July 1987 to 30 June 1990, and another from 1 July 1990. The results show a halving in the hazard from 1 July 1987, but an insignificant change in 1990.

8 Some concluding remarks

The literature on statistical methods for predicting HIV disease is vast, and this overview represents a selected view of techniques used in recent work. Methods for prediction are constantly being updated and extended as new, and sometimes unexpected, information comes to light. Statistical theory and methods can easily outstrip the available information and it is important that extensions to existing methods and new approaches are driven by increasing knowledge of the epidemic.

It is becoming apparent that techniques must be able to incorporate the evolution of knowledge and uncertainties about the epidemic in more sophisticated ways than performing sensitivity analyses, which remain essential. In particular, backcalculation is now being used to incorporate increasing knowledge of HIV prevalence, whilst at the same time allowing for increased uncertainty and nonstationarity of the incubation period. Sometimes this has led to a fully Bayesian framework for prediction. It is also essential for planning purposes to have available estimates of the numbers of individuals at different stages of HIV disease, or interval CD4 counts.

I have not discussed directly the implications of the recent broadening in the definition of AIDS in the US to include all individuals with CD4 cell counts below 200. CD4 cell count is characterised by its variability both within and between individuals, and this variability may well be of biological importance. In analysis, it is important to distinguish the different sorts of things the counts are to be used for. If CD4 is to be used as a basis for definitional change, it is essential to analyse longitudinal data on CD4 at a number of levels:

(i) describing population variability with a view to comparing two or more groups,

(ii) describing individual trajectories with a view to correlating with outcome (such as a diagnosis of AIDS), and as a basis for comparing groups,
and

(iii) monitoring individual trajectories to detect signals of sudden change
or deterioration.

Special difficulties include severe imbalance in the data, very short individual 'time series' and unequally spaced observations. These issues are
receiving attention from AIDS researchers, who can draw on existing statistical methods for the analysis of variability (see, for instance, Cox and Solomon
(1986,1988), Solomon (1985)) as well as developing new, computer-intensive
methods for modelling complex data.

References

Aboulker, J.-P. and Swart, A.M. (1993) 'Preliminary analysis of the Concorde trial',
The Lancet **341**, 889–890.

Anderson, R.M. (1989) 'Editorial review: mathematical and statistical studies of
the epidemiology of HIV', *AIDS* **3**, 333–346.

Anderson, R.M., Blythe, S.P., Gupta, S. and Konings, E. (1989) 'The transmission dynamics of the human immunodeficiency virus type 1 in the male homosexual community in the United Kingdom: the influence of changes in sexual
behaviour', *Phil. Trans. Roy. Soc. Lond. B* **325**, 45–98.

Anderson, R.M. and May, R.M (1991) *Infectious Diseases of Humans: Dynamics
and Control*, Oxford University Press, Oxford.

Bacchetti, P., Segal M. and Jewell, N. (1992) 'Uncertainty about the incubation
period of AIDS and its impact on backcalculation'. In *AIDS Epidemiology:
Methodological Issues*, N. Jewell, K. Dietz and V. Farewell (eds.), Birkhäuser,
Boston.

Bacchetti, P., Segal M. and Jewell, N. (1993) 'Backcalculation of HIV infection
rates', (with discussion), *Statist. Sci.* **8**, 82-119.

Becker, N.G., Watson, L.F. and Carlin, J.B. (1991) 'A method of nonparametric
back-projection and its application to AIDS data. *Stat. Med.* **10**, 1527–42.

Becker, N. (1992) Assessing the extent of the HIV epidemic: methods and achievable results. *Proceedings of the XVIth International Biometrics Conference*
Hamilton, New Zealand.

Becker, N.G. and Marschner, I. (1993) A method for estimating the age-specific
relative risk of HIV infection from AIDS incidence data. *Biometrika* **80**, 165–
178.

Becker, N.G. and Motika, M. (1993) Smoothed nonparametric backprojection of
AIDS incidence data with adjustment for therapy. *Math. Biosci.* **118**, 1–23.

Becker, N.G. and Watson, L.F. (1992) In *AIDS epidemiology: methodological issues*, Jewell, N., Dietz, K. and Farewell, V., (eds.) Birkhäuser, Boston.

Brookmeyer, R. and Gail, M.H. (1988) 'A method for obtaining short-term projections and lower bounds on the size of the AIDS epidemic', *J. Am. Statist. Assoc.* **83**, 301–8.

Brookmeyer, R. and Damiano, A. (1989) 'Statistical methods for short-term projections of AIDS incidence', *Stat. Med.* **8**, 23–34.

Brookmeyer, R. and Liao, J. (1990a) 'Statistical modelling of the AIDS epidemic for forecasting health care needs', *Biometrics* **46**, 1151–63.

Brookmeyer, R and Liao, J. (1990b) 'The analysis of delays in disease reporting', *Am. J. Epidemiol.* **132**, 355–65.

Brookmeyer, R (1991) 'Reconstruction and future trends of the AIDS epidemic in the United States', *Science* **253**, 37–42.

Brookmeyer, R and Liao, J. (1992) 'Statistical methods for reconstructing infection curves'. In *AIDS Epidemiology: Methodological Issues*, N. Jewell, K. Dietz, and V. Farewell (eds.), Birkhäuser, Boston.

Cleveland, W.S. (1979) 'Robust locally weighted regression and smoothing scatterplots', *J. Am. Stat. Assoc.* **74**, 829–836.

Cox, D.R. and Davison, A.C. (1989) 'Prediction for small subgroups', *Phil. Trans. Roy. Soc. Lond. B* **325**, 185–7.

Cox, D.R. and Medley, G.F. (1989) 'A process of events with notification delay and the forecasting of AIDS', *Phil. Trans. Roy. Soc. Lond. B* **325**, 135–145.

Cox, D.R. and Oakes, D. (1984) *Analysis of Survival Data*, Chapman and Hall, London.

Cox, D.R. and Solomon, P.J. (1986) 'Analysis of variability with large numbers of small samples', *Biometrika* **73**, 543–554.

Cox, D.R. and Solomon, P.J. (1988) 'On testing for serial correlation in large numbers of small samples', *Biometrika* **75**, 145–148.

Day, N.E., Gore, S.M., McGee, M.A. and South, M. (1989) 'Predictions of the AIDS epidemic in the UK: the use of the back projection method', *Phil. Trans. R. Soc. Lond. B* **325**, 123–134.

De Angelis, D., Day, N.E., Gore, S.M., Gilks, W.R. and McGee, M.A. (1993) 'AIDS: the statistical basis for public health', *Stat. Meth. Med. Res.* **2**, 75–91.

Dietz, K. (1992) 'Dynamic AIDS models – have they explained anything?' In *Proceedings of the XVIth International Biometrics Conference*, Hamilton, New Zealand.

Diggle, P.J., Fazekas de St Groth, C. and Solomon, P.J. (1990) 'Application of empirical Bayes to monitoring of the AIDS epidemic in Australia. In *Projections of Acquired Immune Deficiency Syndrome in Australia using data to the end of September 1989*, P.J. Solomon, C. Fazekas de St Groth and S.R. Wilson, NCEPH Working Paper Number 16, Australian National University.

Farewell, V.T., Aalen, O.O., De Angelis, D. and Day, N.E. (1994) 'Estimation of the rate of diagnosis of HIV infection in HIV infected individuals', *Biometrika* **81**, 287–294.

Frydman, H. (1992) 'A nonparametric estimation procedure for a periodically observed three state Markov process, with application to AIDS', *J. Roy. Statist. Soc. B* **54**, 853–866.

Gail, M.H. and Rosenberg, P. (1992) 'Perspectives on using backcalculation to estimate HIV prevalence and project AIDS incidence'. In *AIDS Epidemiology: Methodological Issues*, N. Jewell, K. Dietz, and V. Farewell (eds.), Birkhäuser, Boston.

Harris, J.E. (1990) 'Reporting delays and the incidence of AIDS', *J. Am. Stat. Assoc.* **85**, 915–924.

Heisterkamp, S.H., Jager, J.C., Ruitenberg, E.J., Van Druten, J.A.M. and Downs, A.M. (1989) 'Correcting reported AIDS incidence: a statistical approach', *Stat. Med.* **8**, 963–976.

Isham, V. (1988) 'Mathematical modelling of the transmission dynamics of HIV infection and AIDS: a review', *J. Roy. Statist. Soc. A* **151**, 5–30.

Isham, V. (1989) 'Estimation of the incidence of HIV infection', *Phil. Trans. Roy. Soc. Lond. B* **325**, 113–121.

Isham, V. (1993) 'Stochastic models for epidemics, with special reference to AIDS', *Ann. Appl. Prob.* **3**, 1–27.

Jewell, N. (1990) 'Some statistical issues in studies of the epidemiology of AIDS', *Stat. Med.* **9**, 1387–1416.

Jewell, N., Dietz, K. and Farewell, V. (eds.) (1992) *AIDS epidemiology: methodological issues*, Birkhäuser, Boston.

Keiding, N. (1991) 'Age-specific incidence and prevalence: a statistical perspective', *J. Roy. Statist. Soc. A* **154**, 371–412.

Lawless, J. and Sun, J. (1992) 'A comprehensive backcalculation framework for the estimation and prediction of AIDS cases'. In *AIDS Epidemiology: Methodological Issues*, N. Jewell, K. Dietz, and V. Farewell (eds.), Birkhäuser, Boston.

Longini, I.M. (1990) 'Modeling the decline of CD4$^+$ T-lymphocyte counts in HIV-infected individuals', *J AIDS* **3**, 930–1.

Longini, I.M., Byers, R.H., Hessol, N.A. and Tan, W.Y. (1992) 'Estimating the stage-specific numbers of HIV infection using a Markov model and backcalculation', *Stat. Med.* **11**, 831–843.

Longini, I.M., Clark, W.S. and Karon, J.M. (1993) 'Effect of routine use of therapy in slowing the clinical course of Human Immunodeficiency Virus (HIV) infection in a population-based cohort', *Am. J. Epidemiol.* **137**, 1229–1240.

Mariotto, A. (1989) 'Rate of growth of AIDS epidemic in Europe: a comparative analysis', *Phil. Trans. Roy. Soc. Lond. B* **325**, 175–178.

McCullagh, P. and Nelder, J.A. (1989) *Generalized Linear models*, second edition, Chapman and Hall, London.

McCormick, A. (1989) 'Estimating the size of the HIV epidemic by using mortality data', *Phil. Trans. Roy. Soc. Lond. B* **325**, 163–173.

McNeil, A. (1993) *Statistical Methods in AIDS Progression Studies with an Analysis of the Edinburgh City Hospital Cohort*, PhD Thesis, University of Cambridge.

National Working Group on HIV Projections (1992) *Estimates and Projections of the HIV epidemic in Australia, 1981–1994*, Technical Report 1, National Centre in HIV Epidemiology and Clinical Research, University of New South Wales.

Pagano, M., Tu, X.M., DeGruttola, V. and MaWhinney, S. (1995) 'Regression analysis of censored and truncated data: estimating reporting delay distributions and AIDS incidence from surveillance data', *Biometrics*, to appear.

Petric, A. (1992) *Survival of Australian AIDS patients*, Honours Thesis, University of Adelaide.

Raab, G.M., Gore, S.M., Goldberg, D.J. and Donnelly, C.A. (1994) 'Bayesian forecasting of the human immunodeficiency virus epidemic in Scotland', *J. Roy. Statist. Soc. A* **157**, 17–30.

Reeves, G. (1989) 'The overall distribution of survival times for UK AIDS patients', *Phil. Trans. Roy. Soc. Lond. B* **325**, 147–151.

Report of a Working Group (Chairman, Sir David Cox) (1988) *Short-term Prediction of HIV Infection and AIDS in England and Wales*, HMSO, UK.

Report of a Working Group (Chairman, Professor N.E. Day) (1990) *Acquired Immune Deficiency Syndrome in England and Wales to end 1993: Projections using Data to end September 1989*, PHLS.

Report of a Working Group (1993) *Acquired Immune Deficiency Syndrome and HIV-related Disease in Scotland*, The Scottish Office, Home and Health Department.

Rosenberg, P. (1990) 'A simple correction of AIDS surveillance data for reporting delays', *J AIDS* **3**, 49–54.

Rosenberg, P.S. and Gail, M.H. (1991) 'Backcalculation of flexible linear models of the human immunodeficiency virus infection curve', *Appl. Stat.* **40**, 269–282.

Rosenberg, P.S., Gail, M.H. and Pee, D. (1991) 'Mean square error of estimates of HIV prevalence and short-term AIDS projections derived by backcalculation', *Stat. Med.* **10**, 1167–1180.

Rosenberg, P.S., Gail, M.H. and Carroll, R.J. (1992) 'Estimating HIV prevalence and projecting AIDS incidence in the United States: a model that accounts for therapy and changes in the surveillance definition of AIDS', *Stat. Med.* **11**, 1633–55.

Rosenberg, P.S., Levy, M.E., Brundage, J.F., Petersen, L.R., Karon, J.M., Fears, T.R., Gardner, L.I., Gail, M.H., Goedert, J.J., Blattner, W.A., Ryan, C.C., Vermund, S.H. and Biggar, R.J. (1992) 'Population-based monitoring of an urban HIV/AIDS epidemic: magnitude and trends in the district of Columbia', *JAMA* **268**, 495–503.

Rothenberg, R., Woelfe, M., Stoneburner, R., Milberg, J., Parker, R. and Truman, B. (1987) 'Survival with the acquired immunodeficiency syndrome', *New Engl. J. Med.* **317**, 1297–1302.

Satten, G. and Longini, I.M. Jr. (1994) 'Estimation of incidence of HIV infection using cross-sectional marker surveys', *Biometrics* **50**, 675–688.

Solomon, P.J. (1985) 'Transformations for components of variance and covariance', *Biometrika* **72**, 233–239.

Solomon, P.J., Doust, J.A. and Wilson, S.R. (1989) *Predicting the Course of AIDS in Australia and evaluating the effect of AZT: a first report*, NCEPH Working Paper Number 3, Australian National University.

Solomon, P.J. and Wilson S.R. (1990) 'Accommodating change due to treatment in the method of back projection for estimating HIV infection incidence', *Biometrics* **46**, 1165–1170.

Solomon, P.J., Wilson, S.R., Swanson, C.E. and Cooper, D.A. (1990a) 'Effect of zidovudine on survival of patients with AIDS in Australia', *Med. J. Austral.* **153**, 254–257.

Solomon, P.J., Wilson, S.R., Swanson, C.E. and Cooper, D.A. (1990b) 'Predicting the course of AIDS in Australia', *Med. J. Austral.* **153**, 386–394.

Solomon, P.J., Attewell, R.A., Freeman, E.B and Wilson, S.R. (1991) *AIDS in Australia: Reconstructing the epidemic from 1980 to 1990 and predicting future trends in HIV disease*, NCEPH Working Paper Number 29, Australian National University.

Solomon, P.J. and Wilson, S.R. (1992) 'Predicting AIDS deaths and prevalence in Australia', *Med. J. Austral.* **157**, 121–125.

Solomon, P.J. and Wilson, S.R. (1993a) 'Comment on *Bacchetti, Segal and Jewell: Backcalculation of HIV infection rates*', *Statist. Sci.* **8**, 112–114.

Solomon, P.J. and Wilson, S.R. (1993b) 'Prediction of new cases of disease or infection for small subgroups', *Biometr. J* **35**, 333–341.

Taylor, J.M.G. (1989) 'Models for the HIV infection and AIDS epidemic in the United States', *Stat. Med.* **8**, 45–58.

Wilkie, A.D. (1989) 'Population projections for AIDS using an actuarial model', *Phil. Trans. Roy. Soc. Lond.* B **325**, 99–112.

Wilson, S.R. and Solomon, P.J. (1994) 'Estimates for different stages of HIV disease', *Comp. Appl. Biosci.* **10**, 681–683.

Wilson, S.R. Fazekas de St Groth, C. and Solomon, P.J. (1992) 'Sensitivity analyses for the backcalculation method of AIDS projections', *J AIDS* **5**, 523–527.

Zeger, S.L., See, L-C. and Diggle, P.J. (1989) 'Statistical methods for monitoring the AIDS epidemic', *Stat. Med.* **8**, 3–21.

Staged Markov Models Based on CD4+ T-Lymphocytes for the Natural History of HIV Infection

Ira M. Longini Jr, W. Scott Clark, Glenn A. Satten, Robert H. Byers and John M. Karon

1 Introduction

The natural history of HIV infection has been viewed as a staged process since the early years of the epidemic. The Walter Reed staging system was devised in 1986 (Redfield *et al.* 1986), and a number of other staging systems have been used since then. A staged Markov model is a natural mathematical device for modeling such a process. The Markov model has been used in five basic areas of HIV/AIDS research:

1. To describe the natural history of HIV infection (Longini *et al.* 1989a,b, Longini 1990, Longini *et al.* 1991);

2. to evaluate the effect of covariates on stage-specific progression rates, such as therapy (Longini *et al.* 1993);

3. to predict the stage-specific course of the HIV epidemic in selected populations (Longini *et al.* 1992) and in the USA as a whole (CDC 1992, Brookmeyer 1991);

4. to estimate HIV incidence from infection surveys (Satten and Longini 1994);

5. to provide estimates for HIV transmission models used to estimate transmission probabilities (Longini *et al.* 1989b) and to investigate the dynamics of the HIV epidemic (Hethcote *et al.* 1991a,b, Jacquez *et al.* 1988, Koopman *et al.* 1991).

The purpose of this paper is to review the progress that has been made in areas 1–3, and to describe further refinements of the Markov modeling approach.

In Section 2, we give the general mathematical framework for the model, and this is followed by a description of how to fit the model to data in Section 3. An application of the model to data from the San Francisco Men's

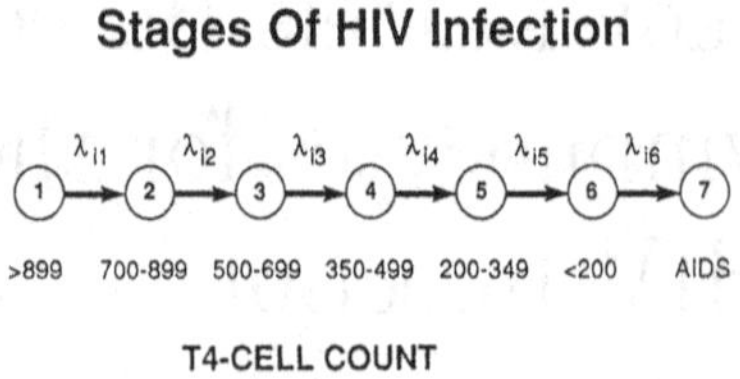

Stages Of HIV Infection

>899   700-899   500-699   350-499   200-349   <200   AIDS

T4-CELL COUNT

Figure 1. The modeled flows through the stages of HIV infection, where λ_{ik} is the monthly progression rate for a person with cofactor status i, who is in stage k.

Health Study (SFMHS) is presented in Section 4. In Section 5, we give the mathematical details on how to couple the staged Markov model with the back calculation method. We apply the stage-specific back calculation to the state of New Jersey in Section 5.2, and to the entire United States in Section 5.3. Various extensions of the model are given in Sections 6 and 7. Finally, a discussion is given in Section 8.

2 Model for disease progression

The material presented in this section and the next is largely a summary of work that has appeared as a sequence of papers (Longini *et al.* 1989a,b, Longini 1990, Longini *et al.* 1991). We define seven irreversible stages of HIV infection based on T4-cell count (Figure 1). Persons in stages 1–6 are infected but AIDS free, and those in stage 7 have an AIDS diagnosis. Stages 1–6 are modeled as transient states and stage 7 as an absorbing state. The stage-specific, monthly progression (i.e., hazard) rate is $h_{ik}(t)$ for a person who is in stage k ($k = 1, \ldots, 6$) with covariate level i ($i = 1, \ldots, I$), at calendar time t. The natural history of HIV infection is described by the transition probabilities, $p_{ijk}(\tau, t)$, $j \leq k$, and $\tau \leq t$; that is, the probability that a person who is in stage j at time τ will be in stage k at time t given that he has covariate level i between times τ and t. We will consider the case where the progression rates are piece-wise constant of the form

$$h_{ik}(t) = \begin{cases} \lambda_{ik} & 0 \leq t < t^* \\ \lambda_{ik}^* & t^* \leq t < \infty \end{cases} \quad (k = 1, \ldots, 6, \ i = 1, 2.) \tag{1}$$

The transition probabilities are, for $0 \leq \tau \leq t < t^*$,

$$p_{ijk}(\tau, t) = g_{ijk}(\tau, t; \lambda_{ij}, \ldots, \lambda_{ik}), \tag{2}$$

for $0 \leq \tau < t^* \leq t$,

$$p_{ijk}(\tau, t) = \sum_{r=j}^{k} g_{ijr}(\tau, t^*; \lambda_{ij}, \ldots, \lambda_{ir}) g_{irk}(t^*, t; \lambda_{ir}^*, \ldots, \lambda_{ik}^*), \tag{3}$$

from the Chapman-Kolmogorov equations, and for $t^* \leq \tau \leq t$,

$$p_{ijk}(\tau, t) = g_{ijk}(\tau, t; \lambda_{ij}^*, \dots, \lambda_{ik}^*), \qquad (4)$$

where, when $k \leq 6$,

$$g_{ijk}(\tau, t; \lambda_{ij}, \dots, \lambda_{ik}) = \begin{cases} e^{-\lambda_{ij}(t-\tau)} & \text{if } j = k, \\ \dfrac{(-1)^{k-j} (\prod_{r=j}^{k-1} \lambda_{ir}) \sum_{r=j}^{k} e^{-\lambda_{ir}(t-\tau)}}{\prod_{\ell=j}^{k} {}_{\ell \neq r}(\lambda_{ir} - \lambda_{i\ell})} & \text{if } j < k \end{cases} \qquad (5)$$

and when $k = 7$,

$$g_{ij7}(\tau, t; \lambda_{ij}, \dots, \lambda_{i6}) = \begin{cases} 1 & \text{if } j = 7, \\ \dfrac{(-1)^{6-j} (\prod_{r=j}^{6} \lambda_{ir}) \sum_{r=j}^{6} [1 - e^{-\lambda_{ir}(t-\tau)}]}{\lambda_{ir} \prod_{\ell=j}^{6} {}_{\ell \neq r}(\lambda_{ir} - \lambda_{i\ell})} & \text{if } j < 7 \end{cases} \qquad (6)$$

where $\lambda_{ij} \neq \lambda_{ik}$, $j \neq k$, $i = 1, 2$. Standard methods for Markov processes are used to derive expressions for the mean waiting times in various stages.

Our first measure of the impact of covariates on progression rates is the hazard ratio $\theta_{ijk}(t) = h_{ik}(t)/h_{jk}(t)$, $i \neq j$, when comparing the effects of covariate level i to that of j. Our second measure of the impact of covariates is based on the probability that a person who enters some stage $k < 7$ at time τ has been diagnosed with AIDS by time $t > \tau$. The risk ratio of interest is $\phi_{ijk}(\tau, t) = p_{ik7}(\tau, t)/p_{jk7}(\tau, t)$, $i \neq j$. It is important to note that $\lim_{t \to \infty} \phi_{ijk}(\tau, t) = 1$, for fixed τ, because 7 is an absorbing state.

3 Fitting the model to the data

The Markov model is fitted to data via maximum likelihood (ML) methods. We estimate the parameters by formulating the likelihood function on each person's passage through the stages of infection. Let r $(r = 1, 2, \dots, n)$ denote the index for each of the n persons in the cohort. Let $m_r + 1$ be the number of observation times for the rth person. Then, the data on the rth person is in the form of the triplets

$$[\tau_r, y_r, i_r] = [(\tau_{r0}, y_{r0}, i_{r0}), (\tau_{r1}, y_{r1}, i_{r1}), \dots, (\tau_{rm_r}, y_{rm_r}, i_{rm_r})], \qquad (7)$$

where $\tau_{rj}, y_{rj}, i_{rj}$ are the time, stage and covariate level, respectively, of the rth person at the jth observation. The contribution that the rth person makes to the likelihood function is

$$L_r[\mathbf{h(t)}] = \prod_{k=0}^{m_r - 1} p_{i_{rk} y_{rk} y_{rk+1}}(\tau_{rk}, \tau_{rk+1}), \qquad (8)$$

where $p_{ijk}(\tau, t)$ are from (1–6). The likelihood function over the n persons is

$$L[\mathbf{h(t)}] = \prod_{r=1}^{n} L_r[\mathbf{h(t)}]. \qquad (9)$$

The maximum likelihood estimates (MLEs) of the parameters $h(t)$ are found by maximizing (9) via the Newton-Raphson algorithm. The asymptotic multivariate normality properties of MLEs and the delta method are used to construct confidence intervals for the $\theta_{ijk}(t)$ and the mean first passage times, as well as other statistics of interest. Bootstrap confidence intervals are calculated for the $\phi_{ijk}(\tau, t)$.

3.1 Persistence criteria

T4-cell counts exhibit considerable intra-individual variability. Thus, the observed T4-cell count at an exam may not reflect the actual stage of infection. Some sort of smoothing in needed. In order to stabilize the counts we employed standard clinical criteria for classifying persons into stages (Redfield *et al.* 1986). The idea is that HIV disease is a progressive, monotonic process reflected in a mean decline of T4 cells over time. Thus, we do not classify persons into a stage unless they are persistently in that stage or move to an even more advanced stage. If exams are spaced approximately six months apart, then our definition of persistence is that a person is persistently in a stage k at time t, if he or she is still in that stage or a higher stage (i.e., $j \geq k$) at the time $t + 6$. Persons who have measurements that go up are simply held in their current state until progression by the above criteria occurs. See Longini *et al.* (1993) for details on how the persistence criterion was implemented. In this case, the mean first passage time to go from stage 1 to $k > 1$ is the sum of the mean times in stages 1 through $k - 1$.

4 Application to data from the San Francisco Men's Health Study

The material presented in this section is based on Longini *et al.* (1993). We are first interested in estimating the progression rates, and assessing the effects of prophylactic therapy on these progression rates. We use data from the San Francisco Men's Health Study (SFMHS), a prospective study of a random sample of 1,045 homosexual and bisexual men who were 25-54 years old at the time of enrollment, which occurred during June 1984-January 1985 (Winklestein *et al.* 1987). The men were examined approximately every six months, and tested for HIV infection. They were also asked to detail their therapy history since their last visit. We placed each man who reported zidovudine and/or pentamidine use since his last visit in the treated group for that period of time. If other therapies were employed, then the men were left in the no therapy group. Thus, in this paper, the term 'therapy' refers only to the use of zidovudine and/or pentamidine. Our conceptualization of how therapy affects progression is that zidovudine alone may slow or temporarily

Year	Percentage by drug category				Number examined[a]
	Zidovudine	Pentamidine	Both	Either	
1985	0.0	0.0	0.0	0.0	253
1986	0.3	0.0	0.0	0.0	204
1987	6.4	0.0	0.0	6.4	202
1988	15.8	0.0	0.0	15.8	137
1989	25.3	15.5	12.3	28.5	148
1990	45.0	28.8	24.8	49.0	221
1991	54.7	28.3	26.4	56.6	88[b]

[a]Number of men who had one or more exams during the given year.
[b]Number of men who had one or more exams during the three month period of Jan.–March 1991

Table 1. Percentage of HIV-1[+] men who have used zidovudine and pentamidine in a particular year, the San Francisco Men's Health Study (from Longini *et al.* 1993)

arrest the progression from higher to lower T4-cell counts and that zidovudine and pentamidine, either separately or jointly, delay the development of AIDS.

From the time of enrollment through March 1991, 428 HIV-infected men had at least two seropositive exams with T4-cell counts taken. Among these men, 385 were seropositive at their first exam, and 43 seroconverted during the study. For HIV-infected men, there was an average of 8.3 exams per man, and a total of 3,561 exams for which T4-cell tests were performed. The percentages of HIV-infected men who used zidovudine at any time during each year increased steadily from 6.4 percent in 1987 to nearly 57 percent in 1991; most who used pentamidine also used zidovudine at the same time (Table 1). In 1991, for example, 93 percent of those using pentamidine were also using zidovudine. The percentage of men who had used zidovudine increasing steadily with the clinical progression of HIV infection (Table 2). Only about four percent of the men with T4-cell counts of at least 500 were on therapy. However, this percentage increased to nearly 41 percent for those who have an AIDS diagnosis.

4.1 Progression rates without covariates

In this case, $h_{ik}(t) = \lambda_k$, and $k = 1, \ldots, 6$, where λ_k is simply the progression rate for a person who is in stage k. The vector of progression rates to be estimated is $\boldsymbol{\lambda} = [\lambda_1, \ldots, \lambda_6]$. Table 3 shows the parameter estimates without stratification by therapy use or calendar time. The estimated mean waiting time from seroconversion to when the T4-cell count persistently drops into

k	count	Zidovudine	Pentamidine	Both	Either
1	> 899	0.0	0.0	0.0	0.0
2	700–899	1.4	0.5	0.5	1.4
3	500–699	3.7	0.5	0.5	3.7
4	350–499	7.2	1.1	1.1	7.2
5	200–349	20.2	8.8	7.4	21.6
6	0–199	35.3	22.1	19.5	37.9
7	AIDS	36.2	25.6	21.0	40.8

Table 2. Percentage of men who ever had used zidovudine and pentamidine by stage of infection in the San Francisco Men's Health Study, 1987–1991 (From Longini *et al.* 1993).

Stage k	T4-cell count	Transition rate $\hat{\lambda}_k$ (SE) months^{-1}	Mean waiting time $\hat{\mu}_k$ (SE) years	Cum. waiting time[a] (SE) years
1	> 899	0.0483 (0.0046)	1.7 (0.2)	1.7 (0.2)
2	700–899	0.0577 (0.0039)	1.4 (0.1)	3.1 (0.2)
3	500–699	0.0344 (0.0020)	2.4 (0.1)	5.5 (0.2)
4	350–499	0.0418 (0.0025)	2.0 (0.1)	7.5 (0.3)
5	200–349	0.0497 (0.0029)	1.7 (0.1)	9.2 (0.3)
6	0–199	0.0805 (0.0045)	1.0 (0.1)	10.2 (0.3)

[a]Mean waiting time from seroconversion to when the subject passes from stage k to $k + 1$.

Table 3. Estimated parameters, λ, and mean waiting times, μ, in each stage of infection ignoring therapy and calendar time, San Francisco Men's Health Study June 1984 through March 1991 (From Longini *et al.* 1993). Standard error (SE)

the 350–499 range, is estimated as 5.5 ± 0.2 years. The mean waiting time from seroconversion to when the T4-cell count is less than 200 is estimated as 9.2 ± 0.3 years, and the estimated mean AIDS incubation period is 10.2 ± 0.3 years.

Stage k	T4-cell count	Transition rates $\hat{\lambda}_{ik}$ (SE) in months^{-1}		Therapy effects[a] $\hat{\theta}_k(t)$ 95% CI	
		No therapy	Therapy[a]		
4	350–499	0.0314 (0.0047)	0.0233 (0.0054)	0.74	0.45–1.22
5	200–349	0.0580 (0.0085)	0.0386 (0.0055)	0.67	0.46–0.96
6	0–199	0.1281 (0.0158)	0.0481 (0.0069)	0.38	0.27–0.53

[a]Only persons with T4 cell counts below 500 were evaluated for therapy effects.

Table 4. Estimated transition rates and hazard ratios for men in stages 4–6 after January 1, 1988, from the San Francisco Men's Health Study, June 1984 through March 1991 (From Longini *et al.* 1993). Standard error (SE), confidence interval (CI).

4.2 Progression rates with therapy, controlling for calendar time

In order to control for the effect of time related biases, we stratified our analysis on calendar time. The stratification date was $t^* =$ January 1, 1988, since few men were on therapy prior to that time and it divides the analysis time interval roughly in half. The covariate is $i = 1$ for therapy and $i = 2$ for no therapy. To simplify notation, we write $\theta_k(t) = \theta_{12k}(t)$ and $\phi_{12k}(\tau, t) = \phi_k(\tau, t)$, and then the comparisons between treated and untreated persons are for the time on or after January 1, 1988, i.e., $\theta_k(t) = \lambda^*_{1k}/\lambda^*_{2k}$. Since few men with T4-cell counts of at least 500 were on therapy, we could not estimate the effect of therapy for the first three stages. Thus, the vectors of progression rates to be estimated are $\boldsymbol{\lambda}_1 = [\lambda^*_{14}, \lambda^*_{15}, \lambda^*_{16}]$, for those on therapy, and $\boldsymbol{\lambda}_2 = [\lambda_{21}, \ldots, \lambda_{26}, \lambda^*_{21}, \ldots, \lambda^*_{26}]$, for those not on therapy. Table 4 shows the parameter estimates, for $k = 4, 5, 6$, when therapy is taken into account on or after January 1, 1988. The estimated risk ratio for therapy for those in stage 4 is $\hat{\theta}_4(t) = 0.74$, and thus, therapy reduced the progression rate from stage 4 to 5 by a factor of 0.26 (95 percent confidence interval (CI) -0.22 to 0.55); for those in stage 5, $\hat{\theta}_5(t) = 0.67$, and thus, therapy reduced the progression rate from stage 5 to 6 by a factor of 0.33 (95 percent CI 0.04–0.54); and for those in stage 6, $\hat{\theta}_6(t) = 0.38$, and thus, therapy reduced the progression rate from stage 6 to 7 by a factor of 0.62 (95 percent CI 0.47–0.73).

Table 5 gives the estimated therapy risk ratios $\hat{\phi}_k(\tau, t)$, for developing AIDS 6, 12, 18, and 24 months after entering stages 4, 5, and 6. For those in stage 4, the estimated therapy risk ratio at six months is $\hat{\phi}_4(\tau, \tau + 6) = 0.17$. Thus, therapy in stage 4 reduces the estimated probability of AIDS in six months by a factor of 0.83 (95 percent CI 0.46–0.94). However, the

446   *Longini* et al.

Stage k	Time since entering stage in months $t - \tau$	Risk $\hat{p}_{ik7}(\tau,t)$ (SE) No therapy	Therapy	Risk ratio $\hat{\phi}_k(\tau,t)$	95% CI
4	6	0.006 (0.002)	0.001 (0.001)	0.17	0.06–0.54
	12	0.036 (0.010)	0.009 (0.003)	0.25	0.07–0.58
	18	0.091 (0.021)	0.026 (0.009)	0.29	0.09–0.61
	24	0.164 (0.033)	0.053 (0.018)	0.32	0.11–0.65
5	6	0.093 (0.024)	0.028 (0.008)	0.30	0.10–0.61
	12	0.267 (0.054)	0.095 (0.024)	0.36	0.13–0.66
	18	0.439 (0.069)	0.182 (0.041)	0.41	0.17–0.71
	24	0.584 (0.072)	0.276 (0.057)	0.47	0.22–0.75
6	6	0.536 (0.076)	0.251 (0.041)	0.47	0.29–0.72
	12	0.785 (0.069)	0.439 (0.061)	0.56	0.38–0.78
	18	0.900 (0.049)	0.579 (0.069)	0.64	0.47–0.82
	24	0.954 (0.031)	0.685 (0.069)	0.72	0.55–0.86

Table 5. Estimated risk ratios $\phi_k(\tau,t) = p_{1k7}(\tau,t)/p_{2k7}(\tau,t)$ for AIDS for men entering stages 4–6 after January 1, 1988, from the San Francisco Men's Health Study, June 1984 through March 1991 (From Longini *et al.* 1993). Standard error (SE), confidence interval (CI).

estimated probabilities of progressing to AIDS in six months are small, i.e., 0.001 and 0.006 for those on and not on therapy, respectively. By 24 months, the estimated probabilities of progressing to AIDS from stage 4 have increased to 0.053 and 0.164 for those on and not on therapy, respectively. Therapy in stage 4 reduces the estimated probability of AIDS 24 months after entering stage 4 by a factor of 0.68 (95 percent CI 0.35–0.89); therapy in stage 5 reduces the estimated probability of AIDS in six months by a factor of 0.70 (95 percent CI 0.39–0.90) and in 24 months by a factor of 0.53 (95 percent CI 0.25–0.78); and therapy in stage 6 reduces the estimated probability of AIDS in six months by a factor of 0.53 (95 percent CI 0.28–0.71) and in 24 months by a factor of 0.28 (95 percent CI 0.14–0.45).

4.3 Progression rates with therapy, without controlling for calendar time

Our findings that zidovudine and pentamidine have a strong effect in a population-based cohort on the progression of the clinical course of HIV infection have important implications for understanding and quantifying the size and dynamics of the HIV epidemic in the United States. Estimates of numbers of persons on therapy along with the estimated hazard ratios θ_k and progression rates λ_k are needed to make forecasts as outlined below. In this case, we need to estimate the impact of increasing therapy use in the HIV-infected population on the baseline AIDS incubation period, which is composed of the progression rates of all infected persons not on therapy. Thus, we estimate the θ_ks by comparing the progression rates of those who were on therapy to those who were not, including, for the latter group, the faster progressing persons prior to January 1, 1988. These estimates are $\hat{\theta}_4 = 0.43$, $\hat{\theta}_5 = 0.45$, $\hat{\theta}_6 = 0.34$ (analysis not given here), and they are incorporated into the projections given in the next section.

4.4 Assessing fit

In order to assess how well the Markov model fits the data, we carried out a comparison of observed vs. expected (from the fitted model) percentage of men in the stages of infection over six years of follow-up. Table 6 gives the observed percentages of men in each stage of infection. In order to build the table, a hypothetical time 0 was created for each man at the entry time for seroprevalent men and the seroconversion time for seroconverters. We used the persistence criteria (in Section 3.1) to assign men to stages at exam times. We then extrapolated the percentages of men in each stage at one-year intervals through six years of follow-up. In Table 6, 18.9 percent of the men were assigned to stage 1 upon entry or seroconversion, while 31.3 percent were in stage 3. Only 2.3 percent had AIDS upon entry. Then, after six years of follow-up, there was only 1.5 percent in stage 1, and 54.4 percent had gone on to have an AIDS diagnosis. There is very little difference between the observed and expected percentages. This demonstrates that the model fits the data quite well.

5 Back-calculation of the stage-specific numbers of HIV infected

The material in this section is based on Longini *et al.* (1992). The probability that a susceptible person becomes infected in the time interval $[t, t + dt]$ is $\gamma(t)dt + o(dt)$, where $\gamma(t)$ is a family of HIV infection probability density functions (pdf) with parameters $\phi = (\phi_1, \ldots, \phi_m)$. Thus, the rate that persons

Stage		Years of follow-up						
		0	1	2	3	4	5	6
1	Obs.	18.9	9.3	5.2	3.9	2.4	1.4	1.5
	Exp.	–	10.9	6.0	3.2	1.8	1.0	0.5
2	Obs.	22.0	14.8	10.9	6.3	5.9	4.2	2.2
	Exp.	–	16.0	11.0	7.1	4.6	2.7	1.5
3	Obs.	31.3	27.4	24.9	18.8	15.4	14.2	11.4
	Exp.	–	31.5	28.1	23.5	18.8	14.1	10.0
4	Obs.	15.4	23.6	20.4	19.8	15.6	13.9	12.5
	Exp.	–	19.0	22.2	22.0	18.7	14.9	11.7
5	Obs.	7.5	11.5	15.2	19.8	19.4	12.5	11.4
	Exp.	–	10.8	13.0	14.2	13.5	12.5	10.7
6	Obs.	2.6	6.2	6.7	8.1	10.0	11.6	6.6
	Exp.	–	4.5	5.7	6.7	6.7	6.6	5.8
7[a]	Obs.	2.3	7.2	16.7	23.3	31.3	42.2	54.4
	Exp.	–	7.3	14.0	23.3	35.9	48.2	59.8

[a]Cumulative percentage with AIDS diagnosis.

Table 6. Observed and predicted percentages of men in each stage after one through six years of follow-up, from the San Francisco Men's Health Study

flow into stage 1 in Figure 1 is

$$\lambda_0(t) = \gamma(t)/\int_t^\infty \gamma(\tau)d\tau. \tag{10}$$

We add a stage 8 which is deceased. In addition, we model treatment effects as follows: Treatment, on a population level, starts at time t_1 with a proportion p_1 of the HIV-infected persons receiving treatment. At time $t_2 > t_1$, a total proportion $p_2 > p_1$ of the HIV-infected persons receive treatment. Thus, an additional proportion $p_2 - p_1$ of the HIV-infected persons receive treatment on or after time t_2. This process continues, so we summarize the treatment history in the population from time 0 to T by the sequence $\{t_j, p_j\}$, $j = 1$, 2, ..., where $0 < t_1 < t_2 < \ldots < t_n < \ldots < T$, and $0 < p_1 < p_2 < \ldots < p_n < \ldots \leq 1$. We define T_I as the random variable for the AIDS incubation period. Then we wish to find $f_I(\tau, t)$, $t > \tau$, which is the pdf of T_I for a person infected at time τ and developing AIDS at time t. Then, we use (4) for the functional form of $p_{ijk}(\tau, t)$. The pdf of T_I for an HIV-infected person not receiving treatment is

$$f_I(\tau, t) = p_{216}(\tau, t)\lambda_6, \ \tau < t. \tag{11}$$

The pdf for a person receiving treatment at time t_0 $(t_0 > \tau)$ when he or she enters stage $j_0 < 7$ is

$$f_I(\tau, t) = \begin{cases} 0 & t < t_0 \\ p_{21j_0}(\tau, t_0)[p_{1j_06}(t_0, t)]\lambda_{16} & t \geq t_0 > \tau. \end{cases} \tag{12}$$

For a whole population of HIV-infected persons, we have a mixture of the pdfs given in (11, 12) with mixing parameters p_1, p_2, ... To derive the mixture of pdfs, we assume that infection takes place at time $\tau \in L_m = [t_m, t_{m+1})$, and that AIDS diagnosis occurs at time $t \in L_n = [t_n, t_{n+1})$, where $n > m$. Thus, L_m and L_n are the intervals in which a person becomes infected and develops AIDS, respectively. In general, the time line is

$$0 < t_1 < \ldots < t_m \leq \tau < t_{m+1} < \ldots < t_n \leq t < t_{n+1} < \infty.$$

Then, the mixture pdf for the AIDS incubation period is

$$\begin{aligned} f_I(\tau, t) \ = \ & (1 - p_n)p_{216}(\tau, t)\lambda_{26} + p_m p_{116}(\tau, t)\lambda_{16} \\ & + \sum_{j=m+1}^{n} \left((p_j - p_{j-1}) \sum_{r=1}^{6} [p_{21r}(\tau, t_j)p_{1r6}(t_j, t)\lambda_{16}] \right) \end{aligned} \tag{13}$$

for $\tau \in L_m$ and $t \in L_n$. The first term on the right side of the equality in (13) gives the AIDS incubation period for HIV-infected persons who do not receive treatment by time t_n. The second term gives the AIDS incubation period for persons who receive treatment on or after time t_m. The third term gives the AIDS incubation period for persons who receive treatment in increasing numbers between times t_{m+1} and t. Note that for these three terms we have

$$(1 - p_n) + p_m + \sum_{j=m+1}^{n} (p_j - p_{j-1}) = 1. \tag{14}$$

5.1   Stage-specific numbers of persons infected with HIV

We let $a(t)$ be the pdf for new cases of AIDS at time t. Then, $a(t)$ is the convolution $\gamma * f$, which is

$$a(t) = \int_0^t \gamma(\tau) f_I(\tau, t) d\tau, \ 0 \leq \tau < t < \infty, \tag{15}$$

where $f_I(\tau, t)$ is given in (13). We define N as the cumulative number of persons who will ever become infected, and then the expected AIDS incidence during $[t, t + dt]$ is $x(t)dt$, where

$$x(t) = a(t)N. \quad \text{(Note that } N = \int_0^\infty x(t)dt). \quad (16)$$

We define $n(t)$ as the cumulative number of persons infected with HIV, up to time t, and we have

$$n(t) = N \int_0^t \gamma(\tau)d\tau. \quad (17)$$

Now we define $n_k(t)$ as the number of HIV-infected persons in stage k at time t. We derive $n_k(t)$ by using the same logic used above for (13) as follows:

$$\begin{aligned} n_k(t) &= N\Big((1 - p_n) \int_0^t \gamma(\tau)p_{21k}(\tau, t)d\tau \\ &+ \sum_{j=1}^n (p_j - p_{j-1}) \sum_{r=1}^k [p_{1rk}(t_j, t) \int_0^{t_j} \gamma(\tau)p_{21r}(\tau, t_j)d\tau] \\ &+ (p_n - p_{n-1}) \int_{t_n}^t \gamma(\tau)p_{11k}(\tau, t)d\tau\Big), \end{aligned} \quad (18)$$

for $t \in L_n$, $k = 1, \ldots, 7$, and where $p_0 = 0$.
For stage 8, we have

$$n_8(t) = n(t) - \sum_{k=1}^7 n_k(t). \quad (19)$$

We use the method of back calculation to obtain MLEs, $\hat{\phi}$ (thus, $\hat{\gamma}(t) = \gamma(t)|_{\phi=\hat{\phi}}$) and $\hat{N}$, from the observed AIDS incidence over the time $0 \le t \le T$, where t is measured in months. The ML procedure also provides the estimated variance-covariance matrix of $\hat{\phi}$ and $\hat{N}$. We then find the estimates $\hat{n}_k(t)$ by evaluating (18) at $\hat{\gamma}(t)$ and $\hat{N}$. We use a conditional argument (see Longini *et al.* 1992) to estimate the asymptotic variances of $\{\hat{n}_k(t)\}$.

5.2   Back-calculation for the state of New Jersey

We applied the above described methods from Section 4 to AIDS incidence data from the state of New Jersey. Figure 2 shows the quarterly reported AIDS incidence (adjusted for reporting delays) for the cohort from January 1980 up to January 1993 ($T = 1/93$). We used the generalized log-logistic distribution for $\gamma(t)$. The cumulative distribution function is

$$\begin{aligned} \int_0^t \gamma(\tau)d\tau &= 1 - (1 + \lambda e^{-z(t)})^{-1/\lambda}, \\ \text{and } z(t) &= [\log(t) - \mu]/\sigma, \ t \ge 0, \end{aligned} \quad (20)$$

Back Calculation of New Jersey AIDS Incidence

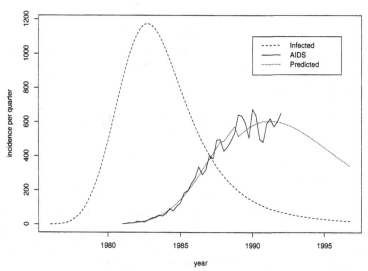

Figure 2. Observed AIDS incidence up to January 1993, and modeled HIV and AIDS incidence up to January 1996, in New Jersey. We assume that the HIV epidemic started in January 1976, and that effective treatment began in January 1987.

where μ is a location parameter, σ a scale parameter, and λ is a shape parameter. When $\lambda \to 0$, we have a Weibull distribution, and when $\lambda = 1$, we have the log-logistic distribution.

For the AIDS incubation distribution, we used the progression rates from Table 3 for persons not on treatment. For those on treatment, we use the θs given in Section 4.3. (Note that $\lambda_{1k} = \theta_k \lambda_{2k}$). We use an estimate $\hat{\lambda}_{27} = 0.043$ for the progression rate from AIDS to death of a person not on therapy, and the estimate of $\hat{\theta}_7 = 0.770$ for a person with AIDS who is on therapy.

We fitted equation (15) to the AIDS incidence data assuming that the HIV epidemic started in the cohort on 1/1/76. National data are available on the approximate proportions of late-stage HIV-infected persons who received zidovudine. We estimate that 2.2 percent of HIV-infected men received zidovudine starting in January 1987, i.e., $(t_1, p_1) = (1/87, 0.022)$. Table 7 provides the complete treatment history. Conditional on the above preset values, the MLEs of ϕ are $\hat{\mu} = 4.501 \pm 0.012$, $\hat{\sigma} = 0.223 \pm 0.007$, and $\hat{\lambda} \approx 0$; and the MLE for N is $30,131 \pm 260$.

From Figure 2 we see that the back-calculation provides an adequate fit of the reported AIDS incidence. Reported AIDS incidence began to level off

Time Point	Date t_j	Proportion p_j
1	1/87	0.022
2	1/88	0.110
3	1/89	0.300[a]

[a]Proportion after 1/89

Table 7. Estimated proportion of HIV-Positive persons receiving zidovudine in New Jersey

after 1988, and the model predicts that AIDS incidence will remain relatively flat through the mid-1990s. From Figure 2 we also see that the modeled peak in HIV incidence occurred in 1983. Table 8 shows the stage-specific numbers of infected persons by year and stage. Note the estimated number of mildly immunosuppressed persons, i.e., T4-cell count > 500, peaked in 1985, and that the number of severely immunosuppressed persons, i.e., T4-cell count < 200 and/or AIDS, is estimated to have peaked around eight years later in 1992–1993. Figure 3 gives the predicted stage-specific numbers infected, $\{\hat{n}_k(t)\}$ to January 1, 1997.

5.3   Back-calculation for the United States

National forecasts for the entire USA, for the period 1992–1994, were recently carried out using two somewhat different methods (CDC 1992). Three groups were provided with AIDS incidence data broken down by exposure category e.g., men who have sex with men, injecting drug use. One group was led by R. Brookmeyer (Brookmeyer 1991) employing a three stage semi-Markov model for the AIDS incubation period. The first stage was equivalent to stages 1–5 in Figure 1, i.e., antibody positive with T4-cell count of at least 200, and the second stage was for equivalent to stage 6 in Figure 1, AIDS-free with T4 count below 200. The third stage was AIDS. A second group led by P.S. Rosenberg (Rosenberg *et al.* 1992), did not employ a staged model for AIDS incubation period. The third group was led by R.H. Byers, of the U.S. Centers for Disease Control and Prevention (CDC), and the method employed was that of Longini *et al.* (1992) which is described in Section 5 of this paper. All three approaches yielded similar estimates of the current numbers of HIV-infected persons and projections of AIDS incidence through 1994. We will give a brief description of the results based on the third group here.

The sequences of the proportions on treatment, $\{t_j, p_j\}$, were estimated from population-level data and by exposure group. For surveillance purposes,

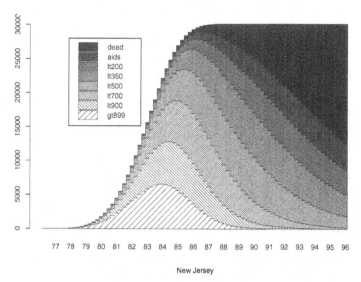

Back Calculated Stages of HIV Infection

New Jersey

Figure 3. Predicted quarterly stage-specific numbers of HIV infected in New Jersey.

the CDC now classifies all persons who have a T4-cell count below 200, but who do not have a 1987-AIDS diagnosis as having severe immunosuppression (SI). The back calculation yields an estimate of about 1,000,000 persons currently infected in the United States. The short term projections for SI and AIDS are given in Table 9. Both SI and AIDS incidence is expected to level off at about 60,000 new cases per year in the short term, and we can expect about 120,000 prevalent persons with SI in the near future.

6   Markov model with back-flows

An alternative to using the persistence criteria for assigning the stages of HIV infection, would be to allow the Markov model to flow backwards, and simply assign persons directly to whatever stage they are observed to be in (Lawless and Yan 1991). This approach has inherent problems when dealing with unsmoothed T4-cell counts, since it does not control for random errors. Nonetheless, it is of interest to fit such a model to the data since it provides some insight into when persons are observed to be in particular stages. The transition rates for an instantaneous transition from stage j to k are now defined as λ_{jk}, and only transitions to neighboring stages are possible, as shown in Figure 4. The transition probabilities are most easily found using

Year	Stage					
	1–3	4–5	6	7	8	1–8
	T4-cell count					
	> 500	200–500	< 200	AIDS	Deceased	Cum. Total
1976	0	0	0	0	0	0
1977	10	0	0	0	0	10
1978	137	1	0	0	0	138
1979	694	8	0	0	0	702
1980	2,217	49	2	1	0	2,269
1981	5,291	194	10	4	1	5,500
1982	10,084	572	37	19	6	10,718
1983	15,752	1,357	107	64	26	17,306
1984	20,358	2,686	256	174	83	23,557
1985	22,070	4,544	520	398	224	27,756
1986	20,704	6,673	911	783	520	29,591
1987	17,598	8,657	1,400	1,349	1,060	30,064
1988	14,106	10,140	1,915	2,041	1,925	30,127
1989	10,896	11,036	2,372	2,708	3,118	30,130
1990	8,185	11,413	2,726	3,237	4,569	30,130
1991	6,015	11,178	2,958	3,705	6,277	30,131
1992	4,340	10,498	3,067	4,042	8,184	30,131
1993	3,086	9,533	3,064	4,225	10,223	30,131
1994	2,169	8,433	2,971	4,252	12,306	30,131
1995	1,510	7,310	2,813	4,140	14,358	30,131
1996	1,041	6,237	2,615	3,920	16,318	30,131

Table 8. Stage-specific predicted numbers of HIV-infected persons on January 1 in the state of New Jersey

Year	Prevalent SI	Incident SI	Incident AIDS
1992	115,000	60,000	58,000
1993	120,000	59,000	61,000
1994	125,000	60,000	62,000
1995	130,000	–	–

Table 9. Estimates of the prevalence and incidence of severe immunosuppression (SI) and the incidence of AIDS in the United States for 1992–1994 (Source: CDC 1992)

Stages Of HIV Infection

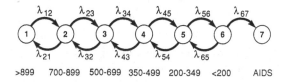

>899   700-899   500-699   350-499   200-349   <200   AIDS

T4-CELL COUNT

Figure 4. The modeled flows through the stages of HIV infection, for the model with back flows, where λ_{jk} is the monthly transition rate from stage j to k.

To stage k	T4-cell count cells/μl	Mean first passage time $\hat{\mu}_k^f$ years	95% CI	Mean persistent passage time $\hat{\mu}_k$ years	95% CI
2	700–899	0.6	[0.4,0.7]	1.7	[1.3,2.1]
3	500–699	1.3	[1.1,1.6]	3.1	[2.7,3.5]
4	350–499	2.6	[2.2,3.0]	5.5	[5.1,5.9]
5	200–349	4.4	[3.9,5.0]	7.5	[6.9,8.1]
6	0–199	7.3	[6.5,8.3]	9.2	[8.6,9.8]
7	AIDS	[a]		10.2	[9.6,11.8]

[a]Mean first and persistent passage times are the same for the AIDS stage.

Table 10. Estimated mean first passage and mean persistent cumulative waiting times from stage 1 San Francisco Men's Health Study, June 1984 through March 1991

matrix methods (Chiang 1980), and the parameters are estimated using ML methods as described above.

One statistic of interest is the first passage time (FPT), i.e., the time it takes to progress from stage 1 to a particular subsequent stage for the *first* time. The mean FPT to go from stage 1 to stage $k > 1$ will be denoted by μ_k^f. For example, μ_4^f is the mean time it takes to go from stage 1 to having T4-cell count below 500 (but greater than 349) for the first time, and μ_7^f is the AIDS incubation period. These FPTs will be considerably shorter than the persistent passage times (PPT) that were calculated from the monotonic process using the persistence criteria described in Section 3.1.

Table 10 shows the estimated mean FPTs and PPTs (repeated from Table

3) from the SFMHS. The estimated FPT to when the T4-cell count drops into the 350–499 range is estimated to be only 2.6 years, but it takes an average of 5.5 years to arrive persistently to that stage. The estimated FPT to when the T4-cell count drops below 200 is estimated as 7.3 years, compared with an estimated mean PPT of 9.2 years.

An approach which avoids *ad hoc* smoothing of T4-cell counts is to model the error in these counts using a hierarchical regression model. As before, let y_{rj} be the observed stage of individual r at time τ_{rj}; however, this observed stage may differ from the 'true' stage, which we denote as $\tilde{y}_{rj}$. Due to measurement error, the sequence of observed stages $\{y_{rj}\}$ is generally not a Markov process, even if we assume that the 'true' stages do follow a Markov process. However, for each individual r, Satten and Longini (1993) propose a Markov model for $\{y_{rj}\}$ by assuming that

$$Pr[\{y_{rj}, j = 1, \ldots, m_r\}|\{\tilde{y}_{rj}, j = 1, \ldots, m_r\}] = \prod_{j=0}^{m_r} Pr[y_{rj}|\tilde{y}_{rj}], \qquad (21)$$

$$Pr[\{\tilde{y}_{rj}, j = 1, \ldots, m_r\}] = \pi(\tilde{y}_{r0}) \prod_{j=0}^{m_r-1} p_{\tilde{y}_{rj}, \tilde{y}_{rj+1}}(\tau_{rj}, \tau_{rj+1}), \qquad (22)$$

where $\pi(y)$ is the distribution of initial stages, and where, for simplicity, we ignore covariates. The transition probabilities on the right side of (22) are given in Section 2. Suitable models for (21) can be obtained by assuming a within-stage distribution for the true T4-cell count (e.g., uniform within stages) and a 'measurement error' distribution (e.g., log-normal) relating the true T4-cell count to the observed count. Note that we assume that the 'measurement error' is composed of both laboratory variation in T4-cell measurements plus short-time-scale fluctuations in the T4-cell count which are not directly related to the HIV infection. Satten and Longini (1993) give a full discussion of fitting this model using the marginal distribution of T4-cell counts.

7 Back-calculation from cross-sectional marker surveys

In Section 5, we described the back-calculation method for estimating the HIV infection pdf from AIDS incidence data. The inherent weakness of this method is that it provides virtually no information about current HIV incidence. This is because the AIDS incubation distribution has a mean length of about ten years. Obviously, current AIDS incidence data contains little information about infections that occurred in the last couple of years. However, if cross-sectional information on a marker, such as T4 cells, were collected then even a single survey would contain a great deal of information about HIV incidence, i.e., infected persons with high T4-cell counts are much more likely to have been currently infected than those with low T4-cell counts. Satten and Longini (1994) have developed methods for calculating past and current HIV incidence, based on the Markov model in Section 2, from repeated cross sectional surveys of T4-cell counts. This method is also being extended for use of other markers such as β_2-microglobulin.

8   Discussion

In this paper, we have presented a method for modeling the natural history of HIV infection based on the premise that the basic pathogenic process is essentially a staged process. A further premise is that the staged process is Markovian. We have found little evidence that the process is not Markovian. The staged Markov model fits the data well and provides a consistent description of the important aspects of the natural history of HIV. For example, the hazard function for the AIDS incubation distribution, i.e., a generalized gamma distribution, (Longini *et al.* 1989b) has a similar shape to the empirically estimated hazard function.

One consequence of the staged assumption is that interventions, such as therapy, that reduce the progression rates to some non-zero value only slow progression to the absorbing state of interest, but do not prevent eventual absorption. Thus, risk or hazard ratios for AIDS or death which compare the the effectiveness of treatment started in a early stage will approach one with increasing time. This is important to keep in mind when assessing the long-term effectiveness of therapies such as zidovudine in preventing AIDS or death in clinical trials or observational studies. The recent Concorde trial (Aboulker and Swart 1993) reports diminishing long-term effectiveness of the early-stage use of zidovudine in preventing serious illness or death. One would expect this effect based on the above argument, but the Concorde results should be further scrutinized in this light. Our results for the effectiveness of therapy, Section 4.2, are entirely consistent with many of the previous clinical trials for zidovudine and pentamidine (Longini *et al.* 1993).

Finally, the estimates of the prevalence and incidence of SI in the United States in Table 9 are based on the persistence criteria. Thus, for example, we are predicting that there are currently 120,000 persons with persistent SI in the United States, but this does not not necessarily include all those HIV-infected persons who had a single T4-cell count below 200. We see from Table 10 that the mean PPT to stage 6 is estimated to be 9.2 years, while the corresponding mean FPT is 7.3 years. Thus, there is a far greater number of HIV-infected persons in the United States that have had a least one T4-cell count less than 200. Brookmeyer (1991) does not use persistence criteria, and

458 Longini et al.

estimates the current persons with SI in the United States to be 190,000. It would seem prudent to base the definition of SI on some form of persistence criterion.

Acknowledgements

This research was supported by the Division of HIV/AIDS, Centers for Disease Control and Prevention. The data analyzed in Section 4 were provided by the San Francisco Men's Health Study, which is supported by contract no. N01-AI-82515 from the National Institute of Allergy and Infectious Diseases.

References

Aboulker, J-P. and Swart, A.M. (1993) 'Preliminary analysis of the Concorde trial', *Lancet* **341**, 889–890.

Brookmeyer, R. (1991) 'Reconstruction and future trends of the AIDS epidemic in the United States', *Science* **253**, 37–42.

Centers for Disease Control and Prevention. (1992) 'AIDS case projection and estimates of HIV-infected immunosuppressed persons in the United States, 1992–1994', *MMWR, No. RR-18*, 1–27.

Chiang, C.L. (1980) *An Introduction to Stochastic Processes and their Applications*, second edition, Krieger, New York.

Hethcote, H.W., Van Ark, J.W. and Longini, I.M. (1991a) 'A simulation model of AIDS in San Francisco: I. Model formulation and parameter estimation', *Math. Biosci.* **106**, 203–222.

Hethcote, H.W., Van Ark, J.W. and Karon, J.M. (1991b) 'A simulation model of AIDS in San Francisco: II. Simulations, therapy, and sensitivity analysis', *Math. Biosci.* **106**, 223–247.

Jacquez, J.A., Simon, C.P. and Koopman, J.S. (1988) 'Modeling and analyzing HIV transmission: The effect of contact patterns', *Math. Biosci.* **92**, 119–199.

Koopman, J.S., Longini, I.M., Jacquez, J.,*et al.* (1991) 'Assessing risk factors for HIV transmission', *Am. J. Epidemiol.* **133**, 1199–1209.

Lawless, J.F. and Yan, P. (1991) 'Some statistical methods for for followup studies of disease with intermittent monitoring'. In *Multiple Comparisons in Biostatistics: Current Research in the Topics of C.W. Dunnett*, F.M. Hoppe (ed.), Marcel Dekker, New York, 427–446.

Longini, I.M., Clark, W.S., Byers, R.H., Lemp, G.F., Ward, J.W., Darrow, W.W., and Hethcote, H.W. (1989a) 'Statistical analysis of the stages of HIV infection using a Markov model', *Stat. Med.* **8**, 831–843.

Longini, I.M., Clark, W.S., Haber, M. and Horsburgh, R. (1989b) 'The stages of HIV infection: Waiting times and infection transmission probabilities. In

Mathematical and Statistical Approaches to AIDS Epidemiology, Lecture Notes in Biomathematics, **83** C. Castillo-Chavez (ed.), Springer-Verlag, New York, 112–137.

Longini, I.M. (1990) 'Modeling the decline of CD4$^+$ T-lymphocyte counts in HIV-infected individuals', *JAIDS* **9**, 930–931.

Longini, I.M., Clark, W.S., Gardner, L.I. and Brundage, J.F. (1991) 'The dynamics of CD4$^+$ T-lymphocyte decline in HIV-infected individuals: A Markov modeling approach', *JAIDS* **4**, 1141–1147.

Longini, I.M., Byers, R.H., Hessol, N.A. and Tan, W.Y. (1992) 'Estimating the stage-specific numbers of HIV infection using a Markov model and back-calculation', *Stat. Med.* **11**, 831–843.

Longini, I.M., Clark, W.S. and Karon, J. (1993) 'The effect of routine use of therapy on the clinical course of HIV infection in a population-based cohort', *Am. J. Epidemiol.* **137**, 1229–1240.

Redfield, R.R., Wright, D. and Tramont, E. (1986) 'The Walter Reed staging system classification for HTLV-III/LAV infection', *New Eng. J. Med.* **314**, 131–132.

Rosenberg, P.S., Gail, M. and Carroll, R.J. (1992) 'Estimating HIV prevalence and projecting AIDS incidence in the United States: a model that accounts for therapy and changes in the surveillance definition of AIDS', *Stat. Med.* **11**, 633–655.

Satten, G.A. and Longini, I.M. (1993) 'Markov chains with measurement error: estimating the 'true' course of a marker of HIV disease progression', submitted.

Satten, G.A. and Longini, I.M. (1994) 'Estimation of incidence of HIV infection using cross-sectional marker surveys', *Biometrics* **50**, 675–688.

Winkelstein, W., Lyman, D.M., Padian, N., *et al.* (1987) 'Sexual practices and risk of infection by the human immunodeficiency virus', *JAMA* **257**, 321–325.

Invited Discussion

N.E. Day

AIDS: Modelling and Predicting

The three authors are to be warmly congratulated on their substantial, yet complementary, papers on an issue of major public health moment – how to get to grips quantitatively with the HIV-AIDS epidemic. Advances in the treatment of HIV disease are proving disappointing, more disappointing now (mid 1993) in fact than at any time in the past several years. Vaccine development too has been largely a succession of false dawns. Primary prevention, however, is demonstrably achievable, as seen by the shape of the HIV epidemic curve in male homosexual populations in much of the developed world, and injecting drug users in at least some communities. Individuals have an underrated capacity to respond to credible information, clearly witnessed in other chronic disease areas by the sharp declines in lung cancer and cardiovascular disease seen in, for example, the US, Britain and Australasia. The most pressing public health need in AIDS is for accurate estimates of the rate at which HIV transmission is occurring in different subsections of the community, defined by age, sex, geography and particularly transmission category. Only then can public health messages be appropriately shaped and directed, and more importantly, be made credible to the subpopulations concerned. There is little point in urging young adults to refrain from sexual pleasure if the message is not clearly substantiated by the facts. HIV disease is, however, a complex temporal process; there is a wide gap between the observations we can currently make on the disease in the population and the conclusions that one would like to draw about the pattern of HIV infection. It is this gap which statistical and mathematical modelling addresses, and the effectiveness of public health messages will depend heavily on the credibility of the modelling techniques.

These two papers are of increasing concentration of focus. Dr Solomon provides a wide and illuminating review of the current state of epidemiological modelling, while the paper by Longini *et al.* is focussed specifically on staged Markov models, and the problems caused by measurement error. Dr Solomon concentrates correctly on back calculation methods and their elaboration both in the face of treatment induced uncertainties over the incubation period distribution, and with the increasing epidemiological information that is becoming available, particularly on HIV prevalence. It has become clear that the back calculation approach has the potential to incorporate new types of information on the distribution of HIV in the population as they emerge, yet is not overly dependent on fixing the values of parameters for which information is essentially absent. For estimates of the past, present and immediate future, back calculation methods, by using what is available and not needing what is not available, provide the best chance of giving accurate results. By contrast, transmission models take a more cosmological approach, describing the logically necessary shape of the epidemic over an ordered time axis, but rather vague on the here and now. Dr Solomon glides swiftly over multi stage models, which are the prime focus of attention of Dr Longini and his colleagues. It is logical to consider HIV disease as a continuous time Markov process, and the development of back calculation methods for a seven stage Markov model is highly elegant. The resulting figures for the New Jersey epidemic should become a classic as an illustration of how one wants to model, describe and predict what is happening in a population. The problem with adopting Markov models in this context is, of course, the inherent measurement error in the observations on which Markov staging is based, and this topic is addressed by the authors.

Given the evident success of the modelling methods presented to produce quantitatively coherent descriptions of the HIV epidemic in different populations, and with confirmation that resulting predictions are accurate, reservations may seem out of place. There are, however, two points I would make. First, much of the elegance derives from assumptions that seem unlikely to hold, as in 'Assuming the times spent in the different stages are independent random variables with densities $f_i(u|s)$' or 'The simple adjustment for treatment is essentially equivalent to taking $\rho_1(s) = \theta\rho_0(s)$ for known, constant θ, which is the proportional effect of treatment on the baseline hazard.' In the first case the independence assumption would appear unlikely, and in the second case there is strong evidence that the effect of treatment is not to effect a constant change in hazard. These assumptions can, of course, be loosened, and extra parameters introduced to provide grater realism. But then 'such detailed modelling of the effects of treatment would depend largely on the available data and information.' Exactly. As Dr Solomon points out early in her paper, by far the major source of error is from model errors. The emphasis then needs to be on assessing the real degree of uncertainty in the quantification process, and resulting estimates, and this requires putting in the extra parameters which make the models murkier and less tractable. It would be interesting to see a realistic estimate of the uncertainty surrounding the estimates of Figure 3 of the paper by Longini *et al.* This figure is the result of back calculation using AIDS incidence data. Reduction in the uncertainty will not come from further model development but from additional information, which brings me to my second point. Both papers focus on how best to use available information. Statisticians have a broader role, however, which is to elucidate precisely what further information will have the greatest impact on reducing uncertainty. Little attention is given in these papers to the questions of perhaps greatest statistical importance, namely what aspects of the HIV epidemic are estimated with the worst precision, what is the consequence of this lack of precision for public health, and how can this lack be rectified?

The public health control of the HIV epidemic depends heavily on credible quantitative modelling. This credibility depends in turn on the clarity with which the underlying uncertainty is described, and the level of uncertainty follows directly from the scope and reliability of the information on which the modelling is based. Generation of the requisite information should be the next major concern of statisticians.

Response from P.J. Solomon

Professor Day has highlighted important distinctions that need to be made between the purposes of statistical analysis and quantitative predictions, and mathematical and biological modelling.

It is essential for predictions that external information, such as surveys of HIV prevalence, are incorporated in modelling and analysis of HIV disease. For instance, I mentioned in my paper a number of approaches being taken to backcalculation for estimating past HIV incidence, and others are presented elsewhere in this volume.

The publication, during the workshop, of the preliminary results from the Concorde trial leaves the question of the effects of zidovudine on the incubation period for AIDS and length of life wide open. The management of opportunistic infections could be the main reason for lengthening incubation periods, and there are biological theories too. It is important to note that irrespective of the precise nature of the effects of treatments, estimates are required of the numbers of people at different stages of HIV disease, and particularly of those eligible for treatment. The issue of whether CD4 cell counts are useful for this purpose (and other purposes) is of course extremely important and relevant.

Adjustments made for the effects of treatment on the incubation distribution do not usually distinguish the possible effects of prophylaxis for *Pneumocistis carinii* and other opportunistic infections and antiviral treatment, as the data are not in general available with which to do this on a population basis. Moreover, it is often not possible to separate statistically other temporal effects. Consequently, the term 'treatment' tends to be used to represent what is really an 'average' temporal effect, although it is generally assumed that the effects of treatments are a major component of the observed nonstationarity.

It is interesting that in recent analyses of the Australian AIDS data, substantially *worse* fits to the observed data are obtained by incorporating a simple treatment adjustment into the backcalculation method (Solomon and Wilson 1990), which is in contrast to the UK experience. For example, for a semi-Markov model for the incubation distribution (Wilson and Solomon 1991), quadratic exponential h constrained to 150 per quarter, a one-year treatment effect in advanced-stage HIV disease, and quarterly data, the deviance increases from 43 (no treatment effect) to 57.

Short Term Projections by Dynamic Modelling in Large Populations: a Case Study in France and The Netherlands

S.H. Heisterkamp and A.M. Downs

Short and medium term projections of AIDS incidence and HIV back-projections can be estimated using different techniques. The simplest technique for projection of AIDS cases is extrapolation by curve fitting applied to past AIDS incidence data, corrected for reporting delays. A severe criticism of this method is the total dependency of the projections on the chosen function for the curve. A second technique which incorporates more knowledge of the transmission mechanisms of the epidemic, uses the incubation time distribution, sometimes including data on early treatment with anti-viral drugs, to back-project the HIV incidence from the delay corrected AIDS incidence, and projects forwards the minimum expected AIDS incidence. Projections depend on the form of the chosen incubation time distribution, and moreover, the interplay of behavioural change, early treatment and other interventions all make the use of the back-projection method more difficult in the future. If still more information is used on the mechanism of the epidemic, i.e. not only incubation time distribution but also assumptions on the spread of infection through the population, more detailed projections can be made by the use of deterministic or stochastic models on restricted risk groups and relatively small populations e.g. Switzerland, San Francisco or Amsterdam. In this paper, a model developed earlier for the risk group of homo/bisexual men in Amsterdam (Heisterkamp et al. 1992) is adapted for the inclusion of early treatment effects and used for the projection of AIDS and HIV incidence for the same transmission group although for a risk group on a larger scale. As populations we used the risk group of homo/bisexual men in Île de France (IDF), Provence, Alpes and Côte d'Azur (PACA), France as a whole and in the Netherlands.

Parameters of local interest, such as effective infectivity, and the numbers initially at risk, are estimated for each local epidemic. The influence of the uncertainty of the observations, especially in the case of adjusting for reporting delay, is discussed. As the latest observed (and adjusted) AIDS reports are the most influential with regard to the projections, and as these are also the most uncertain, these observations are downweighted in the Poisson likelihood. The weights are inversely proportional to the variance of the adjusted AIDS incidence, which is the estimated ratio of observed and adjusted incidence. For example in IDF, adding the latest observations from 1990 onwards does not alter the projections significantly until 1994. So applying these weights makes the projections indeed insensitive to adding or deleting observations.

As the assumption on homogeneous mixing is certainly violated in such large populations, the effect of such violation on the parameter estimates of the model is being investigated by simulation. It appears that the estimates of the initial numbers at risk are only affected to a slight extent, i.e. are slightly negatively biased. However the estimate of the effective infectivity is biased upwards. The total effect on projections is a slight underestimation of the epidemic by a 4–5%. Comparing the estimates for the whole of The Netherlands, and by splitting up into Amsterdam and non-Amsterdam, gives similar estimates. The application of early treatment with anti-viral drugs is included in the model, although little is known about the extent to which these drugs are used as well as the effect such treatment has on the survival of the AIDS patients. We assumed an lengthening of the time to AIDS of 1 year as a result of the use of these anti-viral drugs.

The question of the meaning of the parameter, representing initial number at risk, was solved by simulation. Simulating independent epidemics with a small number at risk, 2000, and high effective infectiousness ($\simeq 0.7$) and a large epidemic (20000 at risk) with respectively half, quarter and an eighth of that level of infectiousness reveals that the estimates for infectiousness were not affected and that the estimate for the number at risk reflects the number in the high-risk group, apart from the case where the low infectiousness was 0.35 (estimated at risk 2240). The projections two years ahead remain accurate.

We conclude that as an instrument of projection of AIDS and HIV this model and the statistical tools involved (Poisson likelihood and overdispersion) is suitable, although it may result in a slight underestimation of the epidemic by a 4-5%.

References

Heisterkamp, S.H., de Haan, B.J., Jager, J.C., van Druten, J.A.M. and Hendriks, J.C.M. (1992) 'Short and medium term projections of the AIDS/HIV epidemic by a dynamic model with an application to the risk group of homo/bisexual men in Amsterdam', *Stat. Med.* **11**, 1425–41.

Bayesian Prediction of AIDS cases and CD200 Cases in Scotland

G.M. Raab

1 Scottish data

Scotland has a comprehensive system for recording both AIDS diagnoses and the numbers of HIV positive individuals under immunological monitoring who have low CD4 counts. The CD4 Collaborative Group (1992) provide data anually on new CD200 cases under monitoring in Scotland. A case becomes CD200 when two consecutive CD4 counts below 200 are obtained (the date of the first count defines the date of diagnosis) or when an AIDS defining diagnosis is reached.

Various investigations provide information on the likely incidence of new infections in Scotland since the start of the epidemic. They all point to an epidemic with a sharp peak of new infections in 1983 and 1984 and a steep decline thereafter. The total size of the HIV infected population can be estimated from the numbers of known HIV infections and the proportion of AIDS and CD200 cases who have their first HIV test around the time of their AIDS or CD200 diagnosis. Estimates in the range 1800–4000 were considered possible.

An Edinburgh study of a clinical cohort (McNeil 1993), along with results from elsewhere, allow us to define a range of possible incubation distributions to use in predicting new AIDS and CD200 cases. Incubation distributions of the Weibull and Gamma families were used. A treatment effect was incorporated from 1989 onwards, when pre-AIDS therapy was widely used.

2 Sensitivity analyses

Initial back-projections investigated the sensitivity of the predictions to the various features of the incubation distribution and the infection curve. These included back-projections where the infection curve was estimated for a fixed incubation distribution. This has been the common form of back projection since it was first used for AIDS data (Brookmeyer and Gail 1986). These showed that, for a fixed total size of the epidemic, the predictions were insensitive to the precise shape of the epidemic provided the peak is within a given two to three year period. We also found that the number of new infections

466

assumed for recent years (in our case after 1989) has very little effect on the short-term AIDS predictions.

Further back-projections were carried out which assumed a known infection curve and estimated the parameters of the incubation distribution (including the effect of treatment). The Weibull distributions which these back-projections estimated had hazard functions which increased steeply from 10 years after sero-conversion in a way which appeared to contradict recent evidence on the hazard function (Gail and Rosenberg 1992, Bachetti *et al.* 1992). In contrast the estimates obtained from the Gamma incubation distributions appeared reasonable. Thus Gamma distributions, rather than Weibull, were used to describe the incubation distribution.

3 Bayesian prediction

This preliminary work allowed us to construct priors for the incubation distribution and for the infection curve. The prior for the incubation distribution was obtained by considering all gamma distributions over a range of parameter values and then restricting this set to those with 4,6 and 8 year progression rates within specified ranges. All such incubation curves were considered to have equal prior probability. A prior was also assigned to the increased average survival for the whole cohort after 1989. This included values from one to four years for the additional AIDS-free or CD200-free years. Because of the insensitivity of the predictions to the precise shape of the epidemic the shape was taken as fixed and a prior assigned to the total size (H) of the HIV epidemic to 1989.

These priors were combined with the data on incident cases, assuming a Poisson distribution for the number of cases occurring each year with a mean defined in terms of the parameters of the infection curve and the incubation distribution. The prior and posterior were calculated over a grid of values within the appropriate ranges of the parameter space. This gave posterior confidence sets (calculated from the highest posterior density regions) for the parameters of the infection curve and the incubation distributions as well as for predictions of new cases for the next four years.

The posterior distributions for H calculated from CD200 cases and from AIDS cases each had a mode of between 2,000 and 2,500 infections to 1989. The posterior confidence sets for the predicted incident AIDS and CD200 cases are shown in Figure 1. Further details of these results are presented in Raab *et al.* (1993).

468   Raab

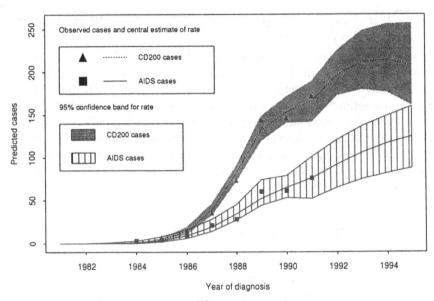

Year of diagnosis

Figure 1

References

Bachetti P.R., Segal M.R. and Jewell N.P. (1992) 'Perspectives on using backcalculation to estimate HIV prevalence and project AIDS incidence'. In *AIDS Epidemiology: Methodological Issues*, N.P. Jewell, K. Dietz and V.T. Farewell (eds.), 39–61.

Brookmeyer R. and Gail M.H. (1986) 'Minimum size of the AIDS epidemic in the United States', *Lancet* **2**, 1320.

CD4 collaborative group (1992) 'Use of monitored CD4 counts: predictions of the AIDS epidemic in Scotland', *AIDS* **6**, 213–22.

Gail M.H. and Rosenberg P.S. (1992) 'Uncertainty about the incubation period of AIDS and its impact on back projection'. In *AIDS Epidemiology: Methodological Issues*, N.P. Jewell, K. Dietz and V.T. Farewell (eds.), 1–38.

McNeil A.(1993) *Statistical Methods in AIDS Progression Studies with an Analysis of the Edinburgh City Cohort*, PhD Thesis, University of Cambridge.

Raab G.M., Gore S.G., Goldberg D.J. and Donnelly C. (1993) 'Bayesian forecasting of the HIV epidemic in Scotland', submitted.

Discussion

HETHCOTE There is real danger in considering the HIV and AIDS epidemics on a country-wide basis, as Raab has done, without first ensuring that the patterns throughout the country are consistent. It can be seen with the USA, that combining epidemics that are at very different stages can produce misleading results.

REPLY We have looked separately at the epidemic in intra-venous drug users and in homo-sexual/bi-sexual men (the only groups for which we have adequate numbers to date). Although we have not done a full Bayesian analysis for the separate groups, the preliminary back-projection work which we carried out suggested that the HIV infection curve had a similar form for both of these groups, although the peak was rather less pronounced for the homo-sexual/bi-sexual group. The back-projection results showed that the projections obtained separately for these two groups were very similar to those for the combined cases. Where the shape of the infection curve is the same for the two groups, it seems likely that we can use an averaged estimate of the incubation distribution. We do appreciate, however, that if this were not the case it would be dangerous to treat the two epidemics as if they were one.

Some Scenario Analyses for the HIV Epidemic in Italy

Mario Abundo and Carla Rossi

1 Introduction

Forecasting the evolution of the AIDS epidemic in different situations is a primary problem which has to be solved in order to perform cost-benefit analyses and evaluate different policies which can be adopted to control the epidemic.

Several mathematical and statistical models have been proposed for these purposes in recent years. Most of them are deterministic models which try to take into account very complex situations. Others are statistical models which simply try to fit data and extrapolate the observed beaviours (some references can be found in Rossi (1991)). The most suitable approach to modelling AIDS epidemic is via stochastic models, based on an understanding of the transmission dynamics of HIV.

In the following, a stochastic compartmental model, recently proposed (Rossi 1991), is used to perform some scenario analyses and evaluate the impact of different policies.

The model used here concentrates, in particular, on the proportion of stayers, s_t, throughout, i.e. the proportion of individuals of the population who are not at risk of infection by HIV, either through behaviour or by possible immunity, and on the proportion of infected individuals who can be considered removed from the transmission process due to their 'prudent' behaviour.

The flow chart and the equations of the model can be found in Rossi (1991). In the present contribution we concentrate on the influence on the behaviour of the epidemic of the parameters s_0 and ν_{ij}, where ν_{12}, ν_{23}, ν_{32} and ν_{21} are four parameters that represent the effects of screening and associated treatment programmes.

We assumed the incubation period divided into three stages:

- latent phase (CD4 cell appoximately constant, no HIV antibodies);

- first incubation phase (CD4 cell counts above 400, HIV antibodies);

- second incubation phase (CD4 cell counts between 400 and 200, HIV antibodies).

470

$$\nu_{12} = \nu_{23} = \nu_{32} = \nu_{21} = 0$$

s_0	$Y_{\max}$	$T_{Y_{\max}}$	$Z_{\max}$	$T_{Z_{\max}}$	TD
0.92	6.0	(10–12)	2.0	(16–18)	80
0.95	3.0	(16–18)	1.1	(22–24)	47
0.98	0.4	(48–50)	0.2	(54–56)	0.2

$$\nu_{12} = 0.0026; \ \nu_{23} = 0.018; \ \nu_{32} = 0.018; \ \nu_{21} = 0.0012$$

s_0	$Y_{\max}$	$T_{Y_{\max}}$	$Z_{\max}$	$T_{Z_{\max}}$	TD
0.92	4.8	(10–12)	1.2	(16–18)	58
0.95	2.2	(16–18)	0.6	(24–26)	28

$$\nu_{12} = 0.0026; \ \nu_{23} = 0.018; \ \nu_{32} = 0.018; \ \nu_{21} = 0.0024$$

s_0	$Y_{\max}$	$T_{Y_{\max}}$	$Z_{\max}$	$T_{Z_{\max}}$	TD
0.92	4.0	(10–12)	1.1	(18–20)	51
0.95	1.5	(20–22)	0.6	(26–28)	27

Table 1. Values of some summary indices: $Y_{\max}$ = maximum number of infectives (% of the whole population), $T_{Y_{\max}}$ = time corresponding to $Y_{\max}$ (years since the beginning of the epidemic), $Z_{\max}$ = maximum number of AIDS cases (% of the whole population), $T_{Z_{\max}}$ = time corresponding to $Z_{\max}$ (year since the beginning of the epidemic), TD = Total number of deaths (in thousands for million)

Thus the whole period was approximated by the sum of three independent exponentially distributed periods, with parameters given by: 0.1143, 0.0026, 0.018, assuming one week as the unit of time.

2 Some scenario analyses

To obtain numerical simulation results we used values of the demographic parameters given by the official statistics for Italy, for the mortality rate of AIDS patients and infection rate μ_{12}, the estimates provided by the Epidemiological Unit of Latium (Perucci, C., personal comunication). Mortality rates during the incubation period have been estimated averaging the mortality rate of intravenous drug users and the mortality rate of the remaining population (the first is about 10 times the second (Perucci *et al.* 1990)). Using one week as unit time, several trajectories of the processes were simulated choosing some suitable values for s_0 and the ν_{ij}, i.e. the parameters which can be modified by control policies and information campaigns.

As observed in Rossi (1991), one peculiar effect of increasing the s_0 parameter is the delay induced in the epidemic waves corresponding to $Y = Y_1 + Y_2 + Y_3$ (total number of infectives) and Z_3 (AIDS cases), as well as the reduction of the values of the correspondings peaks. This information can be summarized using the following indices: Y_{max} = maximum number of infectives (% of the whole population), $T_{Y_{max}}$ = time corresponding to Y_{max} (years since the beginning of the epidemic), Z_{max} = maximum number of AIDS cases (% of the whole population), $T_{Z_{max}}$ = time corresponding to Z_{max} (year since the beginning of the epidemic), TD = Total number of deaths in forty years (in thousands per million).

The values of these indices are reported in Table 1.

3 Concluding remarks

On the basis of the scenario analyses we can observe that:

- the influence of small variations in s_0 values is much greater than the influence of variations in ν values;

- s_0 has a much higher impact in delaying the spread of the epidemic.

We can conclude that the best intervention for controlling the spread of the epidemic should be directed towards the susceptibles via information campaigns. This kind of intervention could, in fact, produce an increase in the s_0 value, while, interventions directed towards seropositives, in particular through compulsory screening programmes (as was suggested in Italy), do not seem to be very effective as, even with a high proportion of removals from infectives ($\nu_{21} = 0.0012$ means that about 31% of the infectives in compartment 3 are removed before reaching compartment 4 and $\nu_{23} = 0.018$ means that 50% of the infectives in compartment 4 are removed before reaching compartment 5) the differences with respect to the case with $\nu = 0$ are not so high.

References

Perucci, C.A., Davoli, M., Rapiti, E., Abeni, D., Forastiere, F. (1990) 'The impact of illicit drug use on cause specific mortality of young adults in Rome, Italy', technical report, Epidemiological Unit of Latium Region, Rome, Italy.

Rossi, C. (1991) 'A stochastic mover-stayer model for HIV epidemic', *Math. Biosci.* **107**, 521–545.

Relating a Transmission Model of AIDS Spread to Data: Some International Comparisons

Brian Dangerfield and Carole Roberts

1 Introduction

The first phase in researching AIDS epidemiology using transmission models was characterised by a need to promote understanding of the dynamics of the epidemic and provide a template around which to specify data collection needs. Unlike the back-calculation and curve fitting approaches, there was no need to directly relate model output to data: comparisons between different model runs offered insight and understanding. Transmission models became more complex with the incorporation of heterogeneity in sexual behaviour, variable infectiousness and various forms of mixing between partners.

Transmission modelling has more to offer than a capability to make projections of the likely course of the epidemic. For instance, it is incontrovertibly the best way to assess the effects of various interventions which may help in mitigating the extent of the epidemic. However, the inherent complexity involved in formulating a transmission model which embraces all three main groups of susceptibles (homosexuals, intravenous drug users and heterosexuals) has meant that, in the main, transmission models have been restricted to the homosexual risk group. By one criterion this is appropriate for in the United Kingdom, United States and several countries in Western Europe, the homosexual population has contributed the largest proportion of the cumulative total of AIDS cases thus far reported. Where exceptions to the single risk-group transmission models exist, they are far from parsimonious in the number of independently specified parameters. The scope for relating models containing scores of parameters to time-series data is extremely limited.

It is the relating of a model to time-series data on reported AIDS cases which marks the second phase of epidemiological research using transmission models. There seems no *a priori* reason why the structure of a model of the spread of HIV and AIDS in the homosexual population should differ as between one country and another. What will differ, of course, are the parameters, including those which are incorporated in order to specify behavioural changes which might have occurred in the risk group involved.

Our recent research has focused on this second phase of transmission modelling work. The research has three main objectives:

473

474 Dangerfield and Roberts

(i) an international comparison of the parameter values obtained as a result of fitting a model to time-series data from a number of different countries;

(ii) a comparison of the optimised parameter values with those derived from clinical studies and sample surveys;

(iii) a comparison with the projections made by the two other approaches to modelling AIDS epidemiology insofar as they offer projections disaggregated by risk group.

2 Relating the model to data

The current research involves optimising the parameters of a model of AIDS spread in the homosexual population by fitting it to data on reported cases of AIDS in this particular population. A reporting delay is estimated discarding those cases reported as diagnosed in the last 18 months in order to overcome some of the problems relating to right-censored data. The lags between diagnosis and report are fitted to a negative exponential distribution and the resultant value is adopted as a parameter which is not a member of the set to be optimised. This set consists of:

(i) the size of the susceptible population;

(ii) the mean number of different partners per unit time (refined by a factor which mimics changing behaviour);

(iii) the probability of passing on HIV infection, specified as three separate probabilities which relate to distinct phases in the natural history of HIV infection over the long incubation period;

(iv) the durations of the second and third phases of the assumed three-stage incubation distribution.

3 Results

Table 1 shows the estimated timing of the peak incidence in (i) HIV infection and (ii) AIDS, together with (iii) an estimate of the prevalence of HIV at the end of 1992. These results were obtained using data on AIDS incidence in homosexuals to the end of 1992. (This data is provided by the WHO-EC Collaborating Centre on the basis of physicians' reports.) The analysis involved optimising the parameters of a transmission model of AIDS spread in the homosexual population (Dangerfield and Roberts, 1989; Roberts and

Country	HIV	AIDS	Prevalence
United Kingdom	1987 (3)	1995 (1)	12700
France	1987 (4)	1994 (1)	24600
FR Germany	1987 (2)	1993 (3)	11800
The Netherlands	1987 (2)	1992 (4)	3400
Switzerland	1988 (1)	1996 (4)	2700

Table 1. Estimated timings for peaks in HIV and AIDS incidences and estimated HIV prevalence (nearest hundred) at end-1992

Country	Phase 1	Phase 2	Phase 3
United Kingdom	0.0627	0.0164	0.136
France	0.0780	0.0287	0.104
FR Germany	0.0762	0.0208	0.134
The Netherlands	0.0795	0.0194	0.101
Switzerland	0.0710	0.0431	0.162

Table 2. Comparison of the optimised infectiousness parameters

Dangerfield, 1990). The fitting process uses an iterative heuristic search algorithm applied to the multi-dimensional parameter space. One thousand iterations (runs) of the model, which consists of 70+ equations and a run length of 16.5 years, takes 58 seconds on a 486-DX PC running at 50 MHz. The simulated time step is 16^{-1} years.

Further results from the analysis of the European data are given in Table 2. These concern the three probabilities corresponding to the three phases of the natural history of HIV disease. We find that the hypothesis of a sharp climb in infectivity towards the onset of AIDS is not refuted by the study.

The use of the search routine for estimating model parameters is at an early stage and further refinements can be anticipated. With this caveat in mind, however, we currently expect to see an annual total of around 1200 new cases of AIDS reported in the UK homosexual/bisexual exposure group over the next 3-4 years. This arises from our simulations of the fitted model which show an incipient peak in the incidence of AIDS for this exposure group.

4 Comparisons with other studies

Table 3 shows some comparisons of estimated HIV prevalence with other studies in the UK, The Netherlands and Switzerland. It should be noted that these other studies were conducted with earlier datasets. Revised estimates for England and Wales, for example, will soon be available when the working

Country	Our estimate	Other estimate	Reference
United Kingdom	12900 (end 1990)	15500 (end 1990)	PHLS (Day) Report (1990) (Upper projection England and Wales)
Netherlands	3800 (end 1990)	4000–5000 (end 1990)	Van den Boom *et al.* (1992)
Switzerland	2700 (end 1991)	1890 (end 1991)	Bailey (1993)

Table 3. Some comparisons of estimated HIV prevalence with other studies (Homosexual exposure group)

group responsible for the Day Report publishes its latest findings.

References

Bailey, N.T.J. (1993) 'An improved hybrid HIV/AIDS model geared to specific public health data and decision-making', *Math. Biosci.* **117**, 221–237.

Dangerfield, B.C. and Roberts, C.A. (1989) 'A Role for System Dynamics in Modelling the Spread of AIDS', *Trans. Inst. Msmt. and Crtl.* **11**, 187–195.

Public Health Laboratory Service (1990) *Acquired Immune Deficiency Syndrome in England and Wales to end 1993: projections using data to end September 1989 (Day Report)*, Communicable Disease Surveillance Centre, London.

Roberts, C.A. and Dangerfield, B.C. (1990) 'Modelling the epidemiological consequences of HIV infection and AIDS: a contribution from operational research', *J. Opl. Res. Soc.* **41**, 273–289.

Van den Boom, F.M., Jager, J.C. *et al.* (1992) *AIDS up to the Year 2000*, Kluwer, Dordrecht.

Estimation of the Rate of HIV Diagnosis in HIV-Infected Individuals

V. T. Farewell, O. O. Aalen, D. De Angelis and N. E. Day

Individuals who are infected with the HIV virus, may or may not have had a positive HIV antibody test. From a public health point of view it is important to know the rate at which infected individuals have their infection diagnosed, that is, when they have their first positive antibody test. We will call this the rate of HIV diagnosis. Only HIV diagnosis prior to one year before AIDS diagnosis will be considered, since HIV tests close to AIDS diagnosis may possibly be closely linked to disease development.

One approach to estimating the rate of HIV diagnosis, is through information on the time of first HIV-diagnosis among individuals who develop AIDS. Such information has been made available for England and Wales by the Public Health Laboratory Service (PHLS) AIDS Centre at the Communicable Disease Surveillance Centre. For the period 1981–91, data are available on the number of AIDS cases diagnosed in each quarter, and reported by mid 1992, and, furthermore, on the number who had an earlier HIV-diagnosis, and on the quarter of this diagnosis.

We have defined an extended backcalculation method to incorporate the HIV diagnosis information. Three exposure groups are considered: homo/bisexuals, injecting drug users, heterosexuals. For the first two groups the infection curve is assumed to have a quadratic exponential form up to a specified time (the knot) and constant thereafter; the knot has been taken at the beginning of 1987 and 1988 respectively. For the heterosexuals a quadratic exponential infection curve has been used.

A Weibull incubation period is assumed for the homo/bisexuals and heterosexuals, and a gamma incubation period for the injecting drug users. The availability of treatment from the beginning of 1988 is modelled by reducing the incubation time hazard by a given factor from this time.

It is assumed that testing was generally available by mid 1984. Tests prior to one year before diagnosis are assumed to be unrelated to later development of disease.

The general model is illustrated in the figure. The rate of HIV infections is $h(t)$. The rate, or hazard, of HIV diagnosis is $\alpha(t)$, possibly dependent on calendar time t. The incubation time hazard $\beta(.,.)$ is dependent on infection time T_I and time since infection $t - T_I$, and it is assumed to be the same

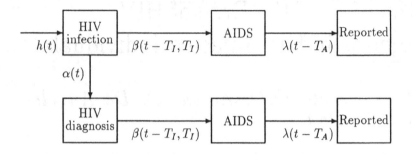

Figure 1. Model for HIV diagnosis

for those with and without an HIV diagnosis prior to one year before AIDS diagnosis. The reporting time hazard $\lambda(.)$ is dependent on time since AIDS diagnosis $t - T_A$, but assumed independent of calendar time, and equal for those with and those without an early HIV diagnosis.

The usual information used in backcalculation corresponds to the entries into the *combined* 'reported states', while here we exploit information on the entries into these two states separately, counting only the HIV-diagnoses prior to one year before AIDS diagnosis.

Initially, a constant rate α of HIV diagnosis from mid 1984 was assumed. Estimates have been derived by maximum likelihood for a discrete version of the model. For infected individuals the estimated HIV diagnosis rate may be transformed into a yearly proportion of HIV-diagnosis. With 95% confidence intervals this is estimated to be 16.1% (15.2, 17.1) for homo/bisexuals, 17.1% (13.1, 20.9) for injecting drug users and 9.3% (7.0, 11.6) for heterosexuals. The results were reasonably consistent with external information for the first and third group, but not for the injecting drug users. In this case there may be a high mortality from causes other than AIDS, which should be taken into consideration.

HIV diagnosis information about AIDS cases does not improve the precision of the infection curve estimates to any great extent. A considerable improvement may, however, be achieved if one has information on the total number of people diagnosed with HIV infection, that is, the total number who have passed through the vertical transition in the figure up to a certain time. Based on voluntary confidential laboratory reports, estimates have been made of the number of HIV infected individuals in England and Wales who were diagnosed prior to January 1, 1992, and who did not develop AIDS by January 1, 1993. The original model may easily be extended to incorporate this information. Model estimates changed somewhat, but the precision of the estimated rate of HIV diagnosis as well as the predicted infection curve improved considerably.

The underlying assumptions in the model may be relaxed or modified in various ways. The HIV diagnosis rate has been allowed to vary over calendar time, yielding slight or moderate estimated variation. Variation with time since infection has been briefly investigated for the homo/bisexuals. The impact of varying the treatment effect has also been studied for this group, leading only to slight changes in the estimated rate of HIV diagnosis.

For further details of our work see Aalen *et al.* (1994), Farewell *et al.* (1994).

References

Aalen O.O., Farewell V.T., De Angelis D. and Day N.E. (1994) 'On the use of HIV diagnosis information in monitoring of the AIDS epidemic', *J. Roy. Statist. Soc. A* **157**, 3–16.

Farewell V.T., Aalen O.O., De Angelis D. and Day N.E. (1994) 'Estimation of the rate of diagnosis of HIV infection in HIV-infected individuals', *Biometrika* **81**, 287–294.

Discussion

LONGINI Without better data on HIV infection levels, we can say almost nothing about current infection rates. However, better data can be incorporated into techniques such as those presented here.

ADES In relation to the work described here, is there any information available on the factors influencing individuals' decisions to seek an HIV test?

GORE In answer to Ades' question, there is information available in HIV testing rates on the awareness of a population to the issues surrounding HIV and AIDS. For example, the introduction of anonymous surveillance for HIV infection in prisons can produce a doubling of the rate at which individuals seek an informed HIV test.

Effects of AIDS Public Information on HIV Infections among Gay Men

David P. Fan

This paper shows that the time trend of HIV infections among gay men could be forecast from persuasive information in the press. The principal methodologies are detailed in Fan (1993). The mainstream press was likely to be a good gauge of the persuasive information acting on the public for AIDS related topics because the news media could be used to forecast time trends of public opinion and behavior for over a dozen topics (e.g. Fan 1988, Fan and McAvoy 1989, Fan 1993). The analysis began with the electronic retrieval from the NEXIS commercial database of the texts of 2462 out of 8728 AIDS stories in the New York Times and the Washington Post from January 1, 1981 to February 12, 1992. The chosen stories contained the word 'AIDS' within five words of one of the word roots 'disease', 'illness' or 'immune'. The 8.0 million characters of retrieved text were scored by computer using the InfoTrend computer programs previously described (Fan 1988). The algorithm depended on the occurrence of key words, their orders in paragraphs and the distances between them. For the scoring, the analyst enters a topic specific dictionary and a set of word relationship rules, usually about 50 in number. The resulting scores are in the form of numbers of paragraphs containing user specified ideas at specific times.

The computer first discarded all paragraphs except those containing the word 'AIDS or the word pair 'acquired immune'. Then, the AIDS paragraphs were scored by machine for their views on HIV transmission through: sex, blood, nonsterile needles, the mother, casual contact, not through casual contact, and miscellaneous including mosquitos. In addition, the text was also scored for whether the target population was gay men or heterosexuals, for whether the disease was lethal, and for whether a person could avoid infection through sex, needles or blood. In all cases, there were no relevant paragraphs before the end of 1982 when AIDS was defined as a disease.

The scores for modes of transmission were entered into the model of ideodynamics (Fan 1993) to compute the media share devoted to each of the modes. The results showed that sex occupied about a quarter of the discussion on modes of transmission in 1983 but increased to almost half by 1992. Simultaneously, there was a drop in concern about the blood route, from about 40% to under a quarter. There was not much change in coverage for any of the other transmission pathways.

After the end of 1982, there was a rapid rise in paragraph scores for the ideas that AIDS was a fatal disease, that AIDS was a threat to the gay/bisexual and heterosexual populations, and that AIDS could be avoided by a person's own actions in the areas of sex, blood contact, and contaminated needles. The only important difference for these six ideas was a pause in prominent coverage of the threat to heterosexuals from late 1983 through mid 1985.

The news media scores were used in the ideodynamic equations to compute time trends of opinions for the six positions. For all ideas, the awareness was zero before 1983 and then rapidly rose to majority awareness within a year and 90% knowledge by 1985. The one exception was a lag in the perception of heterosexual risk corresponding to a lull in press coverage of this idea. For all six topics, the Root Mean Squared Deviation (RMSD) between opinion time trends computed from the media and those constructed from surveys was 11.4%. For all computations, only one parameter was used in the model, the persuasibility constant describing the ability of one press paragraph to sensitize one percent of those not already aware within one day. As expected, the 11.4% was higher than the 3-8% observed in the past because a common, compromise persuasibility constant was used to fit all six sets of time trends. The ability to use the same constant for all cases indicates that the persuasive forces of the different types of information were approximately the same.

The ideodynamic model was then used to predict sexual behavior among the gay subpopulation by assuming that high risk activities would be decreased by mass media information on the lethal outcome of the disease, on the ability to avoid infection by a person's own behavior and on the high risk to gays. The same equation was used as for opinion and could fully account for the drop in the proportion of San Francisco gays engaging in unsafe sex from 59% in 1984 to a plateau value around 30% in 1987 and 1989. That is, the predicted line was within the measurement errors in the reference survey data. In addition to the persuasibility constant describing the ability of the media to change behavior, there was a parameter reflecting the inherent urge to engage in unsafe sex and another one describe the natural tendency toward no sex or toward safe behavior.

The model was further extended to predict HIV infection among gays assuming that infected and noninfected individuals have the same behavior until the infected individuals develop the overt symptoms of AIDS at which point they are assumed to stop transmitting the disease. Public information is modeled to move some members of both of subpopulations from a state of high risk activity to one of safe behavior. Infection is modeled to occur when infected and noninfected persons engage in unsafe sexual activities together. The calculation began in 1981 with Brookmeyer's (1991) first backcalculated value of HIV infection by the sexual route among gay men. The computation continued every 24 hours to February 12, 1993 and included both birth and death due to AIDS and other causes. Beside the three constants used for the behavior calculation, there was one more describing the likelihood of infection upon joint unsafe behavior by infected and noninfected persons.

An HIV infection time trend computed with the addition of this infection parameter was compared to Brookmeyer's (1991) yearly backcalculations for HIV infection from 1981 to 1989. The RMSD between the predicted and backcalculated values was approximately 1%.

Therefore, it is possible to use a single parsimonious mathematical model to unify time trends data from a number of sources: mass media information, attitude and knowledge surveys, behavior surveys, and HIV incidence and prevalence obtained from backcalculations.

References

Brookmeyer, R. (1991) 'Reconstruction and future trends of the AIDS epidemic in the United States', *Science* **253**, 37–42.

Fan, D.P. (1988) 'Predictions of public opinion from the mass media'. In *Computer Content Analysis and Mathematical modeling*, Greenwood Press, Westport, CT.

Fan, D.P. (1993) 'Quantitative estimates for the effects of AIDS public education on HIV infections', *Int. J. Biomed. Comput.* **33**, 157–177.

Fan, D.P. and McAvoy, G. (1989) 'Predictions of public opinion on the spread of the disease of AIDS: Introduction of new computer methodologies', *J. Sex Res.* **26**, 159–187.

Discussion

GOVE** In the work presented by Fan, all the public opinion graphs seem to vary from 'disbelief' to 'belief'. Does the data analysis algorithm allow for mis-information or incorrect information? Is there room in the model for a 'don't know' state that people initially leave and then can revert to if not re-exposed to the information?

REPLY The data analysis algorithm does not correct for mis-information and incorrect information since the goal was to model public responses. The public can obviously be persuaded by erroneous messages. For the sake of parsimony, the model used did not include the 'don't knows'. However, the calculations can easily be modified to account for such a group.

Changes in Sexual Behaviour and HIV Control

Chinma O. Uche and Roy M. Anderson

The effect of changes in sexual behaviour of a population stratified into high and low sexual activity classes on the temporal trends of HIV/AIDS is evaluated, using a simple mathematical model (Anderson *et al.* 1989), to obtain the activity class on which control programmes should be targeted. The initial population parameters are such that the introduction of infection into the population results in epidemics in both activity classes (Uche and Anderson 1993a): particular focus is on a population with initial mean rate of partner change of the high and low sexual activity classes given as 200 and 2.5 respectively and transmission probability 0.1. The simple deterministic model, with constant recruitment rate of susceptibles into the population, is used to examine individually the effect of varying the mean rate of partner change of the high activity class from 200 to 10, the mean rate of partner change of the low activity class from 3.0 to 1.75 and the transmission probability from 0.5 to 0.025. The proportion of the total recruitment rate into the high activity class is in all cases fixed at 1/11.

Assuming fully assortative mixing, two peaks in seroprevalence of infection were realised. It was observed that changes in the mean rate of partner change of the high activity class from 200 to 10 reduced the the magnitude of the first peak by 2.6% from 8.7% and delayed the time of its occurance by only 12.4 years with no effect on the magnitude (difference of about 0.4%) or the time of occurance of the second peak. Changes in the mean rate of partner change of the low activity class did not seem to affect the first peak seroprevalence of infection, with very disproportionate effects on the second peak. A reduction of the mean rate of partner change of the low activity class from 3.0 to 2.5 reduced the peak seroprevalence of infection by 12.6% from 62.8% delaying its occurance by about 40.2 years, while a reduction from 2.5 to 2.0 delays the time of occurance of the second peak by about 118 years (giving ample time for the development of an effective AIDS therapy) reducing the peak value by 19.8% from 50.2%. Nonlinear effects of changes in the transmission probability were obtained. An increase in the transmission probability from 0.1 to 0.5, which is possible in populations with sexually transmitted diseases, increases the first and second peak values of the seroprevalence of infection by 0.33% and 46% from 8.67% and 50.2% for the mean rates of partner change in the low and high activity classes of 2.5 and 200; hastening the times of occurance of each peak by 1 and 115 years respectively. By contrast, a reduction of the transmission probability by 0.025 from 0.1, through the use

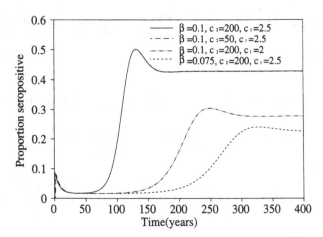

of condoms, reduces the magnitude of the second peak by 25% from 50.2% while delaying its occurance by 196 years.

The relative merit of reducing the mean rate of partner change of the high activity class by 150 from 200, the mean rate of partner change of the low activity class by 0.5 from 2.5 and the transmission probability by 0.025 from 0.1 were considered in terms of their effect on the seroprevalence of infection and cost of implementation. The reduction in the transmission probability gave the greatest reduction in the seroprevalence of infection while the reduction in the mean rate of partner change of the high activity class gave the least (see Figure). The effectiveness of using condoms to substantially reduce the magnitude of the epidemic depends on the target class and the pattern of mixing. More detailed considerations of these and other related factors like the magnitude and timing of changes in sexual behaviour for non-assortative mixing are discussed elsewhere (Uche and Anderson 1993b).

References

Anderson, R.M., Blythe, S.P., Gupta, S., and Konings, E. (1989) 'The transmission dynamics of the human immunodeficiency virus type 1 in the male homosexual community in the United Kingdom: the influence of changes in sexual behaviour', *Phil. Trans. Roy. Soc. Lond. B* **325**, 45–98.

Uche, C.O. and Anderson, R.M. (1993a) 'The endemic equilibrium of HIV/AIDS: Effect of rates of partner change and patterns of mixing', manuscript.

Uche, C.O. and Anderson, R.M. (1993b) 'Temporal effects of changes in sexual behaviour on HIV dynamics', manuscript.

The Time to AIDS in a Cohort of Homosexual Men

Jan C.M. Hendriks, Graham F. Medley, Godfried J.P. van Griensven and Hans A.M. van Druten

The incubation period of AIDS is a key characteristic in understanding the HIV and AIDS epidemic, both clinically and epidemiologically. The incubation period distribution (IPD) provides information about the probability of progression to AIDS as it changes with time since infection with HIV. The IPD also provides the link between the HIV infection rate and the occurrence of AIDS cases over time, and is an essential feature in back calculation procedures (Brookmeyer and Gail 1988). Knowledge of the IPD creates the opportunity to make more reliable projections (Hendriks *et al.* 1992), which are necessary for health-care planning.

Cohort study data relating to development of AIDS are inevitably incomplete in dates of seroconversion (infection) or development of AIDS, or both. This incompleteness has inspired a variety of approaches. We used a multiple imputation procedure, with four related models, each covering different assumptions, to investigate the sensitivity of the estimated IPD regarding the imputation method. The imputation procedure was used to provide the unobserved interval between seroconversion and enrolment for those individuals who were already HIV infected at enrolment. We can exclude observations relating to individuals who received antiviral and or prophylactic treatment designed to delay the onset of AIDS. The results obtained from data such as these will be valuable in future to aid the understanding of the effects of new therapies on the evolution of the AIDS epidemic.

The IPD was estimated using data available at February 1990 from all homosexual and bisexual men with HIV seropositive blood samples ($n = 348$; aged 25–45 years), who were part of a larger cohort study in Amsterdam. All 348 participants were grouped into one of the following four categories: (1) seroconverted during study and AIDS-free at their last visit ($n = 68$); (2) seroconverted and developed AIDS during study ($n = 11$); (3) seropositive at enrolment and AIDS-free at their last visit ($n = 219$); (4) seropositive at enrolment and developed AIDS during study ($n = 50$). The 27 men who received zidovudine treatment (mostly in randomized controlled trials) were included in groups 1 and 3, using the first date of zidovudine treatment as the date of the last visit. In this study period PCP prophylaxis was not used in any AIDS-free cohort member.

The number of seroconversions per quarter-year between 1985 and 1990 of homosexual and bisexual men from the Amsterdam cohort, who entered the study between October 1984 and May 1985 (55 out of all 79 seroconversions during the study) shows the time-dependent pattern of probability of HIV infection. We found that a Weibull distribution mirrors this pattern and we used this distribution to provide the elongation of the observed part of the incubation period. The parameters of the truncated Weibull distribution were chosen so that the probability of seroconversion between 1 January 1980 and 1 January 1985 is 50% and between 1 January 1980 and 1 January 1990, is 90%. In concordance with data from a Hepatitis B cohort study, the start of the HIV epidemic was put at 1 January 1980.

In this Weibull elongation model, the infection distribution can be regarded as the force of infection from the population on an individual. In this way, date of an individuals' enrolment into the study is treated as a covariate that alters the imputed seroconversion date of that individual. Another covariate, that has been used in this context is CD4 count at enrolment.

To investigate the sensitivity of the results to the elongation model, we also used an exponential elongation model. This model assumes that the probability of infection rises exponentially from the start of the HIV epidemic and is largest immediately before enrolment. This model is more appropriate when men are more likely to participate in the study if they have been infected recently.

The imputed elongation period (from either the truncated exponential or the truncated Weibull distribution) was added to the AIDS-free period actually observed in the cohort to give an AIDS-free period for each individual seropositive at entry. Thus, direct, non-parametric analysis (Kaplan-Meier) of survival to AIDS is possible. The Weibull and gamma distributions were also fitted to these data by maximum likelihood. The probability of not developing AIDS (p) after infection is estimated simultaneously (Bachetti 1990). It appeared that all estimates of p had large confidence intervals, and because p is expected to be small, it was assumed to be zero.

The choice of the elongation model or the IPD affects the median by 1.5 years or < 0.5 year, respectively. Within each elongation model both distributions fit equally well to the Kaplan-Meier estimator. After 10 years' incubation the Weibull and gamma IPD diverge, with the gamma distribution predicting a longer tail. The associated hazard functions of these four IPDs revealed that, although all functions of the hazard rate are increasing, there is a noticeable abatement in the rate of increase when the gamma distribution is used.

After controlling for therapy, the true natural history of AIDS in homosexual men may be better described by a slowing of the hazard approximately 5 years after infection (Bachetti 1990), so that the gamma IPD might be preferable to the Weibull IPD, although both agree equally with the Kaplan-Meier estimator. This study (Hendriks *et al.* 1993) suggests that after 7 years 33% (95% CI: 26–37%) will have progressed to AIDS, when no treatment is involved and 50% will develop AIDS within 9.2 years (95% CI: 8.3–10.3). This is in agreement with other studies, especially with the more recent ones. The probability of being diagnosed with AIDS during the 12 months after being AIDS-free for 7 years is 12%.

Acknowledgements

Supported by grant number 91-56 of the Netherlands Ministry of Welfare, Health and Cultural Affairs (Ministerie van Welzijn, Volksgezondheid en Cultuur).

References

Bachetti, P. (1990) 'Estimating the incubation period of AIDS by comparing population infection and diagnosis patterns', *JASA* **412**, 1002–1008.

Brookmeyer, R. and Gail, M.H. (1988) 'A method for obtaining short-term projections and lower bounds on the size of the AIDS epidemic', *JASA* **83**, 301–308.

Hendriks, J.C.M., Medley, G.F., Heisterkamp, S.H., van Griensven, G.J.P., Bindels, P.J.E., Coutinho, R.A. and van Druten, J.A.M. (1992) 'Short term projections of HIV prevalence and AIDS incidence'. *Epidemiol. Infect.* **109**, 149–160.

Hendriks, J.C.M., Medley, G.F., van Griensven, G.J.P., Coutinho, R.A., Heisterkamp, S.M. and van Druten, J. A. M. (1993) 'The treatment-free incubation period of AIDS in a cohort of homosexual men', *AIDS* **7**, 231–239.

Lui, K.-J., Darrow, W.W., Rutherford III, G.W. (1988) 'A model-based estimate of the mean incubation period for AIDS in homosexual men', *Science* **240**, 1333–1335.

Operational Models for the Care of HIV and AIDS Patients

A.K. Shahani, S.C. Brailsford and R.B. Roy

HIV infection is a major threat to the health of most nations in the world. Prevention of the spread of HIV requires major behavioural changes and the current evidence points to rather a gloomy picture. Prevention through vaccination is a hope for the future for developed countries but this hope has to be sustained with the knowledge that for the developing countries the expected large cost of vaccination would be a very major problem. Further, the travelling patterns of people mean that people from various countries will continue to be in contact. HIV infection is thus a challenging problem and efforts of a variety of people can contribute to the control of this threat.

The control of HIV infection and the care of HIV patients have to meet the challenges of complexity, uncertainty, variability, and limited resources. The modelling approach of Operational Research has grown from dealing with these challenges. This paper is mainly concerned with operational models for the care of HIV patients. The models can also provide some information for evaluating the effects of proposed preventive measures. The models can help two groups of users: Health Planners concerned with resource allocation and budgeting can use the models to obtain information about resource usage and costs over time; Clinical Staff interested in effective patient care and in the monitoring of resources used for patient care can obtain helpful quantitative information from the models.

Starting with an infected person, the natural history of HIV infection is characterised by uncertainty and variability. Clinical staff need quite detailed information about patients. These and other considerations resulted in the choice of simulation modelling which were developed by a team of Health and Operational Research professionals. Data from Bournemouth, Sheffield, and San Francisco helped in the development and testing of the models.

This summary describes the modelling work which uses three descriptions of the natural history of HIV infection.

- A simple three state model;

- a model with a World Health Organisation classification;

- a model which uses the Centers for Disease Control (CDC 1987) classification in which CD4 cell count is not used.

The simple model may be adequate for an overall planning purpose. At the clinical level the CDC classification is useful.

In the simulation models an infected person is taken through time and the disease states experienced by the individual are noted. The individuals are described in suitable terms such as by age, sex, and sexual behaviour. The information can be gathered for a given cohort of patients or new patients in various states of the disease, including newly infected, can be added. Treatment of the patients requires resources and these are grouped under the headings: personnel, drugs, facilities. The costs of the resources used can be specified in appropriate units such as time and money.

Transitions between disease states are governed by probabilities and random variables. The model with the CDC classification needs a large amount of information and there is insufficient data for the necessary information. We have provided the user with an easy way of giving expert opinion about the necessary probabilities and random variables. The user can choose from Weibull or Gamma variates and specify the mean and one percentage point. Two percentage points, instead of a mean and a percentage point, can also be specified. The user can choose the group of patients to be studied and choose any new patients that should be added. The user can specify the resources that are necessary and allocate the resources to various disease states. The user can control the time for which the simulation will be run.

The models calculate the disease status as represented by the states of the natural history model of the people. Examples for the CDC model are: Number of infected people without symptoms over time, number of people with persistent Generalised Lymphadenopathy over time, and the number of deaths over time. The resources used and the costs incurred are also calculated as functions of time. Examples are: Total time spent per week by a senior registrar or consultant for looking after HIV patients over a specified period of time, total cost of a particular drug used over time, and total cost of all resources used over time. This information can be looked at in graphical or tabular form. The available information is listed in a helpful manner and the user can select the information that is needed for a particular purpose.

The models can be used to note the likely disease profiles and resource use for actual patients in a particular clinical department. An appropriate method of linking the patient data system in the department to the models would be needed for this purpose. The models can be used on standard microcomputers.

Further details are given in Brailsford *et al.* (1992) and Shahani *et al.* (1993).

We acknowledge the financial and other help given by the University of Southampton and the Wessex Regional Health Authority for this modelling work.

References

Brailsford, S.C., Shahani, A.K., Roy, R.B. and Sivapalan, S. (1992) 'Simulation modelling for HIV infection and AIDS', *Int. J. Biomed. Comput.* **31**, 73–88.

Centers for Disease Control (1987) 'Revision of the CDC surveillance case definition of the Acquired Immunodeficiency Syndrome', *Morbidity and Mortality Weekly Report* **36**, suppl. 15, 15–155.

Shahani, A.K., Brailsford, S.C. and Roy, R.B. (1993) 'Operational models for the care of HIV and AIDS patients'. Preprint No. OR51, Faculty of Mathematical Studies, University of Southampton.